Children's Well-Being and Mental Health in an Educational Context

Children's Well-Being and Mental Health in an Educational Context

Guest Editor

Sanja Tatalović Vorkapić

MDPI

Basel • Beijing • Wuhan • Barcelona • Belgrade • Novi Sad • Cluj • Manchester

Guest Editor
Sanja Tatalović Vorkapić
Faculty of Teacher Education
in Rijeka
University of Rijeka
Rijeka
Croatia

Editorial Office
MDPI AG
Grosspeteranlage 5
4052 Basel, Switzerland

This is a reprint of the Special Issue, published open access by the journal *Children* (ISSN 2227-9067), freely accessible at: https://www.mdpi.com/journal/children/special_issues/SC2C6JCUOH.

For citation purposes, cite each article independently as indicated on the article page online and as indicated below:

Lastname, A.A.; Lastname, B.B. Article Title. *Journal Name* **Year**, *Volume Number*, Page Range.

ISBN 978-3-7258-7837-6 (Hbk)
ISBN 978-3-7258-7838-3 (PDF)
https://doi.org/10.3390/books978-3-7258-7838-3

Contents

About the Editor

Sanja Tatalović Vorkapić

Sanja Tatalović Vorkapić, Ph.D., is a full professor at the Faculty of Teacher Education, University of Rijeka. She has published 230 scientific papers, 7 scientific monographs and 9 manuals. She has held numerous invited lectures. She has led six projects and is currently leading two scientific projects. She served as the vice-dean for science, development and quality assurance on two occasions and is currently the main editor of the scientific journal *Educational Topics* within her faculty. She was awarded the Award for the Best Scientist in Social Sciences in the ac. year 2013/2014 and the Award for Excellence in Teaching in the ac. year 2016/2017. She is the Head of the School Psychologist Division of the Croatian Psychological Association.

children

MDPI

Review

School Refusal Behavior in Japan: The Impact of COVID-19 on Children

Daisuke Matsubara [1,2], Kazuhiko Kotani [1,*] and Hitoshi Osaka [2]

1 Division of Community and Family Medicine, Jichi Medical University, Tochigi 329-0498, Japan; 99081dm@jichi.ac.jp
2 Department of Pediatrics, Jichi Medical University, Tochigi 329-0498, Japan; hosaka@jichi.ac.jp
* Correspondence: kazukotani@jichi.ac.jp; Tel.: +81-285-44-2111

Abstract

School refusal behavior, defined as a child's prolonged voluntary absence from school for reasons unrelated to illness and/or economic hardship, is a growing concern in Japan. The COVID-19 pandemic has worsened this issue by disrupting children's lives. This review summarizes the prevalence, contributing factors, and health implications of school refusal, particularly in the context of COVID-19. A literature review of government reports and PubMed-indexed studies indicates that school refusal in Japan has been rising for eleven years, reaching a record 340,000 cases in 2023. Middle school students (6.7%) were the most affected, followed by elementary school students (2.1%). The pandemic intensified school-related, family-related, and child-related risk factors. School closures disrupted routines, reduced peer interactions, and increased social isolation, contributing to higher rates of anxiety and depression. Reports of suicides and mental health disorders among children have also surged. Family stressors, including economic hardship and parental mental health struggles, further exacerbate school refusal. Additionally, remote learning has widened socioeconomic disparities in access to education, leaving vulnerable children at greater risk. Addressing school refusal requires a multifaceted approach involving schools, families, healthcare providers, and policymakers. School-based interventions, mental health approach, and flexible educational programs would be essential. The Japanese government's "COCOLO Plan" represents progress toward a more inclusive education system, and a comprehensive, interdisciplinary strategy is needed. Ensuring all children receive the necessary support to reengage with education is critical to overcoming the long-term challenges posed by school refusal.

Keywords: childhood; COVID-19; disparity; mental health; wellbeing

1. Introduction

Japan is facing a unique challenge of a super-aging society with a low birth rate, possibly reflecting future trends in many other countries [1]. The annual number of births in Japan has been declining for nine consecutive years, reaching its lowest level in 2023 with total fertility rate of 1.20 [1]. Interestingly, in contrast to the declining number of children, school refusal behavior is a growing issue in Japan and worldwide [2,3]. Defined as a child's prolonged voluntary absence from school for reasons unrelated to physical illness and/or economic reasons, it has had social and psychological implications [3]. While various factors contribute to school refusal behavior, the COVID-19 pandemic has amplified this by affecting children's health, social structures, and educational experiences [2]. The impact of

 https://doi.org/10.3390/children12091105

COVID-19 on this status indicates the points necessary for the future plan, which should be reviewed in the period when we live with COVID-19. In spite of the significance of school refusal, this topic has been rarely reviewed in Japan. Thus, this review summarizes the important points such as the prevalence, contributing factors, and health implications of school refusal in Japan, particularly in relation to COVID-19.

We conducted a literature review using available government reports and peer-reviewed studies that were searched via PubMed until 31st December 2024. The focus to select literature was on school refusal behavior and its relationship with the COVID-19 pandemic. While this manuscript aims to summary the situation in Japan, many key sources were published in Japanese. For English-language studies, we thoroughly selected those that were thematically relevant to the focus of this manuscript. In addition, several Japanese studies provided references to international trend, which helped to contextualize Japan's situation and could aid to establish a deeper understand of this essential topic in other countries. In this way, this narrative review was made. A summary of references we selected is provided in Table 1.

Table 1. Summary of references selected in the review.

Authors (Ref. No.)	Year	Summary
Ministry of Health, Labor, and Welfare, Japan (Ref. [1])	2023	Japan's official annual demographic statistics highlighting a record low total fertility rate of 1.20 in 2023, which showed the demographic backdrop against which school refusal is increasing.
Ministry of Education, Culture, Sports, Science, and Technology, Japan (Ref. [2])	2023	Japan's official annual report on school absenteeism, including details on prevalence, reasons for absenteeism, and the sharp increase during COVID-19, with breakdowns by school level and absence duration.
Kearney CA (Ref. [3])	2008	A review article defining school absenteeism and refusal behaviors in youth, which discussed prevalence, etiological factors, and frameworks for intervention, forming the conceptual basis for the review.
Dee TS (Ref. [4])	2024	A report from the Proceedings of the National Academy of Sciences of the United States of America, describing chronic absenteeism trends in U.S. schools, showing a near doubling during the pandemic to 28.3%.
Lester KJ, Michelson D (Ref. [5])	2024	A review paper, exploring the phenomenon of emotionally based school avoidance in the post-COVID-19 era, which highlighted the 'perfect storm' of risk factors exacerbated by pandemic disruptions.
Rahman MA et al. (Ref. [6])	2023	A large multi-country study on chronic absenteeism in 71 nations, examining prevalence and associated factors.
de Figueiredo CS et al. (Ref. [7])	2021	A review paper exploring the multifactorial impact of COVID-19 on children's and adolescents' mental health, which integrated biological, environmental, and social influences relevant to school refusal.
Ministry of Education, Culture, Sports, Science, and Technology, Japan (Ref. [8])	2021	Japan's official annual report tracking physical fitness trends among Japanese children, which noted declines during COVID-19 due to reduced physical activity and disrupted routines.

Table 1. *Cont.*

Authors (Ref. No.)	Year	Summary
Saito M et al. (Ref. [9])	2022	An original article assessing mental health in Japanese schoolchildren during school closures, which found disrupted sleep, eating habits, and physical activity patterns.
National Center for Child Health and Development, Japan (Ref. [10])	2023	Japan's national center report summarizing the overall health impact of COVID-19 on Japanese children, which included mental, physical, and lifestyle changes observed during the pandemic.
Ministry of Health, Labor and Welfare, Japan (Ref. [11])	2024	Japan's official annual report on child suicide in Japan, which highlighted a sharp increase in suicides among children during the pandemic.
Racine N et al. (Ref. [12])	2021	A meta-analysis of global studies on depression and anxiety in children and adolescents during COVID-19, which found doubled prevalence compared to pre-pandemic estimates.
Roumeliotis N et al. (Ref. [13])	2024	A Canadian population-based study reporting increased youth hospitalizations for mental health issues during the pandemic, which highlighted conditions such as anxiety, personality disorders, and suicidality.
Madigan S et al. (Ref. [14])	2023	A systematic review and meta-analysis of pediatric ED visits for suicide attempts, self-harm, and ideation, which found significant increases during the pandemic.
Okajima, I et al. (Ref. [15])	2022	An original article from Japan linking COVID-19-related sleep problems and anxiety to loneliness, which identified an indirect link to school refusal feelings among adolescents.
Hiraoka D, Tomoda A (Ref. [16])	2020	An original article from Japan on parenting stress during school closures, which found heightened stress linked to disrupted routines and caregiving demands.
Bourion-Bédès S et al. (Ref. [17])	2023	An original article from France examining stress levels in parents during the first lockdown, which identified socioeconomic and family structure factors as risk modifiers.
El-Osta A et al. (Ref. [18])	2021	A UK cross-sectional survey on the mental health of parents during lockdown, which reported elevated depression and anxiety symptoms linked to childcare and homeschooling burdens.
Achterberg M et al. (Ref. [19])	2021	A Dutch longitudinal study on the mediation effect of perceived stress on parental and child wellbeing, which showed pre-existing negative emotions increased vulnerability to pandemic stress.
Johnson MS et al. (Ref. [20])	2021	A Norwegian longitudinal study following parents during and after the first lockdown, which found declines in clinically significant depression and anxiety over time, suggesting resilience in some families.
Whaley GL, Pfefferbaum B (Ref. [21])	2023	A review article summarizing parental challenges during the pandemic, which discussed risk and protective factors relevant to child outcomes.

Table 1. *Cont.*

Authors (Ref. No.)	Year	Summary
Gender Equality Bureau Cabinet Office, Japan (Ref. [22])	2021	Japan's official white paper on gender equality, including statistics showing a significant increase in domestic violence reports during COVID-19.
Children and Families Agency, Japan (Ref. [23])	2023	Japan's official annual report on child abuse cases, noting a 5% increase in 2023 compared to 2022, with implications for child mental health.
Cohodes EM et al. (Ref. [24])	2021	An original article from the U.S. on parental buffering of stress during COVID-19, which found that supportive parenting can mitigate youth psychological symptoms despite pandemic stressors.
Agostinelli F et al. (Ref. [25])	2022	An economic analysis on the role of schools, peers, and parents in child development during closures, highlighting the unequal effects of shutdowns across families.
Patrinos HA (Ref. [26])	2023	A World Bank analysis quantifying learning loss per week of school closures, which estimated that long closures can result in learning deficits equivalent to nearly one school year.
Goudeau S et al. (Ref. [27])	2021	A review article on how COVID-19 lockdown and remote learning increased the social class achievement gap, which explained mechanisms by which inequalities in resources and support widened.
Nippon Foundation and Mitsubishi UFJ Research and Consulting, Japan (Ref. [28])	2021	A survey assessing the impact of COVID-19 on educational disparities in Japan, which found significant gaps in access to technology and learning resources.
Johnson SB et al. (Ref. [29])	2024	An original article from the U.S. showing developmental score declines in children aged 0–5 years during COVID-19, which affected communication, problem-solving, and personal-social skills.
McDonald B et al. (Ref. [30])	2023	A UK qualitative study on school attendance problems post-pandemic, which captured perspectives of parents and professionals on re-engagement challenges.
Dessain A et al. (Ref. [31])	2024	A systematic review of longitudinal cohort studies on children with ADHD during the pandemic, which found worsening mental health symptoms and functional difficulties.
Tso WWY et al. (Ref. [32])	2022	A Hong Kong survey of families during COVID-19, which identified greater psychosocial risk in children with special educational needs or from vulnerable families.
Yamamoto T et al. (Ref. [33])	2022	A Japanese caregiver survey on children with neurodevelopmental disorders during school closures, which found links between infection prevention difficulties and relationship changes post-reopening.
Matano M et al. (Ref. [34])	2022	A pilot study from Japan on internet-delivered parent–child interaction therapy for children with ASD, which suggested feasibility of remote intervention during pandemic restrictions.

Table 1. *Cont.*

Authors (Ref. No.)	Year	Summary
Ministry of Education, Culture, Sports, Science, and Technology, Japan (Ref. [35])	2023	A Japanese government's 'COCOLO Plan' addressing school refusal, which outlined goals for diverse learning opportunities, early detection, and inclusive school environments.
Department of Defense Education Activity (Ref. [36])	2025	Information from the U.S. DoDEA recognizing homeschooling as a valid alternative to formal school attendance, which provided an international comparison for Japan's evolving policies.

2. The Current Status of School Refusal Behavior in Japan and Worldwide

The Ministry of Education, Culture, Sports, Science and Technology in Japan has reported an increasing number of school refusal cases in middle and elementary school for consecutive eleven years since 2013 [2]. In Japan, school refusal is defined as students who are voluntarily absent from school for over 30 days for reasons unrelated to physical illness and/or economic reasons. The number showed a gradual increase until 2020, but in 2021, during the COVID-19 pandemic, the number showed a sharp increase, reaching over 240,000 cases (2.6%). Its impact remains, reaching over 340,000 cases (3.7%) in 2023, which is the highest recorded number to date. Among them, absent school days of 30–49, 50–89 and over 90 days are 22.4%, 22.7% and 55.0%, respectively. In addition, 4.2% of students experiencing school refusal have not been properly consulted or managed. School refusal is prevalent among middle school students (5.0% in 2021 to 6.7% to 2023), followed by elementary school students (1.3% in 2021 to 2.1% in 2023). The reasons for school refusal include "unmotivated toward school" (32.2%), followed by "anxious or depression mood (23.1%)" and "disturbed daily life (23.0%)" in both elementary and middle schools [2]. These findings could highlight the profound impact of the pandemic on school children.

As there is no clear consensus on the duration of absence that constitutes school refusal, it can be challenging to estimate the actual number of children affected by school-related issues. Similar trends have been observed globally. In the United States, chronic absenteeism nearly doubled during the pandemic, with rates reaching 28.3% among K-12 students [4]. In the United Kingdom, emotion-based school avoidance has risen, now affecting over 22% of students, approximately double the pre-pandemic rate [5]. In 71 lower-middle and high-income nations, the overall population-weighted prevalence of chronic school absenteeism was 11.4% [6]. Globally, the pandemic can influence children's behavior toward school. Economic hardships and limited access to technology created further barriers to education, often preventing children from returning to school after the pandemic.

3. Factors Contributing to School Refusal

School refusal arises from the complex interplay of multiple factors [3,5]. Several methods have been proposed to categorize these factors. For instance, Lester and Michelson suggested three primary categories: school-related, family-related, and child-related factors [5]—which we adopt in this manuscript.

School-related factors include bullying, peer problems, academic difficulties, academic pressures, and poor home-school relationships. Family-related factors encompass parents' physical and mental health problems, divorce or separation, family conflict, and the presence of young carers. Child-related factors include physical and mental health issues, special educational needs, neurodevelopmental disorders, behaviorally inhibited temperament, and low self-esteem [5].

In Japan, family-related problems, such as parent–child relationship, are a major concern among elementary school students, whereas school-related issues, such as poor academic performance or peer problems, predominate among secondary school students [2]. Notably, child-oriented problems such as lethargy or anxiety were significant concerns for both groups, affecting approximately 30% of students. All or some of these factors may have been affected or exacerbated by the negative impact of the COVID-19 pandemic on children across biological, psychological, and social dimensions [5,7].

4. The Impact of COVID-19 on Children

The COVID-19 pandemic has profoundly affected children's lives, with impacts on physical health, mental wellbeing, family dynamics, and societal structures [4–7]. These changes are thought to be associated with school refusal by intensifying the existing challenges and creating new barriers.

4.1. Physical and Mental Health

COVID-19 has altered children's physical and psychological wellbeing [4–8]. Prolonged school closures and lockdowns have disrupted daily routines, leading to increased screen time and reduced physical activity. Physical fitness scores among Japanese children have declined, with many Japanese children experiencing sleep disturbances and weight gain due to sedentary lifestyles [8]. A study from Japan found that school closures resulted in elementary and junior high school students spending more time with their families and sleeping, but their sleep rhythms, eating habits, and physical activities were disrupted [9]. Concurrently, mental health disorders, such as anxiety and depression, have surged. A survey revealed that among Japanese middle and high school students, the number of those who show a depressive mode increased from 6.4% in 2020 to 13.3% in 2023, exacerbated by isolation, loss of extracurricular activities, and uncertainty about the future [10]. Japanese children's suicides, including those in elementary, middle, and high schools, had remained stable at approximately 300–350 cases per year since 2011. But in 2020, during the COVID-19 pandemic, the number increased sharply, exceeding 500 cases annually in 2022 and 2023 [11].

Globally, the prevalence of mental health disorders in children and adolescents has also increased during the COVID-19 pandemic. A meta-analysis revealed that 1 in 4 youth (age of <18 years) experience clinically elevated depression symptoms, while 1 in 5 youth experience clinically elevated anxiety symptoms, which are double the pre-pandemic estimates [12]. Another cross-sectional study of Canadian youth and young adults (age of 6–20 years) found an increase in anxiety with incidence rate ratio (IRR) of 1.11, personality disorders with IRR of 1.21, and suicidality with IRR of 1.10 in females and an increase in eating disorders in both sexes (IRR of 1.66 in females, IRR of 1.47 in males) in the COVID-19-prevalent period [13]. This trend also applied to suicide in children. A systematic review on emergency department visits for all indications among children and adolescents (aged < 19 years) across 18 countries revealed good evidence of an increase for attempted suicide during the pandemic (rate ratio 1.22, 90% Confidence interval (CI) 1.08–1.37), modest evidence of an increase for suicidal ideation (rate ratio 1.08, 90% CI 0.93–1.25), and good evidence of only a slight change in self-harm (rate ratio 0.96, 90% CI 0.89–1.04) [14].

Social isolation during the pandemic further deepened feelings of loneliness and anxiety, affecting children's ability to form and maintain friendships. A study in Japan suggested that COVID-19-related sleep disorders affected feelings of school refusal through the exacerbation of loneliness directly or indirectly [15]. Although the long-term outcome of mental health disorders in children is unclear, the prolonged stress of the pandemic may have contributed to neuroinflammatory changes, influencing the hypothalamic–pituitary–adrenal axis [7].

4.2. Family Dynamics

The pandemic's economic and emotional toll has strained family relationships, creating challenges in providing a supportive environment for children. Parents, particularly mothers, reported heightened stress levels during school closures in Japan [16]. Another study in Japan showed that approximately 40% of parents experienced moderate depression symptoms during the COVID-19 pandemic [10], while this trend was reported similarly in other countries as well [12,17]. An international meta-analysis found that clinically significant depression symptoms and anxiety symptoms during the COVID-19 pandemic were found in 26.9% and 41.9% of mothers of children aged 0–5 years [12]. Clinically elevated depression and anxiety symptoms were more prevalent in older mothers, and clinically elevated anxiety was more common in highly educated mothers [12]. Notably, pre-pandemic vulnerabilities are at higher risk of negative outcomes than those without. A cross-sectional online survey in the United Kingdom suggested that parents with children who requires special needs are at higher risk of loneliness, parent burnout and decreased perception of social support [18]. In addition, a longitudinal study in the Netherlands found that parents with higher levels of negative emotions prior to lockdown were more likely to perceive COVID-19-related stress [19].

Although considerable numbers of parents experienced elevated levels of depression and/or anxiety initially at the pandemic, symptoms often decreased over time. For instance, a two-wave longitudinal study on Norwegian parents found that depression meeting clinical criteria decreased from 23% in the first wave to 16.8% in the second wave, similarly anxiety meeting clinical criteria decreased from 23.3% to 13.8% [20]. While many parents show resilience as a common outcome due to COVID-19 pandemic, family dynamics should be considered in the context of children's health and should be a target of future interventions [21].

Economic instability disproportionately affects low-income families, limiting their ability to access resources necessary for remote learning. The reduced availability of social services and school-based support systems has further compounded the difficulties faced by vulnerable families. Increased domestic tensions during lockdowns have led to an increase in Japanese reports of domestic violence (190,030 cases in 2020, increasing approximately 1.6 times higher than in 2019) and child abuse (225,509 cases in 2023, a 5.0% increase compared to 2022), further destabilizing children's home environments [22,23]. These familial factors could profoundly affect the child–parent relationship, which in turn may positively or negatively affect children's mental wellbeing states [24].

4.3. Societal Impacts

On a broader scale, the COVID-19 pandemic has exposed and exacerbated societal inequalities, particularly in education. Prolonged school closures and lockdowns due to the COVID-19 pandemic may have contributed to these educational disparities [25]. A paper from a World Bank report by Patrinos described the educational impact of the pandemic on school children [26]. The duration of school closures in Japan was over 10 weeks, varying across countries from 0 weeks (Sweden) to over 90 weeks (India). The report by Patrinos estimated that for every week schools were closed, learning levels declined by almost one percent of a standard deviation—meaning that a 20-week closure could reduce leaning outcomes by 0.20 standard deviation, equivalent to nearly one year of schooling [26].

Socioeconomic status also contributed educational gaps during the pandemic, particularly in lower-income countries [25]. Remote learning highlighted disparities in access to technology and digital infrastructure, among children from socioeconomically disadvantaged households [27]. These disparities widened the achievement gap and limited the educational opportunities of students [28]. Since the duration of lockdown and school closures was determined based on public health decisions, we should examine the link between these decisions and their spillover effects—not only on learning outcomes but also on broader human capital factors—which could influence children in various ways.

The impact of the pandemic extended to children's social development, as restrictions on group activities and social gatherings reduced opportunities for meaningful interactions with peers. An oversea study investigating changes in developmental screening scores among American children of 0–5 years of age between the pre-pandemic period (1 March 2018, to 29 February 2020) and the intra-pandemic period (1 June 2020, to 30 May 2022) found significant declines in the communication (−0.029), problem-solving (−0.018), and personal-social (−0.016) domains [29].

4.4. *Direct Impact on School Refusal*

The COVID-19 pandemic has intensified the factors contributing to school refusal. For students already struggling with academic pressure, remote learning environments can lack necessary structure and support, increasing students' feelings of frustration and disengagement. Fear of infection and concern about safety also discouraged many students from returning to in-person schooling, especially those with health vulnerabilities or at-risk family members [30].

The COVID-19 pandemic has had a particularly severe impact on students who are already vulnerable to difficulties in school attendance. These children, including those with pre-existing mental health conditions, neurodevelopmental disorders, or adverse family environments, face heightened challenges due to the disruptions caused by the pandemic [30,31]. A large-scale cross-sectional online survey conducted during the COVID-19 pandemic in Hong Kong, involving families with children aged 2–12 years, found that the risk of child psychosocial problems was higher in children with special educational needs, acute/chronic disease, mothers with mental illness, single-parent families, and low-income families [32]. Another questionnaire survey in Japan of caregivers of children with neurodevelopmental disorders showed that although no relationship was observed between difficulty in infection prevention measures and deterioration in their relationship with parents and friends during school closures, a positive association was found after school reopened [33].

The COVID-19 pandemic has revealed many aspects of social vulnerability, particularly among children in vulnerable situations, which had previously remained unrecognized. The lessons we have learned from this pandemic could serve to prepare for future pandemics and to create a more inclusive society.

5. Interventions, Support, and Future Directions

Addressing school refusal behavior and its associated challenges requires a multifaceted approach. School-based interventions such as counseling services, peer support programs, and teacher training in mental health awareness are essential for identifying and supporting at-risk students [2,5,27]. Schools should foster inclusive environments that accommodate diverse needs and ensure that all students feel valued and supported.

Family support plays a relevant role in addressing school refusal. Providing resources and education to parents can help mitigate family-related stressors. Parenting workshops and family therapy can address the underlying dynamics and strengthen relationships, fostering a supportive home environment for children [34].

At the societal level, government policies must prioritize mental health services and educational equity. Ensuring equal access to technologies and educational opportunities is vital for reducing disparities [35]. Telemedicine and digital tools, which have gained attention during the pandemic, offer valuable options for providing mental healthcare to children who are reluctant to attend in-person consultations [27].

In 2023, the 'COCOLO Plan (Comfortable, Customized and Optimized Locations of learning)' was implemented by the Japanese government as a comprehensive, multi-sector approach to address school refusal in Japan [35]. This plan set forth three clear goals: (1) securing diverse learning opportunities, (2) early detection and support through the "one device per student" initiative, and (3) visualizing school culture to make schools places where "everyone can learn with ease".

The plan promotes support not only for children experiencing school refusal but also for their families by integrating several measures. These include promoting the establishment of in-school education support centers (such as special support rooms), assigning school counselors and school social workers, developing an environment in which students can easily consult with such specialist at any time via online services, supporting education through ICT or collaborating with Non-Profit Organizations and free schools.

It also emphasizes early detection of changes in health and feelings of students through individual devices and early-stage interventions by "team schools" to identify the support needs of students facing difficulties.

This plan is expected to expand various educational options for children experiencing school refusal. For instance, under certain conditions, students attending free schools or learning through ICT-based methods may have their attendance officially recognized. This could bring Japan more in line with international best practices to support diverse learning needs—for example, the U.S Department of Defense Education Activity, which officially recognizes homeschooling as a valid alternative to school attendance [36].

To address the complex and evolving issues of school refusal, future research should focus on several key areas—such as longitudinal studies to evaluate the long-term mental health, educational, and social outcomes of children and families; comparative international studies to examine how different policies/systems/cultures influence school refusal; and biopsychosocial approaches that integrate biological, psychological, and social factors affecting children.

6. Conclusions

The COVID-19 pandemic has impacted school refusal behavior in Japan and worldwide in various ways. Its effects have been pronounced with pre-existing vulnerabilities and those from socially disadvantaged backgrounds. Addressing this issue requires coordinated efforts to provide support through schools, families, and societal systems.

School refusal arises from the complex interplay of multiple contributors, often making it difficult for children to recognize underlying problems. While this can be a challenging experience, it also presents an opportunity for a deeper understanding and stronger relationships for both children and their families. Physicians, healthcare providers, and the government play a crucial role in supporting these children and their families in overcoming these challenges together, just like a team and community, so that they can move toward a future.

Author Contributions: Conceptualization, D.M.; investigation, D.M.; writing—original draft preparation, D.M.; writing—review and editing, K.K. and H.O.; supervision, K.K. and H.O. All authors have read and agreed to the published version of the manuscript.

Funding: This research received no external funding.

Institutional Review Board Statement: Not applicable.

Informed Consent Statement: Not applicable.

Data Availability Statement: The authors declare that data supporting the findings of this study are available in the article.

Acknowledgments: During the preparation of this manuscript, the authors used commercial native checking editing services and ChatGPT-4o for grammar checking. The authors have reviewed and edited the output and take full responsibility for the content of this publication.

Conflicts of Interest: The authors declare no conflicts of interest.

References

1. Ministry of Health, Labour and Welfare, Japan. Annual Report on Vital Statistics. 2023. Available online: https://www.mhlw.go.jp/toukei/saikin/hw/jinkou/kakutei23/index.html (accessed on 5 June 2025).
2. Ministry of Education, Culture, Sports, Science and Technology, Japan. Report on School Absenteeism in Japan. 2023. Available online: https://www.mext.go.jp/content/20241031-mxt_jidou02-100002753_2_2.pdf (accessed on 5 June 2025).
3. Kearney, C.A. School absenteeism and school refusal behavior in youth: A contemporary review. *Clin. Psychol. Rev.* **2008**, *28*, 451–471. [CrossRef]
4. Dee, T.S. Higher chronic absenteeism threatens academic recovery from the COVID-19 pandemic. *Proc. Natl. Acad. Sci. USA* **2024**, *121*, e2312249121. [CrossRef]
5. Lester, K.J.; Michelson, D. Perfect storm: Emotionally based school avoidance in the post-COVID-19 pandemic context. *BMJ Ment. Health* **2024**, *27*, e300944. [CrossRef] [PubMed]
6. Rahman, M.A.; Renzaho, A.M.N.; Kundu, S.; Awal, M.A.; Ashikuzzaman, M.; Fan, L.; Ahinkorah, B.O.; Okyere, J.; Kamara, J.K.; Mahumud, R.A. Prevalence and factors associated with chronic school absenteeism among 207,107 in-school adolescents: Findings from cross-sectional studies in 71 low-middle and high-income countries. *PLoS ONE* **2023**, *18*, e0283046. [CrossRef] [PubMed]
7. de Figueiredo, C.S.; Sandre, P.C.; Portugal, L.C.L.; Mázala-de-Oliveira, T.; da Silva Chagas, L.; Raony, Í.; Ferreira, E.S.; Giestal-de-Araujo, E.; Dos Santos, A.A.; Bomfim, P.O. COVID-19 pandemic impact on children and adolescents' mental health: Biological, environmental, and social factors. *Prog. Neuropsychopharmacol. Biol. Psychiatry* **2021**, *106*, 110171. [CrossRef] [PubMed]
8. Ministry of Education, Culture, Sports, Science and Technology, Japan. Physical Fitness Trends Among Japanese Children. 2021. Available online: https://www.mext.go.jp/sports/content/20211222-spt_sseisaku02-000019583_111.pdf (accessed on 5 June 2025).
9. Saito, M.; Kikuchi, Y.; Lefor, A.K.; Hoshina, M. Mental health in Japanese children during school closures due to the COVID-19. *Pediatr. Int.* **2022**, *64*, e14718. [CrossRef]
10. National Center for Child Health and Development. COVID-19 Impact Report on Child Health. 2023. Available online: https://www.ncchd.go.jp/center/assets/CXCN_repo2023.pdf (accessed on 5 June 2025).
11. Ministry of Health, Labour and Welfare, Japan. Annual Report on Child Suicides. 2024. Available online: https://www.mhlw.go.jp/content/2024-2-1.pdf (accessed on 5 June 2025).
12. Racine, N.; McArthur, B.A.; Cooke, J.E.; Eirich, R.; Zhu, J.; Madigan, S. Global Prevalence of Depressive and Anxiety Symptoms in Children and Adolescents During COVID-19: A Meta-analysis. *JAMA Pediatr.* **2021**, *175*, 1142–1150. [CrossRef]
13. Roumeliotis, N.; Carwana, M.; Trudeau, O.; Charland, K.; Zinszer, K.; Benigeri, M.; Diop, M.; Papenburg, J.; Ali, S.; Yaskina, M.; et al. Mental Health Hospitalizations in Canadian Children, Adolescents, and Young Adults Over the COVID-19 Pandemic. *JAMA Netw. Open* **2024**, *7*, e2422833. [CrossRef]
14. Madigan, S.; Korczak, D.J.; Vaillancourt, T.; Racine, N.; Hopkins, W.G.; Pador, P.; Hewitt, J.M.A.; AlMousawi, B.; McDonald, S.; Neville, R.D. Comparison of paediatric emergency department visits for attempted suicide, self-harm, and suicidal ideation before and during the COVID-19 pandemic: A systematic review and meta-analysis. *Lancet Psychiatry* **2023**, *10*, 342–351. [CrossRef]
15. Okajima, I.; Honda, Y.; Semba, O.; Kiyota, Y.; Tani, Y. Effects of COVID-19-Related Anxiety and Sleep Problems on Loneliness and Feelings of School Refusal in Adolescents. *Front. Psychiatry* **2022**, *13*, 918417. [CrossRef]
16. Hiraoka, D.; Tomoda, A. Relationship between parenting stress and school closures due to the COVID-19 pandemic. *Psychiatry Clin. Neurosci.* **2020**, *74*, 497–498. [CrossRef]
17. Bourion-Bédès, S.; Rousseau, H.; Batt, M.; Beltrand, C.; Machane, R.; Tarquinio, P.; Tarquinio, C.; Baumann, C. Measuring COVID-19 related stress and its associated factors among the parents of school-aged children during the first lockdown in France. *BMC Public Health* **2023**, *23*, 1823. [CrossRef]

18. El-Osta, A.; Alaa, A.; Webber, I.; Riboli Sasco, E.; Bagkeris, E.; Millar, H.; Vidal-Hall, C.; Majeed, A. How is the COVID-19 lockdown impacting the mental health of parents of school-age children in the UK? A cross-sectional online survey. *BMJ Open* **2021**, *11*, e043397. [CrossRef] [PubMed]
19. Achterberg, M.; Dobbelaar, S.; Boer, O.D.; Crone, E.A. Perceived stress as mediator for longitudinal effects of the COVID-19 lockdown on wellbeing of parents and children. *Sci. Rep.* **2021**, *11*, 2971. [CrossRef] [PubMed]
20. Johnson, M.S.; Skjerdingstad, N.; Ebrahimi, O.V.; Hoffart, A.; Urnes Johnson, S. Mechanisms of parental distress during and after the first COVID-19 lockdown phase: A two-wave longitudinal study. *PLoS ONE* **2021**, *16*, e0253087. [CrossRef]
21. Whaley, G.L.; Pfefferbaum, B. Parental Challenges During the COVID-19 Pandemic: Psychological Outcomes and Risk and Protective Factors. *Curr. Psychiatry Rep.* **2023**, *25*, 165–174. [CrossRef]
22. Gender Equality Bureau Cabinet Office, Japan. White Paper on Gender Equality. 2021. Available online: https://www.gender.go.jp/about_danjo/whitepaper/r03/zentai/html/honpen/b1_s00_02.html (accessed on 5 June 2025).
23. Children and Families Agency, Japan. Annual Report on Child Abuse. 2023. Available online: https://www.cfa.go.jp/assets/contents/node/basic_page/field_ref_resources/a176de99-390e-4065-a7fb-fe569ab2450c/5fbbaa2e/20250327_policies_jidougyakutai_32.pdf (accessed on 5 August 2025).
24. Cohodes, E.M.; McCauley, S.; Gee, D.G. Parental Buffering of Stress in the Time of COVID-19: Family-Level Factors May Moderate the Association Between Pandemic-Related Stress and Youth Symptomatology. *Res. Child. Adolesc. Psychopathol.* **2021**, *49*, 935–948. [CrossRef]
25. Agostinelli, F.; Doepke, M.; Sorrenti, G.; Zilibotti, F. When the great equalizer shuts down: Schools, peers, and parents in pandemic times. *J. Public. Econ.* **2022**, *206*, 104574. [CrossRef]
26. Patrinos, H.A. The Longer Students Were Out of School, the Less They Learned. 2023. Available online: https://documents1.worldbank.org/curated/en/099534004242341552/pdf/IDU0807776730889d04a240ad3305c282c112fe8.pdf (accessed on 5 August 2025).
27. Goudeau, S.; Sanrey, C.; Stanczak, A.; Manstead, A.; Darnon, C. Why lockdown and distance learning during the COVID-19 pandemic are likely to increase the social class achievement gap. *Nat. Hum. Behav.* **2021**, *5*, 1273–1281. [CrossRef]
28. Nippon Foundation and Mitsubishi UFJ Research and Consulting, Japan. Impact of the COVID-19 Pandemic on Educational Disparities—Survey Report. 2021. Available online: https://www.nippon-foundation.or.jp/wp-content/uploads/2021/06/new_pr_20210629.pdf (accessed on 5 June 2025).
29. Johnson, S.B.; Kuehn, M.; Lambert, J.O.; Spin, J.P.; Klein, L.M.; Howard, B.; Sturner, R.; Perrin, E.M. Developmental Milestone Attainment in US Children Before and During the COVID-19 Pandemic. *JAMA Pediatr.* **2024**, *178*, 586–594. [CrossRef] [PubMed]
30. McDonald, B.; Lester, K.J.; Michelson, D. 'She didn't know how to go back': School attendance problems in the context of the COVID-19 pandemic-A multiple stakeholder qualitative study with parents and professionals. *Br. J. Educ. Psychol.* **2023**, *93*, 386–401. [CrossRef] [PubMed]
31. Dessain, A.; Parlatini, V.; Singh, A.; De Bruin, M.; Cortese, S.; Sonuga-Barke, E.; Serrano, J.V. Mental health during the COVID-19 pandemic in children and adolescents with ADHD: A systematic review of controlled longitudinal cohort studies. *Neurosci. Biobehav. Rev.* **2024**, *156*, 105502. [CrossRef] [PubMed]
32. Tso, W.W.Y.; Wong, R.S.; Tung, K.T.S.; Rao, N.; Fu, K.W.; Yam, J.C.S.; Chua, G.T.; Chen, E.Y.H.; Lee, T.M.C.; Chan, S.K.W.; et al. Vulnerability and resilience in children during the COVID-19 pandemic. *Eur. Child. Adolesc. Psychiatry* **2022**, *31*, 161–176. [CrossRef]
33. Yamamoto, T.; Tanaka, S.; Yoshizaki, A.; Yoshimura, Y.; Fauzi, A.A.; Syarinaz, A.; Adlan, A.; Jayanath, S.; Hamzah, N.; Fujino, H.; et al. Relationship between children with neurodevelopmental disorders and their caregivers and friends during early phase of COVID-19 school closure in Japan: Association with difficulty in implementing infection prevention measures. *Child. Adolesc. Psychiatry Ment. Health* **2022**, *16*, 78. [CrossRef]
34. Matano, M.; Monden, Y.; Kurane, K.; Kawasaki, M.; Kamo, T. Potential of internet-delivered PCIT for ASD in the COVID-19 era: A pilot study. *Pediatr. Int.* **2022**, *64*, e14699. [CrossRef] [PubMed]
35. Ministry of Education, Culture, Sports, Science and Technology, Japan. COCOLO Plan: Addressing School Refusal in Japan. 2023. Available online: https://www.mext.go.jp/content/20230418-mxt_jidou02-000028870-cc.pdf (accessed on 5 June 2025).
36. Department of Defense Education Activity. Available online: https://www.dodea.edu (accessed on 5 August 2025).

children

MDPI

Article

Psychological Impact of Distance Learning on Children and Adolescents in Saudi Arabia: A Multi-City Analysis of Behavioral and Mental Health Outcomes During the COVID-19 Pandemic

Samah H. Alkhawashki [1,2,†], Maram H. AlTuwairqi [1,2,†], Ahmad H. Almadani [1,2], Atnan A. Almarshedi [3], Rahaf Alasiri [4,5], Noha A. Mobeireek [6], Mishaal R. Alrashoud [7], Noura A. Abouammoh [8], Fatimah S. Alshahrani [9], Areej A. AlFattani [10] and Shuliweeh Alenezi [1,2,*]

1 Department of Psychiatry, College of Medicine, King Saud University, Riyadh 11472, Saudi Arabia
2 SABIC Psychological Health Research and Applications Chair (SPHRAC), Department of Psychiatry, College of Medicine, King Saud University, Riyadh 11451, Saudi Arabia
3 Department of Psychiatry, Prince Sultan Military Medical City, Riyadh 11159, Saudi Arabia
4 King Abdullah International Medical Research Center, Jeddah 22384, Saudi Arabia
5 College of Medicine, King Saudi bin Abdulaziz University for Health Sciences, Jeddah 21498, Saudi Arabia
6 King Abdullah International Medical Research Center, Riyadh 11481, Saudi Arabia
7 Department of Psychiatry, Dammam Medical Complex, Dammam 32253, Saudi Arabia
8 Department of Family and Community Medicine, King Saud University, Riyadh 11451, Saudi Arabia
9 Department of Medicine, King Saud University, Riyadh 11451, Saudi Arabia
10 Biostatistics, Epidemiology and Scientific Computing, King Faisal Specialist Hospital and Research Center, Riyadh 11211, Saudi Arabia
* Correspondence: salenizi@ksu.edu.sa
† These authors contributed equally to this work.

Abstract: Background: The COVID-19 pandemic triggered a global transition to distance learning, which significantly impacted children's mental health. In Saudi Arabia, remote education began on 8 March 2020, lasting between 1.5 to 2.5 years. This study aims to explore the psychological effects of distance learning on children and adolescents, with a focus on mental health challenges and coping mechanisms. Methods: A cross-sectional study was conducted using an online survey distributed to parents of children aged 6 to 18 in the major metropolitan areas of Jeddah and Riyadh. The survey included demographic questions and the Arabic version of the Vanderbilt ADHD Diagnostic Rating Scale, a tool for assessing behavioral challenges, anxiety, and symptoms of attention deficit hyperactivity disorder (ADHD). Results: A total of 71.6% of families reported a positive experience with distance learning. A significant correlation was found between parents' marital status and children's ability to cope with remote education. Interestingly, children without ADHD symptoms experienced three times more negative outcomes than those with ADHD symptoms. However, despite reporting fewer negative experiences, children with ADHD exhibited increased symptom severity and academic difficulties. Of the students, 5.4% were diagnosed with predominantly inattentive ADHD, 1.8% with predominantly hyperactive/impulsive ADHD, and 3.9% with combined ADHD. Additionally, 7.2% of students screened positive for oppositional defiant disorder, 1.5% for conduct disorder, and 6.6% for anxiety or depression. Children from separated or divorced families were more likely to exhibit ADHD symptoms ($p = 0.002$). Children with ADHD symptoms reported a more positive experience with distance learning ($p < 0.05$). Conclusion: This study represents the first comprehensive, multi-city investigation in Saudi Arabia examining the relationship between distance learning, sociodemographic factors, and mental health symptoms in children. The findings highlight the psychological challenges faced by children during the pandemic and emphasize the need for targeted interventions to support both mental health and academic outcomes. These results offer valuable insights for future research and inform strategies to address children's well-being in scenarios involving distance learning.

Keywords: distance learning; virtual schooling; mental health; students; youth; Saudi Arabia

1. Introduction

The COVID-19 pandemic caused widespread disruption, significantly impacting the routines and education of children and adolescents worldwide. One of the most notable changes was the shift to distance learning to maintain physical distancing and manage the spread of the virus [1,2]. This transition was mandated in Saudi Arabia for all K–12 schools and higher education institutions starting 8 March 2020. The duration of remote learning varied between 1.5 and 2.5 academic years, depending on factors such as students' age, vaccination status, and the educational system they were enrolled in, as documented by the Ministry of Education (MOE) in its report on efforts to combat COVID-19 [3].

In the early stages of the pandemic, numerous studies sought to assess the mental health impact of distance learning on students. For example, a survey of 612 adolescents aged 13 to 18 in the United Kingdom reported mental health symptoms in 53.3% of females and 44.0% of males. Anxiety affected 59.6% of males and 47.4% of females, while depressive symptoms were found in 21.9% of males and 19.4% of females [4]. The mental health challenges associated with remote education included anxiety, depression, loneliness, and perceived stress [5,6]. Similarly, in the United States, a study of first-year college students revealed that anxiety prevalence increased from 18.1% to 25.3% and depression from 21.5% to 31.7% within the first four months of the pandemic [7]. In China, a study involving 7143 college students showed a significant correlation between anxiety symptoms and disruptions in daily life and academics [8].

Poor academic performance in the context of distance education was found to be linked with concentration challenges, shorter attention spans, exam-related stress, COVID-19 contagion anxiety, and depressive symptoms [6,9]. Conversely, students with a positive perception of distance learning, family support, and resilience skills were better able to manage educational challenges [6,10].

A survey-based study in Malaysia assessed students' demographics, academic challenges, and perceptions of remote education while screening for mental health issues using the DASS-21. It reported that 29.4% of university students experienced depression, 51.3% anxiety, and 56.5% stress, with older students showing lower prevalence rates [11]. Another large-scale study using the parent version of the Strengths and Difficulties Questionnaire (SDQ) found that remote learning most negatively affected older children and those from Black, Hispanic, or low socioeconomic backgrounds [12]. Similarly, a survey of Mexican parents of children aged 4 to 15 highlighted behavioral issues, sleep disturbances, and increased screen time as critical challenges of distance education [13]. Interestingly, the perceived threat of COVID-19 among students was correlated with their parents' perceptions, and parents' stress levels were positively associated with students' stress [14].

The topic also gained attention among child age groups. For instance, Panchal U. et al. [15] conducted a systematic review study aiming to review the literature on the effects of the lockdown during the COVID-19 pandemic on mental health among children and adolescents. In this study, the results indicated that depressive and anxiety symptoms were common, although the ranges were wide. Other symptoms that were found to be common were irritability and anger. A systematic mixed studies review conducted by Levante, A. et al. [16] showed that the internalizing/externalizing symptoms among children increased during COVID-19, with girls exhibiting more internalizing symptoms. Nonetheless, in a systematic review conducted by Samji H. et al. [17] the authors also concluded higher anxiety and depressive symptoms among children and adolescents during COVID-19, with certain groups, such as older adolescents, more likely affected.

Despite the breadth of international research, there is a gap in large, multi-city studies in Saudi Arabia that explore the psychological impact of distance learning on children and adolescents. This research aims to bridge that gap by examining how remote education during the pandemic has affected students' mental health and educational experiences across different demographics. More concisely, this study aims to answer the question of the psychological effect of distance learning on children and adolescents in Saudi Arabia. The findings will provide valuable insights to inform mental health advocacy and guide the future direction of education, particularly in situations where distance learning becomes necessary.

2. Methods

2.1. Ethical Considerations

The King Saud University—College of Medicine's IRB (application number E-22-6867) granted approval for this study. Parents consented at the survey's start, and completion was required for participation. Participants were informed of the study's purpose and confirmed consent by clicking "yes". Data were encrypted for confidentiality and accessed only by the research team.

2.2. Study Design and Participants

We employed a cross-sectional study design, distributing the e-questionnaire to parents via social media platforms, including WhatsApp. Data collection occurred between October and the end of November 2022. The sample size "n" was calculated to be 335 participants. According to the Saudi Ministry of Education's statistics, this calculation was based on the estimated population of school-aged children in the Riyadh and Jeddah regions, which is approximately 2,000,000. The following formula was used to determine the appropriate sample size:

$$x = Z({}^{c}/{}_{100})^{2} r(100 - r)$$

$$n = {}^{N x}/{}_{((N - 1)E^{2} + x)}$$

$$E = \text{Sqrt}\,[{}^{(N - n)x}/{}_{n(N - 1)}]$$

This formula ensures that the sample size is sufficient to accurately represent the target population, accounting for population variability and desired precision.

Sample Size Calculator by Raosoft, Inc. 6645 NE Windermere Rd, Seattle, WA 98115, USA.

2.3. Inclusion and Exclusion Criteria

The study included parents of male and female children and adolescents aged 6 to 18 years who attended governmental, national, or international schools, including both public and private institutions, within the Riyadh and Jeddah regions of Saudi Arabia.

Children and adolescents with pre-existing mental illnesses, such as anxiety or depression, before the pandemic lockdown were excluded to focus on the impact of distance learning on previously healthy individuals. Additionally, children with diagnosed neurodevelopmental disorders—including Autism Spectrum Disorder (ASD), Attention Deficit Hyperactivity Disorder (ADHD), intellectual disability, and cerebral palsy—were excluded, as were those with chronic health conditions such as diabetes.

2.4. Tools and Procedures

The survey used for the study consisted of an online questionnaire divided into two sections:

1. Sociodemographic and Background Information:

This section collected data on participants' demographics, medical and psychiatric history, educational settings, and the level of school support provided during the pandemic.

2. Vanderbilt Assessment Scale:

This section employed the Vanderbilt Assessment Scale, which has been validated for use in Arabic. This scale was integrated into the survey without copyright restrictions, thanks to its accessibility through the Saudi ADHD Society's online resources [18]. While its primary purpose is to assess the diagnosis of ADHD, it is also designed to screen for additional behavioral and emotional concerns in children 6 years and above [19]. Furthermore, it is important to note that the diagnosis of ADHD cannot be established solely through an assessment scale; hence, the reported ADHD refers to ADHD symptoms rather than a diagnosis. The e-questionnaire contains 54 items with 6 main domains (Figure 1). We confirm that we adhered to the specified criteria throughout our study, following the Scoring Instructions for the NICHQ Vanderbilt Assessment Scales for each diagnostic category:

- Predominantly Inattentive subtype: We verified that participants scored a 2 or 3 on at least 6 out of 9 items on questions 1–9 and achieved a score of 4 or 5 on one or more of the Performance questions (questions 48–55).
- Predominantly Hyperactive/Impulsive subtype: We ensured that participants met the requirement of scoring a 2 or 3 on at least 6 out of 9 items on questions 10–18, in addition to a score of 4 or 5 on one or more of the Performance items (questions 48–55).
- ADHD Combined Inattention/Hyperactivity subtype: Participants were confirmed to meet the above criteria for both inattention and hyperactivity/impulsivity.
- Oppositional-Defiant Disorder (ODD) Screen: Participants were evaluated to meet the requirement of scoring a 2 or 3 on at least 4 out of 8 items on questions 19–26 and a 4 or 5 on any Performance items (questions 48–55).
- Conduct Disorder Screen: We confirmed that participants scored a 2 or 3 on a minimum of 3 out of 14 items on questions 27–40 and met the requirement of a 4 or 5 on the Performance items (questions 48–55).
- Anxiety/Depression Screen: For this category, we ensured participants scored a 2 or 3 on at least 3 out of 7 items on questions 41–47 and a 4 or 5 on any Performance items (questions 48–55).

Each criterion was consistently applied based on the Scoring Instructions for the NICHQ Vanderbilt Assessment Scales to ensure accuracy and adherence to the study's diagnostic parameters.

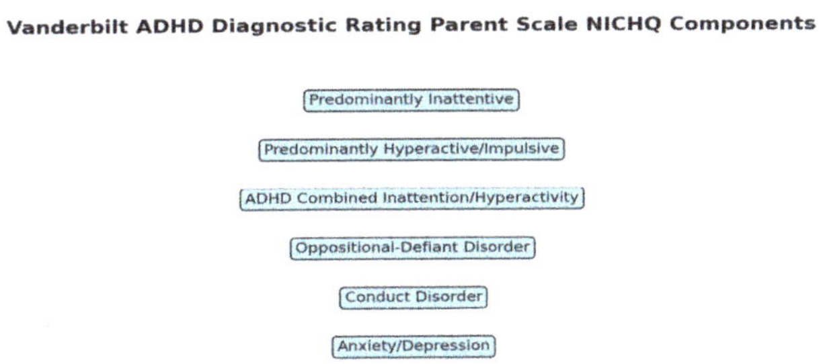

Figure 1. Vanderbilt ADHD Diagnostic Rating Parent Scale NICHQ Components.

2.5. Validation and Data Collection

Parents with more than one child were allowed to complete the survey for each child. To identify multiple responses from the same household while maintaining anonymity, participants provided only the last four digits of their 10-digit family ID number. Data collected during the pilot phase were excluded from the final analysis. On average, it took parents 15 min to complete the survey. Participants self-identified by responding to invitations sent through social media platforms.

2.6. Statistical Analysis

Data were summarized using means ± standard deviations for continuous variables and frequencies with percentages for categorical variables. The Kolmogorov–Smirnov test was used to test the normality of the continuous variables. All statistical analyses were performed using the Statistical Package for Social Studies (SPSS) version 22 (IBM Corp., New York, NY, USA). Responses from the pilot survey were excluded from the final analysis.

Comparisons were made between children exhibiting ADHD symptoms (regardless of subtype) and those without any symptoms. The Chi-square and Fisher's exact tests were used for categorical variables, while *t*-tests were applied for continuous variables. Homogeneity was tested by Levene's test. Multiple logistic regression was performed to evaluate the effect of significant variables on having ADHD diagnosis as a binary response variable (Yes/No). All predictors which were significant in the univariate crosstabulation were included in the model. The regression model was controlled for age as a covariant. A p-value < 0.05 was considered statistically significant.

3. Results

The study involved 335 student participants shown in Table 1, with a mean age of 9.8 SD 3.2 years. Most families (72%) had three or more children, with 91.1% of parents married and 55% with both parents employed. Income varied, with 36.4% earning 10,000–20,000 SAR and 26.8% earning over 30,000 SAR. At the pandemic's start, 48.7% of children were in early primary grades. Remote learning was prevalent, lasting one and a half years for 42.7% and two years for 41.2% of children, while 6.3% experienced schooling delays, primarily due to COVID-19 exposure concerns. Private schools were most common (40.9%), followed by government (36.7%) and international schools (22.4%). School changes affected 19.1% of students. Educational support came from family members in 28.7% of cases and domestic helpers in 9.3%. Almost all families (89.9%) had sufficient electronic devices for home education, with 52.2% rating distance learning as good. Chronic physical illnesses were reported in 4.5% of children, with ADHD and anxiety most frequently noted. A majority (93.7%) were not on medication, though 15% exhibited ADHD symptoms.

Table 1. Characteristics of the students and their parents ("n" = 334).

Variable	Group	Number	%	Variable	Group	Number	%
The number of children in the home "n" = 280	1	54	19.3	What is the reason for the delay? "n" = 21	financial conditions	1	4.8
	2	78	27.9		social conditions	1	4.8
	3	71	25.4		Fear of exposure to the Coronavirus while having a health condition	4	19
	4	48	17.1		Fear of exposure to the Coronavirus and the child's health condition is very good	8	38.1
	5	14	5		Another reason	7	33.3
	>5	15	5.4	School type	government	123	36.7
Parents' marital status "n" = 280	married	255	91.1		private	137	40.9
	separated or divorced	23	8.2		International	75	22.4
	One of the parents is deceased	2	0.7	Has the school changed due to the pandemic?	Yes	64	19.1
The age of the child at the beginning of the pandemic (Mean, SD)		9.8	3.2		No	270	80.6

Table 1. *Cont.*

Variable	Group	Number	%	Variable	Group	Number	%
Parent's employment status Mother and father are working "n" = 280 Only mother works Only father works Mother and father do not work		154	55	Were others, such as grandfather, grandmother, or one of the siblings, used to help the child attend the educational platform?	Yes	96	28.7
		16	5.7		No	239	71.3
		94	33.6	2 Was a maid relied upon to help the child attend the educational platform?	Yes	31	9.3
		16	5.7		No	304	90.7
The total monthly income of the family "n" = 280	<10,000 SR	31	11.1	The presence of sufficient electronic devices for education at home	Yes	301	89.9
	10,000–20,000 SR	102	36.4		No	34	10.1
	20,000–30,000 SR	72	25.7	Assess the overall learning experience of distance learning for your respective child.	very bad	40	11.9
	>30,000 SR	75	26.8		bad	55	16.4
The child's classroom at the beginning of the pandemic—March 2020 "n" = 335	1–3 Primary	163	48.7		acceptable	65	19.4
	4–6 Primary	92	27.5		good	78	23.3
	intermediate	57	17		very good	55	16.4
	secondary	23	6.9		excellent	42	12.5
The child's grade level when attendance or semi-attendance learning began again "n" = 335	1–3 Primary	120	35.8	Did your child suffer from chronic physical illnesses before the pandemic?	No	335	100
	4–6 Primary	111	33.1	Has your child been diagnosed with chronic physical illnesses during the pandemic?	Yes	15	4.5
	intermediate	62	18.5		No	320	95.5
	secondary	42	12.5	What is the diagnosis?	ADHD	5	38
The number of academic years the child studied remotely from March 2020 to March 2022 "n" = 335	half a year	21	6.3		Anxiety	4	31
	one year	33	9.9		get distracted	2	15
	A year and a half	143	42.7		psychosis	1	8
	two years	138	41.2		A combination of distractibility, hyperactivity, learning difficulties, and delay in social communication skills	1	8

Table 1. *Cont.*

Variable	Group	Number	%	Variable	Group	Number	%
Is your child late for school because of Corona? "n" = 335	Yes	21	6.3	Was this assessment done at a time when the child was on meds?	He takes medication	10	3
	No	314	93.7		He does not take medication	314	93.7
If the answer is 1, how many years later? "n" = 21	half a year	11	52.4		I'm not sure	11	3.3
	one year	5	23.8				
	more than one year	5	23.8				

Table 2 presents the findings from the Vanderbilt ADHD Diagnostic Rating Parent Scale. The results show that 5.4% of the children were classified as predominantly inattentive presentation, 1.8% as predominantly hyperactive/impulsive presentation, and 3.9% as combined ADHD presentation. Additionally, 7.2% of students were screened as potentially having oppositional defiant disorder, 1.5% for conduct disorder, and 6.6% for anxiety or depression.

Table 2. Vanderbilt ADHD Diagnostic Rating Parent Scale NICHQ.

	Number	%
Predominantly Inattentive subtype	18	5.4
Predominantly Hyperactive/Impulsive subtype	6	1.8
ADHD Combined Inattention/Hyperactivity	13	3.9
Oppositional-Defiant Disorder Screen	24	7.2
Conduct Disorder Screen	5	1.5
Anxiety/Depression Screen	22	6.6

Table 3 compares the demographic characteristics of students with and without ADHD symptoms, showing that 50 students in the sample exhibited ADHD symptoms. There were no significant differences in the number of children in the household, the child's age, parent's employment status, the length of remote learning, or school delays related to the pandemic. However, significant differences were observed in parental marital status. Specifically, 25.6% of children with ADHD symptoms came from separated or divorced families, compared to only 5.4% of children without ADHD symptoms. Furthermore, a higher proportion of children with ADHD were enrolled in grades 4–6 at the beginning of the pandemic.

Table 4 highlights the academic performance and other characteristics of students with and without ADHD symptoms. No significant differences were found regarding school type, school changes due to the pandemic, or access to electronic devices at home. However, significant differences were observed in the assistance children received for distance learning. Among children with ADHD symptoms, 40% received help from family members, such as grandparents or siblings, compared to 26.8% of children without ADHD symptoms. Additionally, 18% of children with ADHD relied on domestic helpers for assistance, compared to only 7.7% of children without ADHD ($p = 0.032$). Children with ADHD also reported a more positive overall distance learning experience compared to their non-ADHD peers. However, they had a higher likelihood of being diagnosed with chronic physical illnesses during the pandemic. In terms of academic outcomes, children with ADHD symptoms exhibited higher symptom scores and lower academic performance than those without ADHD symptoms.

Table 3. Comparison between students with any ADHD symptom and those without and other demographic characteristics.

		Are There Any ADHD Symptoms				*p* Value *
		No "n" = 284		Yes "n" = 50		
		Number	%	Number	%	
The number of children in the home	1	45	18.8	9	23.1	0.81
	2	68	28.3	9	23.1	
	3	60	25	11	28.2	
	4	40	16.7	8	20.5	
	5	13	5.4	1	2.6	
	>5	14	5.8	1	2.6	
Age	mean SD	9.8	3.2	9.1	3.1	0.353
Parents' marital status	married	225	93.8	29	74.4	0.001 *
	separated or divorced	13	5.4	10	25.6	
	One of the parents is deceased	2	0.8	0	0	
What is the reason for the delay?	financial conditions	1	5.6	0	0	0.701
	social conditions	1	5.6	0	0	
	Fear of exposure to the Coronavirus while having a health condition that makes it vulnerable to complications	4	22.2	0	0	
	Fear of exposure to the Coronavirus and the child's health condition is very good	7	38.9	1	33.3	
	Another reason	5	27.8	2	66.7	

* *p* value was estimated by chi-square or student test.

Table 4. ADHD combines inattention/Hyperactivity of the student by their characteristics.

		Are There Any ADHD Symptoms				*p* Value *
		No "n" = 284		Yes "n" = 50		
		Number	%	Number	%	
School type	government	102	35.9	21	42	0.7
	private	117	41.2	19	38	
	International	65	22.9	10	20	
Has the school changed due to the pandemic?	Yes	52	18.4	12	24	0.337
	No	231	81.6	38	76	
Were others, such as grandfather, grandmother, or one of the siblings2, used to help the child attend the educational platform?	Yes	76	26.8	20	40	0.06
	No	208	73.2	30	60	
Was a maid relied upon to help the child attend the educational platform?	Yes	22	7.7	9	18	0.032 *
	No	262	92.3	41	82	
The presence of sufficient electronic devices for education at home	Yes	254	89.4	46	92	0.8
	No	30	10.6	4	8	

Table 4. *Cont.*

		Are There Any ADHD Symptoms				p Value *
		No "n" = 284		Yes "n" = 50		
		Number	%	Number	%	
Assess the overall learning experience of distance learning for your respective child	very bad	38	13.4	2	4	0.002 *
	bad	51	18	4	8	
	acceptable	54	19	10	20	
	good	69	24.3	9	18	
	very good	44	15.5	11	22	
	excellent	28	9.9	14	28	
Has your child been diagnosed with chronic physical illnesses during the pandemic?	Yes	8	2.8	7	14	0.003 *
	No	276	97.2	43	86	
Total symptom	mean SD	2.6	3.2	8.8	4.7	0.001 *
Average performance	mean SD	0.131	0.211	0.523	0.291	0.001 *

* p value was estimated by chi-square or student test.

The multivariate logistic regression analysis results, summarized in Table 5, further explore factors associated with ADHD symptoms. The analysis found no significant link between age and ADHD symptoms. However, parental marital status was identified as a significant factor, with children from separated or divorced families being more likely to exhibit ADHD symptoms (Odds Ratio [OR] = 4.79, 95% Confidence Interval [CI]: 1.3–12.8, $p = 0.002$). Children with ADHD symptoms also reported a more positive learning experience during distance learning (OR = 5.473, 95% CI: 1.4–21.5, $p < 0.05$).

Table 5. Multiple logistic regression for the associated factors with ADHD Symptoms.

		Odds Ratio	95% C.I. for OR		p Value
			Lower	Upper	
Age		1.008	0.895	1.137	0.89
Parents' marital status	Married **	1			
	separated or divorced	4.79	1.787	12.836	0.002 *
Were others, such as grandfather, grandmother, or one of the siblings, used to help the child attend the educational platform?	No **	1			
	Yes	1.556	0.708	3.421	0.271
Was a maid relied upon to help the child attend the educational platform?	No **	1			
	Yes	1.032	0.322	3.309	0.957
Has your child been diagnosed with chronic physical illnesses such as diabetes, mental disorders such as anxiety or depression, developmental disorders such as autism or ADHD, or mental retardation during the pandemic?	No **	1			
	Yes	2.182	0.479	9.937	0.313
Assess the overall learning experience of distance learning for your respective child	very bad/bad **	1			
	acceptable	5.473	1.392	21.514	0.015 *
	good	3.211	0.781	13.206	0.106
	very good/excellent	6.902	1.831	26.012	0.004 *

* p value < 0.05; ** Reference group.

The analysis also examined whether a diagnosis of chronic physical illnesses or mental disorders during the pandemic was associated with ADHD symptoms. Although the odds ratio (OR = 2.182) was elevated, the association was not statistically significant ($p = 0.31$). No significant associations were found between ADHD symptoms and assistance from family members or domestic helpers with educational platforms. The analysis accounted for multiple children from the same household, identifying 69 children with one to three siblings, where parents completed multiple survey forms. However, the data did not reveal a significant association between having siblings from the same household and ADHD symptoms, and this factor was not further explored in the study.

4. Discussion

This study aimed to evaluate the behavioral and functional effects of distance learning, brought on by the COVID-19 pandemic, on children and adolescents in two major Saudi Arabian cities. Interestingly, our study found that children with ADHD reported a more positive distance learning experience compared to their non-ADHD peers.

The results of our study contrast with previous findings suggesting that students with ADHD typically struggle in remote education environments due to difficulties with attention, time management, and motivation [20,21]. However, our results align with emerging research indicating that certain children with ADHD benefit from the flexibility of remote learning [22]. The home environment may allow them to learn at their own pace, receive tailored support from parents, and avoid overstimulation common in traditional classrooms. Nevertheless, despite the reported positive experience, students with ADHD in our sample exhibited higher symptom severity and lower academic performance, consistent with other studies highlighting the academic challenges ADHD students face even in favorable environments [20].

Our study also found that children with ADHD were five times more likely to be diagnosed with chronic physical illnesses during the pandemic compared to their non-ADHD peers. This aligns with research showing a higher prevalence of chronic health conditions, such as asthma, obesity, and sleep disorders, among individuals with ADHD [23,24]. These comorbid conditions may further complicate the academic and emotional challenges experienced by children with ADHD, underscoring the need for integrated healthcare and educational support.

Furthermore, the findings revealed a significant correlation between parental marital status and ADHD symptoms, with children from separated or divorced families more than six times as likely to display ADHD symptoms compared to those with married parents controlled for their age. These results align with previous studies showing that parents of children with ADHD are more likely to experience marital discord and separation [25]. However, it is unclear whether ADHD symptoms exacerbate marital conflict or result from it. Family stability is recognized as essential in promoting healthy child behavior and mental health [26,27]. Similarly, a study conducted in Italy found that children with married parents experienced fewer traumatic effects during the COVID-19 pandemic, emphasizing the role of family dynamics during stressful times [28].

The emotional challenges for parents and educators during remote learning have been widely documented. Research from Germany, for example, reported heightened levels of stress and anxiety among parents as they took on teaching responsibilities at home, with children requiring intensive supervision to remain engaged in online classes [29]. Similarly, a systematic review by Carrión-Martínez et al. [30] found increased verbal aggression, family tension, and reduced well-being across students, parents, and teachers. The increased household stress identified in these studies aligns with our findings, suggesting that family environments significantly affect children's ability to manage distance learning challenges.

Our study emphasizes the protective role of family support during remote education. Children who received help from siblings or relatives were less likely to exhibit ADHD symptoms than those who relied on domestic helpers. This finding aligns with prior research indicating that family involvement improves academic outcomes and reduces behavioral challenges [31]. Shahali et al. [32] reported that children with learning difficulties performed better academically when provided with structured support and consistent family involvement during the pandemic.

Interestingly, our study found that children with ADHD reported a more positive distance learning experience compared to their non-ADHD peers. This contrasts with previous findings suggesting that students with ADHD typically struggle in remote education environments due to difficulties with attention, time management, and motivation [20,21]. However, our results align with emerging research indicating that certain children with ADHD benefit from the flexibility of remote learning [22]. The home environment may allow them to learn at their own pace, receive tailored support from parents, and avoid overstimulation common in traditional classrooms. Nevertheless, despite the reported positive experience, students with ADHD in our sample exhibited higher symptom severity and lower academic performance, consistent with other studies highlighting the academic challenges ADHD students face even in favorable environments [20]. Our findings emphasize the importance of family involvement and structured support during stressful events like the pandemic. Studies from the U.S. and Europe show that family cohesion and proactive engagement are critical in mitigating adverse outcomes during distance learning [9,33]. Moreover, children who receive consistent support from siblings or parents are more likely to develop resilience and emotional stability [34]. Conversely, reliance on external caregivers, such as domestic helpers, may introduce inconsistencies in children's routines, contributing to behavioral issues. This finding underscores the need for schools and mental health professionals to engage families actively in intervention strategies, especially when managing children with ADHD.

The strength of this study lies in its scope as the first large-scale, multi-city investigation in Saudi Arabia to examine the impact of distance learning on children's mental health. By using the validated Arabic Vanderbilt ADHD Diagnostic Rating Scale, we ensure reliable measurement of behavioral and academic outcomes, contributing to a relatively under-researched area. Additionally, the study highlights the importance of family engagement in helping children manage stress during challenging times.

The findings offer valuable insights for mental health professionals and educators. These findings suggest that flexible learning models and family-centered interventions can improve outcomes for children with behavioral challenges. As the pandemic reshapes educational practices, mental health professionals and policymakers must collaborate to create adaptive learning environments that meet the needs of all students, particularly those with ADHD and other behavioral disorders.

In addition, it emphasizes the need for family-centered interventions and flexible learning environments to support children with behavioral challenges. Further research should explore additional chronic health conditions and investigate how remote learning outcomes vary across different socioeconomic and cultural contexts.

4.1. Practical Implication

This study adds to a growing body of research showing that children with ADHD and other behavioral challenges face unique difficulties during remote learning. In particular, the positive distance learning experience reported by ADHD students in our study suggests that educational policies should explore flexible learning models that accommodate children's individual needs. For instance, remote learning may offer benefits such as reduced distractions and a more structured environment, which can help ADHD students focus better than in traditional classroom settings. However, it also highlights the importance of balancing flexibility with the need for social interaction and hands-on learning. Future research could further investigate the specific features of remote learning environments—such as flexible schedules, personalized attention, and the use of technology to support individualized learning—that may benefit children with ADHD. Additionally, examining the role of parental involvement, peer interaction, and the design of online curricula could provide further insights into how to optimize learning experiences for these students. Understanding these nuances will be critical for developing more inclusive educational strategies and interventions to support children with ADHD in both remote and in-person learning settings.

4.2. Limitations and Prospective Directions

This study contributes to the limited research on the effects of the COVID-19 pandemic on the well-being of school-aged children, but several limitations should be considered. The reliance on an online survey may have excluded families with limited technology access, potentially skewing the sample toward higher-income households. Although the survey was distributed through school platforms, snowball sampling could be attributed to technology gaps or parents being overwhelmed with caregiving responsibilities, limiting the statistical power and scope for follow-up.

While the diverse responses from families in major Saudi cities enhance the study's generalizability, relying solely on parental reports introduces potential bias. This could lead to the Horn effect, where parents of children with severe symptoms might overestimate the negative impact. The absence of teacher input or self-reports from older children further limits the study, especially since no validated self-report tools were available in the local context.

The use of predefined categories, with only a sixth "other" option, may have discouraged detailed reporting of less common conditions. To address these gaps, future research should broaden its scope to include multiple disabilities and allow for comparisons across different age groups.

Given the possibility of selection bias, the findings should be interpreted cautiously. Future studies should seek to integrate parental and teacher perspectives alongside child self-reports to gain a more holistic understanding of the pandemic's impact. A more comprehensive approach would provide insights into the interaction between mental health, family dynamics, and educational outcomes across diverse socioeconomic contexts.

Author Contributions: All authors contributed significantly to the study's design, data acquisition, analysis, and interpretation. They participated in drafting and revising the manuscript for critical intellectual content, approved the final version for publication, and agreed to take accountability for all aspects of the work. All authors have read and agreed to the published version of the manuscript.

Funding: This study was funded by the SABIC Psychological Health Research and Applications Chair, Department of Psychiatry, College of Medicine, Deanship of Postgraduate Teaching, King Saud University.

Institutional Review Board Statement: This study was approved by the Institutional Review Board (IRB) of King Saud University—College of Medicine under application number E-22-6867. To ensure transparency, participants were informed about the study's objectives on the survey's introductory page, and consent was confirmed when participants clicked "yes" to proceed. All data were encrypted to protect participants' confidentiality, and only the research team had access to the data for analysis.

Informed Consent Statement: Informed consent was obtained from all subjects involved in the study. Consent was obtained from parents at the beginning of the e-questionnaire, and parents were required to complete the survey to submit their responses. To ensure transparency, participants were informed about the study's objectives on the survey's introductory page, and consent was confirmed when participants clicked "yes" to proceed.

Data Availability Statement: The data supporting this study's findings are available upon reasonable request from the corresponding author.

Acknowledgments: The authors would like to thank the Deanship of Scientific Research, King Saud University, for their support through the Vice Deanship of Scientific Research Chairs.

Conflicts of Interest: The authors declare that the study was conducted without any commercial or financial relationships that could present a potential conflict of interest.

Abbreviations

ADHD	Attention Deficit Hyperactivity Disorder
GAD 7	Generalized Anxiety Disorder—7 Items
COVID-19	CoronaVirus Disease of 2019
DASS 21	The Depression: Anxiety, and Stress Scale —21 c
ID	Identifying Information

References

1. Qian, M.; Jiang, J. COVID-19 and Social Distancing. *Z. Gesundheitswissenschaften J. Public Health* **2022**, *30*, 259–261. [CrossRef]
2. Hume, S.; Brown, S.R.; Mahtani, K.R. School closures during COVID-19: An overview of systematic reviews. *BMJ Evid. Based Med.* **2023**, *28*, 164–174. [CrossRef] [PubMed]
3. The Saudi MOE Leading Efforts to Combat Coronavirus Pandemic (COVID-19). Available online: https://planipolis.iiep.unesco.org/en/2020/saudi-moe-leading-efforts-combat-coronavirus-pandemic-covid-19-7148 (accessed on 20 November 2023).
4. Viner, R.; Russell, S.; Saulle, R.; Croker, H.; Stansfield, C.; Packer, J.; Nicholls, D.; Goddings, A.-L.; Bonell, C.; Hudson, L.; et al. School Closures during Social Lockdown and Mental Health, Health Behaviors, and Well-Being among Children and Adolescents during the First COVID-19 Wave: A Systematic Review. *JAMA Pediatr.* **2022**, *176*, 400–409. Available online: https://jamanetwork.com/journals/jamapediatrics/article-abstract/2788069 (accessed on 21 January 2024). [CrossRef] [PubMed]
5. Doom, J.R.; Deer, L.K.; Dieujuste, N.; Han, D.; Rivera, K.M.; Scott, S.R. Youth psychosocial resilience during the COVID-19 pandemic. *Curr. Opin. Psychol.* **2023**, *53*, 101656. [CrossRef]
6. Quintiliani, L.; Sisto, A.; Vicinanza, F.; Curcio, G.; Tambone, V. Resilience and Psychological Impact on Italian University Students during COVID-19 Pandemic. Distance Learning and Health. *Psychol. Health Med.* **2022**, *27*, 69–80. [CrossRef] [PubMed]
7. Fruehwirth, J.C.; Biswas, S.; Perreira, K.M. The COVID-19 pandemic and mental health of first-year college students: Examining the effect of COVID-19 stressors using longitudinal data. *PLoS ONE* **2021**, *16*, e0247999. [CrossRef] [PubMed]
8. Cao, W.; Fang, Z.; Hou, G.; Han, M.; Xu, X.; Dong, J.; Zheng, J. The psychological impact of the COVID-19 epidemic on college students in China. *Psychiatry Res.* **2020**, *287*, 112934. [CrossRef]
9. Giusti, L.; Mammarella, S.; Salza, A.; Del Vecchio, S.; Ussorio, D.; Casacchia, M.; Roncone, R. Predictors of Academic Performance during the COVID-19 Outbreak: Impact of Distance Education on Mental Health, Social Cognition and Memory Abilities in an Italian University Student Sample. *BMC Psychol.* **2021**, *9*, 142. [CrossRef] [PubMed]
10. Dändliker, L.; Brünecke, I.; Citterio, P.; Lochmatter, F.; Buchmann, M.; Grütter, J. Educational Concerns, Health Concerns and Mental Health During Early COVID-19 School Closures: The Role of Perceived Support by Teachers, Family, and Friends. *Front. Psychol.* **2022**, *12*, 733683. [CrossRef] [PubMed]
11. Moy, F.M.; Ng, Y.H. Perception towards E-learning and COVID-19 on the mental health status of university students in Malaysia. *Sci. Prog.* **2021**, *104*, 00368504211029812. [CrossRef] [PubMed]
12. Hawrilenko, M.; Kroshus, E.; Tandon, P.; Christakis, D. The Association Between School Closures and Child Mental Health During COVID-19. *JAMA Netw. Open* **2021**, *4*, e2124092. [CrossRef] [PubMed]
13. Reséndiz-Aparicio, J.C. How the COVID-19 Contingency Affects Children. *Bol. Med. Hosp. Infant. Mex.* **2021**, *78*, 216–224. [CrossRef] [PubMed]
14. Garrote, A.; Niederbacher, E.; Hofmann, J.; Rösti, I.; Neuenschwander, M.P. Teacher Expectations and Parental Stress During Emergency Distance Learning and Their Relationship to Students' Perception. *Front. Psychol.* **2021**, *12*, 712447. [CrossRef] [PubMed]
15. Panchal, U.; de Pablo, G.S.; Franco, M.; Moreno, C.; Parellada, M.; Arango, C.; Fusar-Poli, P. The impact of COVID-19 lockdown on child and adolescent mental health: Systematic review. *Eur. Child Adolesc. Psychiatry* **2021**, *32*, 1151–1177. [CrossRef] [PubMed]
16. Levante, A.; Martis, C.; Bianco, F.; Castelli, I.; Petrocchi, S.; Lecciso, F. Internalizing and externalizing symptoms in children during the COVID-19 pandemic: A systematic mixed studies review. *Front. Psychol.* **2023**, *14*, 1182309. [CrossRef] [PubMed]
17. Samji, H.; Wu, J.; Ladak, A.; Vossen, C.; Stewart, E.; Dove, N.; Long, D.; Snell, G. Review: Mental health impacts of the COVID-19 pandemic on children and youth—A systematic review. *Child Adolesc. Ment. Health* **2022**, *27*, 173–189. [CrossRef] [PubMed]
18. Varnham, J. "Clinical Tools". Saudi ADHD Society. 2014. Available online: https://adhd.org.sa/en/adhd/resources/diagnosing-adhd/clinical-tools/ (accessed on 5 November 2014).
19. Wolraich, M.L.; Lambert, W.; Doffing, M.A.; Bickman, L.; Simmons, T.; Worley, K. Psychometric Properties of the Vanderbilt ADHD Diagnostic Parent Rating Scale in a Referred Population. *J. Pediatr. Psychol.* **2003**, *28*, 559–567. [CrossRef]
20. Tessarollo, V.; Scarpellini, F.; Costantino, I.; Cartabia, M.; Canevini, M.P.; Bonati, M. Distance Learning in Children with and without ADHD: A Case-control Study during the COVID-19 Pandemic. *J. Atten. Disord.* **2021**, *26*, 902–914. [CrossRef] [PubMed]
21. He, S.; Shuai, L.; Wang, Z.; Qiu, M.; Wilson, A.; Xia, W.; Cao, X.; Lu, L.; Zhang, J. Online Learning Performances of Children and Adolescents with Attention Deficit Hyperactivity Disorder During the COVID-19 Pandemic. *Inq. J. Health Care Organ. Provis. Financ.* **2021**, *58*, 00469580211049065. [CrossRef]

22. Bobo, E.; Lin, L.; Acquaviva, E.; Caci, H.; Franc, N.; Gamon, L.; Picot, M.C.; Pupier, F.; Speranza, M.; Falissard, B.; et al. Comment les enfants et adolescents avec le trouble déficit d'attention/hyperactivité (TDAH) vivent-ils le confinement durant la pandémie COVID-19? How do children and adolescents with Attention Deficit Hyperactivity Disorder (ADHD) experience lockdown during the COVID-19 outbreak? *L'Encephale* **2020**, *46*, S85–S92.
23. Pan, P. Y.; Bölte, S. The association between ADHD and physical health: A co-twin control study. *Sci. Rep.* **2020**, *10*, 22388. [CrossRef] [PubMed]
24. Sciberras, E.; Lycett, K.; Efron, D.; Mensah, F.; Gerner, B.; Hiscock, H. Anxiety in Children with Attention-Deficit/Hyperactivity Disorder. *Pediatrics* **2014**, *133*, 801–808. [CrossRef]
25. Wymbs, B.T.; Pelham, W.E.; Molina, B.S.G.; Gnagy, E.M.; Greenhouse, J.B. Rate and Pre-dictors of Divorce Among Parents of Youths With ADHD. *J. Consult. Clin. Psychol.* **2008**, *76*, 735–744. [CrossRef]
26. Johnston, C.; Mash, E.J. Families of Children with Attention-Deficit/Hyperactivity Disorder: Review and Recommendations for Future Research. *Clin. Child Fam. Psychol. Rev.* **2001**, *4*, 183–207. [CrossRef] [PubMed]
27. Arfaie, A.; Mohammadi, A.; Sohrabi, R. Relationship Between Marital Conflict and Child Affective-Behavioral Psychopathological Symptoms. *Procedia Soc. Behav. Sci.* **2013**, *84*, 1776–1778. [CrossRef]
28. Spinelli, M.; Lionetti, F.; Pastore, M.; Fasolo, M. Parents' Stress and Children's Psychological Problems in Families Facing the COVID-19 Outbreak in Italy. *Front. Psychol.* **2020**, *11*, 1713. [CrossRef]
29. Letzel, V.; Pozas, M.; Schneider, C. Energetic Students, Stressed Parents, and Nervous Teachers: A Comprehensive Exploration of Inclusive Homeschooling During the COVID-19 Crisis. *Open Educ. Stud.* **2020**, *2*, 159–170. [CrossRef]
30. Carrión-Martínez, J.J.; Pinel-Martínez, C.; Pérez-Esteban, M.D.; Román-Sánchez, I.M. Family and School Relationship during COVID-19 Pandemic: A Systematic Review. *Int. J. Environ. Res. Public Health* **2021**, *18*, 11710. [CrossRef]
31. Sprang, G.; Silman, M. Posttraumatic Stress Disorder in Parents and Youth after Health-Related Disasters. *Disaster Med. Public Health Prep.* **2013**, *7*, 105–110. [CrossRef] [PubMed]
32. Shahali, A.; HajHosseini, M.; Jahromi, R.G. COVID-19 and Parent-Child Interactions: Children's Educational Opportunities and Parental Challenges During the COVID-19 Pandemic. *Soa Chongsonyon Chongsin Uihak J. Child Adolesc. Psychiatry* **2023**, *34*, 133–140. [CrossRef] [PubMed]
33. Thorell, L.B.; Skoglund, C.; de la Peña, A.G.; Baeyens, D.; Fuermaier, A.B.; Groom, M.J.; Mammarella, I.C.; Van der Oord, S.; van den Hoofdakker, B.J.; Luman, M.; et al. Parental experiences of homeschooling during the COVID-19 pandemic: Differences between seven European countries and between children with and without mental health conditions. *Eur. Child Adolesc. Psychiatry* **2021**, *31*, 649–661. [CrossRef] [PubMed] [PubMed Central]
34. Prime, H.; Wade, M.; Browne, D.T. Risk and resilience in family well-being during the COVID-19 pandemic. *Am. Psychol.* **2020**, *75*, 631–643. [CrossRef] [PubMed]

children

MDPI

Article

Attitudes of Adolescents Toward Addictive Substances: Hope and Self-Control as Protective Factors

Serkan Cengiz [1], Mehmet Emin Turan [1] and Eyüp Çelik [2,*]

[1] Department of Psychology, Faculty of Arts and Sciences, Ağrı İbrahim Çeçen University, Ağrı 04100, Türkiye; scengiz@agri.edu.tr (S.C.); meturan@agri.edu.tr (M.E.T.)
[2] Department of Psychological Counseling and Guidance, Faculty of Education, Sakarya University, Sakarya 54050, Türkiye
* Correspondence: eyupcelik@sakarya.edu.tr

Abstract: Background: Experiences of ostracism may be related to attitudes toward substance abuse. However, the protective factors underlying this relationship are still unclear. Therefore, based on the Need-threat and Self-control theory, we aimed to test a model in which self-control and hope mediate the relationship between ostracism and attitudes toward addictive substances. **Methods**: In this model, we highlighted risk factors (ostracism) and protective factors (self-control and hope). This study was a cross-sectional data analysis of 787 students (52.50% boys, 47.50% girls; M_{age} = 15.69, SD = 1.12). **Results:** The results revealed that ostracism was positively associated with attitudes toward addictive substances, and evidence was provided that this relationship was mediated by hope and self-control. Ultimately, the research highlights the link between ostracism and attitudes toward addictive substances, identifying hope and self-control as mediators. **Conclusions**: This study highlights individual risk and protective factors related to attitudes toward addictive substances and offers new perspectives on ways to prevent and reduce adolescents' positive attitudes toward substance use. School counselors and educators should help students strengthen skills such as hope and self-control to prevent them from developing positive attitudes toward substance use in the future.

Keywords: attitudes toward addictive substances; ostracism; self-control; hope; adolescents

1. Introduction

Substance use is among the most serious public health problems, especially during adolescence [1]. During this period, the level of curiosity is high, and young individuals are sensitive to peer pressure, showing a strong tendency to rebel against authority and low self-esteem [2]. These situations can make people vulnerable to substance use and addiction. A comprehensive study worldwide reported that approximately 4.2 million adolescents between the ages of 12 and 17 use substances [3]. Studies in Africa have shown an increasing prevalence of substance abuse among adolescents of approximately 41.6% [4]. The results from the National Survey on Drug Use and Health in the United States have shown that nonmedical use of prescription opioids has increased among adolescents aged 12–17 years [5]. A large-scale study in Europe, including 25 countries, revealed that adolescent cannabis use is increasing [6].

Substance abuse and addiction are quite common among many adolescents in Turkey, as in many other countries [7,8]. However, studies on the prevalence of its use, especially among adolescents, in Turkey are limited because of a lack of coordination between institutions, public health concerns, and cultural factors [9,10]. Substance use is a complex, multifactorial health disorder characterized by a chronic and recurrent nature, affecting almost every family globally [11]. On the other hand, previous studies have focused mostly on the consequences of substance use and attitudes toward addictive substances have not been sufficiently examined. Indeed, attitudes generally precede and influence behavior [12]. A positive attitude indicates a tendency to approach different addictive substances, whereas a negative attitude indicates a tendency to stay away from these substances. Therefore, knowing the risk factors that lead to substance use is important in terms of the early detection of young people at risk of use or the determination of interventions to reduce the risk of future substance use.

1.1. Ostracism and Attitudes Toward Addictive Substances

Among the many antecedents of substance abuse among adolescents, ostracism may be particularly problematic. Ostracism can be situations in which one feels emotionally and physically separate from others [13]. During adolescence, relationships with peers can play an important role in establishing healthy habits. However, compared with other developmental periods, there is a heightened sensitivity to ostracism during adolescence because of factors such as the peak importance of peer groups and the most frequent occurrence of exclusionary behaviors during this period [14].

Individuals who are excluded generally report a sense of meaninglessness, solitude, depressive symptoms, and alienation [15,16]. The perception of ostracism and the resulting threat to basic psychological needs can lead to harmful behaviors, including substance use. Many studies have revealed a significant relationship between ostracism and substance use [17,18]. For example, Levine [19] reported that ostracism poses a risk for cigarette use. One study also reported that isolation from peers increased behavioral responses to cocaine and amphetamines [20].

According to Williams' need-threat model [21], even the simplest form of ostracism is perceived by people as threatening basic needs. In the initial stage, ostracism indicates social danger. A person's reaction to ostracism is reflexive, and the ostracism felt is experienced as social pain. As a result, because of the long-term effects of permanent ostracism, a sudden decline in the mood of individuals may occur, and negative behavioral reactions (e.g., smoking, alcohol, drugs, addictive drug use, etc.) may be observed. The target of ostracism may be attempting to exert control to cope with negative emotions and behaviors or reconnecting with others while maintaining hope. Therefore, we included self-control and hope as potential mediators of the relationship between ostracism and attitudes toward substance abuse.

1.2. The Mediating Role of Hope

Another factor that may affect attitudes toward addictive substance use is the level of hope. Hope is the process of thinking about paths leading to personal goals (pathway thinking) and the ability to think in a way that motivates oneself to reach the goal via these paths (agency thinking) [22]. According to hope theory, the most hopeful individuals are those high in path and action thinking. In contrast, those with low hopes may have difficulty finding available methods to achieve their goals and may be less motivated to achieve what they want. Since greater hope is associated with greater self-confidence, well-being, coping flexibility, and emotion regulation skills [23,24], it can be considered a protective factor in preventing substance use. Gutierrez [25] reported that hope plays a protective role in recovery from withdrawal because it prevents many behavioral and psychological problems in life.

However, hope involves individual ways of thinking and personal motivation and is also affected by communicating with others and interpersonal interactions. Within the framework of the need-threat model [21], ostracism threatens a basic need to belong. This model also emphasizes that individuals respond to ostracism in three sequential stages: reflexive, reflective, and resignation. Hope is one of the characteristics that significantly influences a person's response to ostracism at different stages of the experience of ostracism [26]. Therefore, the state of hope can be affected by ostracism in social environments and, accordingly, affect the psychological state of individuals.

Adolescents may have high levels of hope and low levels of both components. The lack of a sense of belonging and the hopelessness experienced may prevent young people from achieving a role in their social lives and, most importantly, their health identity. This may lead to substance use disorders. Therefore, we suggest that hope is likely to mediate the relationship between ostracism and attitudes toward addictive substances.

1.3. The Mediating Role of Self-Control

Another characteristic associated with attitudes toward addictive substances is self-control. Self-control can be defined as the capacity of a person to control or regulate their emotions, cognition, and behavior [27]. Research has shown that self-control is a strong protective factor in behavioral addiction and health risk behavior [28,29]. Individuals with greater self-control are better able to protect themselves from psychological distress when faced with a stressful situation. In contrast, individuals with low self-control are characterized as impulsive, insensitive, risk-taking, and more narrow-minded. In other words, these individuals enjoy taking risks and engaging in risky behaviors, tend to be self-centered, and have less tolerance [30].

One of the main reasons for the development of low self-control is ostracism [31]. According to the temporal need-threat model, ostracism threatens various psychological needs of individuals, including their sense of control. Considering this approach, in the reflexive stage, individuals affected by ostracism experience social pain when their needs for belonging and control are threatened. In reinforcing thwarted needs, high self-control ability may reactivate prosocial tendencies. Conversely, underdeveloped self-regulatory mechanisms may not adequately process important social stimuli, which may lead to positive attitudes toward substance use.

Gottfredson and Hirschi [32] proposed self-control theory as part of their general theory of crime, suggesting that people are motivated to engage in behaviors that increase their pleasure or decrease their pain. However, criminal and substance use behaviors depend on a person's ability to exercise self-control when appropriate opportunities arise. Low self-control increases the likelihood of engaging in actions such as crime and substance abuse. For these individuals, using addictive substances may seem simple and exciting, especially because individuals cannot see the long-term consequences of their actions and the harm they may cause. Previous researchers have reported that individuals with lower levels of self-control are at greater risk of using alcohol, tobacco, and marijuana [33,34]. In addition to its relationship with attitudes toward addictive substances, recent research has shown that low self-control is also associated with emotional problems such as shyness, loneliness, low self-esteem, and psychological anxiety [35–37]. As a result, adolescents with a lack of self-control are more likely to develop positive attitudes and behaviors toward addictive substances.

1.4. Present Study

One of the important findings from school-based prevention research is that information dissemination interventions help change knowledge or attitudes about addictive substances [38]. However, most current prevention and information programs involve interventions designed for risk behaviors other than school dropout or substance abuse, such as sexual risk behavior, problematic internet, and media use [39,40]. The literature indicates the need for protective mechanisms that can counteract ostracism in adolescence. In addition, most studies on the relationship between ostracism and attitudes toward addictive substances have focused on adults, especially university students, rather than adolescents. Also, a better understanding of the increased sensitivity to interpersonal stressors, such as exclusion from a group, among individuals with positive attitudes toward substance use and evaluating them as protective mechanisms, such as hope and self-control, may have important implications for determining potential treatment strategies. Finally, although the relationships between the variables in the study are theoretically supported in different studies, no studies have been found that include the hypotheses in the current study. To fill these gaps, the current study used a sample of Turkish adolescents to examine the mediating effects of self-control and hope. This study aimed to test the relationships between ostracism and attitudes toward addictive substances and the underlying mechanisms in a sample of adolescents in Turkey. We formulate the research hypotheses as follows:

H_1.: *Ostracism is positively associated with attitudes toward addictive substances.*

H_2.: *Hope mediates the relationship between ostracism and attitudes toward addictive substances.*

H_3.: *Self-control mediates the relationship between ostracism and attitudes toward addictive substances.*

2. Materials and Methods

2.1. Participants

First, the schools where the application would be carried out were selected via a convenience sampling approach, considering their willingness to participate and their accessibility to the researchers. Then, the researchers established some criteria for participation in the study. (i) No history of previous use of addictive substances, (ii) no psychological treatment, (iii) not meeting the criteria for psychosis or a serious personality disorder, and (iv) parental consent to participate in the study. Finally, the G*Power 3.1 program analysis test was performed to determine the number of participants in the current study according to the criteria. The results showed a minimum sample size of 743 for models with an alpha level of 0.05, an effect size of 0.12, and a power level of 0.95. Considering possible data loss, we applied the scales to 800 students. After the exclusion of missing answers and data from 13 individuals who did not meet the normality criteria, the final sample consisted of 787 students. (52.50% females, 47.50% males; M_{age} = 15.69, *SD* = 1.12). The demographic characteristics are shown in Table 1.

Table 1. Demographic characteristics of participants.

Variable	Level	*n*	%
Gender	Female	414	52.50
	Male	373	47.50
Grade	9th	241	30.62
	10th	232	29.48
	11th	280	35.58
	12th	34	4.32
Perceived school success	Below average	118	14.99
	Average	538	68.36
	Above average	131	16.65

Table 1. *Cont.*

Variable	Level	*n*	%
Perceived socioeconomic status	Below average	127	16.14
	Average	580	73.70
	Above average	80	10.16
Age	Minimum	13	
	Maximum	18	
	Mean	15.69	
	SD	1.12	

2.2. Measures

2.2.1. Ostracism Experience Scale for Adolescents (OES-A)

OES-A [41] is an 11-item self-report measure designed to assess an individual's perceptions of being ignored by or excluded from the social group. Each item (e.g., "In general, others treat me as if I am invisible") on the OES-A is answered on a 5-point Likert-type scale varying between 1 (never) and 7 (always). Akın et al. [42] validated the scale in Turkish. Cronbach's alpha coefficient for the OES-A was 0.88 in this study.

2.2.2. Brief Self-Control Scale (BSCS)

The BSBC [43] includes 13 items (e.g., "I can work effectively toward long-term goals.") that are scored on a 5-point Likert-type scale ranging from 1 (not at all like me) to 7 (very much like me). The BSBC is a self-reported measure designed to measure self-control. The BSBC was validated in Turkish by Eroğlu [44]. The Cronbach's alpha coefficient for the BSBC was 0.66.

2.2.3. Hope Scale (HS)

The HS [45] is a commonly used self-reported scale constructed to assess a respondent's level of hope. The HS comprises 12 items (e.g., "I can think of many ways to get out of a jam".) that are rated on an 8-point Likert-type scale ranging from 1 (definitely false) to 5 (definitely true). Turkish validation of the HS indicated satisfactory psychometric properties [46]. The Cronbach's alpha coefficient for the HS was 0.85 in this study.

2.2.4. Attitudes Toward Addictive Substances Scale (ATASS)

The ATASS [47] is a unidimensional self-reported scale developed to assess attitudes toward addictive substances in high school students. The ATASS includes 45 items (e.g., "I think I would be a happier person if I were using an addictive substance"). Each item was rated on a 5-point Likert-type scale varying between 1 (absolutely inappropriate) and 5 (absolutely appropriate). A higher score on the scale represents a greater level of negative attitudes toward addictive substances. The ATASS has shown good evidence of reliability and validity [47]. The Cronbach's alpha coefficient for the ATASS was 0.93 in this study.

2.3. Procedure

The current study was approved by the research ethics committee of the university where the first author works. Informed consent was obtained from school administrators, teachers, families, and students before starting the study. The participants were informed about the nature of the study. We ensured that all the participants were volunteers. We also stated that students could withdraw at any time, even if they started answering the survey items. We told the students that their responses would remain confidential. When determining the period for administering the scales, we considered school exams, academic activities, courses, and project work. In line with this planning, the researchers were present in the classrooms during the application. It took an average of 30 min for the participants to complete all the surveys. We completed the data collection process in 60 days.

2.4. Data Analysis

In this study, multiple linear regression analysis was conducted to see the confounding factors and isolate the relationship of interest. In multiple linear regression, researchers can include many covariates at the same time. In the mediation model of the present study (see Figure 1), we propose that self-control and hope are mediators (M) of the relationship between ostracism (X) and attitudes toward addictive substances (Y). We employed bootstrapping (10,000 samples) to analyze the extent to which ostracism—attitudes toward addictive substance relationships—are mediated by self-control—hope [48]. Kappa-squared (κ2) with 95% bootstrapped confidence intervals were calculated to estimate the effect size for the indirect effect (Preacher and Kelley, 2011). Based on a rule of thumb proposed by Preacher and Kelley [49], the size of κ2, concerning Cohen's criteria for squared correlation coefficients of 0.01, 0.09, and 0.25, refer to small, medium, and large effects, respectively. All analyses were carried out via SPSS v.26 and macro-PROCESS v4.2.

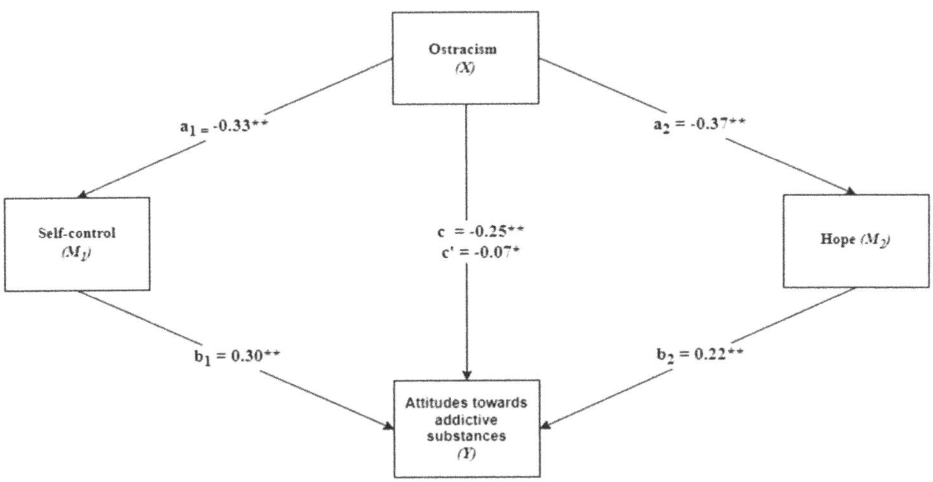

Figure 1. Mediation model (** $p < 0.001$; * $p < 0.05$).

3. Results

3.1. Descriptive Results

Descriptive statistics (e.g., means, standard deviations, normality tests), bivariate correlation coefficients, and internal consistency reliability estimates for the variables of the present study are reported. The values of skewness (range = −0.72 and 0.23) and kurtosis (range = −0.71 and 0.16) fell within the "good" range of a normal distribution with a conventional frame of reference for skewness and kurtosis scores < |1| [50]. The results of the correlation analysis revealed that ostracism was significantly negatively correlated with attitudes toward addictive substances, self-control, and hope. Attitudes toward addictive substances were also significantly positively correlated with self-control and hope. There was a significant positive relationship between self-control and hope. The descriptive statistics and correlations are shown in Table 2.

Table 2. Descriptive statistics and correlations.

Variable	Descriptive Statistics					Correlation			
	M	SD	Skewness	Kurtosis	α	1	2	3	4
1. Ostracism	26.97	10.05	0.23	−0.66	0.88	—	−0.34 **	−0.37 **	−0.25 **
2. Self-control	43.80	8.30	−0.03	−0.24	0.66		—	0.39 **	0.41 **
3. Hope	46.51	12.38	−0.72	0.16	0.85			—	0.36 **
4. Attitudes towards addictive substances	180.21	29.73	−0.60	−0.71	0.93				—

Note. ** $p < 0.01$.

3.2. Mediation Analysis

The results showed that ostracism had a significant positive predictive effect on self-control (β = −0.33, $p < 0.001$) and hope (β = −0.37, $p < 0.001$). Ostracism explained 11% of the variance in self-control and 14% of the variance in hope. Ostracism (β = −0.07, $p < 0.05$), self-control (β = 0.30, $p < 0.001$), and hope (β = 0.22, $p < 0.001$) had significant positive predictive effects on attitudes toward addictive substances. Collectively, these three variables explained 22% of the variance in attitudes toward addictive substances. In addition, the indirect effect of ostracism on attitudes toward addictive substances was statistically significant through self-control (effect = −0.29, 95% CI [−0.40, −0.20]) and hope (effect = −0.24, 95% CI [−0.34, −0.14]). This result shows that self-control and hope mediate the relationship between ostracism and attitudes toward addictive substances (see Tables 3 and 4, and Figure 1).

Table 3. Unstandardized coefficients of the model.

		Outcome Variable			
		M_1 (Self-Control)			
Variable		Coeff.	*SE*	*t*	*p*
Constant	i_{M1}	51.25	0.80	64.12	<0.001
X (Ostracism)	a_1	−0.28	0.03	−9.95	<0.001
		$R^2 = 0.11$			
		$F = 98.90; p < 0.001$			
		M_2 (Hope)			
Constant	i_{M2}	58.82	1.18	50.06	<0.001
X (Ostracism)	a_2	−0.46	0.04	−11.18	<0.001
		$R^2 = 0.14$			
		$F = 125.05; p < 0.001$			
		Y (Attitudes towards addictive substances)			
Constant	by	115.01	7.39	15.57	<0.001
X (Ostracism)	c'	−0.21	0.10	−2.02	<0.05
M_1 (Self-control)	b_1	1.07	0.13	8.43	<0.001
M_2 (Hope)	b_2	0.52	0.09	6.04	<0.001
		$R^2 = 0.22$			
		$F = 72.02; p < 0.001$			

Note. *SE* = standard error. Coeff = unstandardized coefficient. *X* = independent variable; *M* = mediator variable; *Y* = dependent variable.

Table 4. Standardized indirect effects of ostracism on attitudes towards addictive substances.

Path	Effect	*SE*	BootLLCI	BootULCI
Total indirect effect	−0.18	0.02	−0.22	−0.14
Ostracism → self-control → attitudes towards addictive substances	−0.10	0.02	−0.13	−0.07
Ostracism → hope → attitudes towards addictive substances	−0.08	0.02	−0.11	−0.05

Note. Number of bootstrap samples for percentile bootstrap confidence intervals: 10,000.

4. Discussion

The current study revealed that ostracism was associated with attitudes toward substance use. These findings are consistent with other studies associated with substance use [51,52]. Many problematic substance users may have experienced significant disadvantages and ostracism. Furthermore, many studies have shown that ostracism is a risk factor for substance abuse [53,54]. Laws et al. [55] reported that individuals may turn to alcohol as a means of reducing stress due to increased arousal and the negative effects of social rejection. According to the need-threat model [21], ostracism threatens people's need for meaningful existence and belonging. Adolescents spend a significant amount of time with their peers and are therefore highly sensitive to social experiences with them. Adolescents may be overreactive to ostracism, which is a distressing experience [56]. Overreactions and perceived stress to negative experiences such as ostracism may sensitize individuals to positive attitudes toward substance abuse. Thus, youth with increased anxiety and sensitivity to ostracism are more likely to use substances during adolescence than youth with less sensitivity. These findings provide valuable insights into the mechanism of the relationship between ostracism and substance use.

Another study revealed that self-control in adolescents significantly mediated the relationship between ostracism and attitudes toward substance use. This result provides evidence that adolescents with greater self-control skills are less likely to develop positive attitudes toward addictive substances in the face of ostracism. Compared with adults, adolescents have weaker self-control skills [57], so they may be prone to substance abuse when exposed to ostracism. Ostracism has many negative consequences, but few studies have investigated whether self-control helps explain the relationship between ostracism and attitudes toward substance use. Many studies have shown that people often have difficulty controlling impulses when exposed to ostracism [58,59]. According to Gottfredson and Hirschi's [32] self-control theory, people with low self-control tend to be more impulsive and engage in criminal activities. The reason for this tendency is that substance abuse provides instant gratification. Therefore, these deficiencies in self-control can lead to serious problems such as substance addiction and play a serious role in relapse after a period of abstinence.

Our findings also suggest that hope moderates the effect of ostracism on attitudes toward substance use. Consistent with this result, previous research has significantly associated ostracism with hope [60,61]. In terms of the need-threat model [21], the first stage of ostracism is the immediate response stage, where people enter the reflective stage, which involves short-term cognitive or behavioral responses to cope with ostracism. In this context, hope can prevent the negative effects of ostracism in the long term by affecting a person's sense of purpose and positive self-worth. Indeed, hope has been associated with adaptive coping and greater adaptability when faced with stress [62,63]. In addition, hope may be an important component of recovery from substance abuse and may provide willpower in quitting substance use [64]. Research has shown that hope activity and hope pathway scores contribute to drug abstinence [65]. In an experimental study, Koehn and Cutcliffe [66] demonstrated that hope is a resource that contributes positively to clients' mobility, disposition, and activity in substance abuse counseling. In this context, a diminished sense of hope can act as a barrier to recovery in the face of many negative experiences, such as ostracism, and may lead individuals to believe that addictive substances provide them with a better quality of life. When individuals feel hopeful about their future, they are more likely to set meaningful goals and continue their efforts even when faced with setbacks. Interventions that promote hope and self-control can be used to manage ostracism. Additionally, although psychological constructs such as the relationship between ostracism and social media addiction are well documented [67,68], research on the psychological aspects of substance use [69] is limited. The present study may also shed light on the psychological aspect of substance addiction.

5. Limitations and Future Suggestions

This study makes several contributions to the existing research and practice in literature. This study incorporated the need-threat and self-control theory into the relationship between ostracism and attitudes toward substance use and created a new explanatory model for attitudes toward addictive substances. The results show that ostracism can predict attitudes toward substance abuse through the mediating effects of hope and self-control. These findings prove that adolescents who are excluded by peers and others exhibit less social control and hope, which increases their risk of developing deviant substance abuse. This study not only provides an explanatory framework for attitudes toward substance abuse but also contributes significantly to research on variables related to attitudes toward substance abuse.

Moreover, the results of this study provide ideas on how to address attitudes toward substance use in adolescence, especially in Turkish society. Considering the positive effect of ostracism on attitudes toward addictive substances, hope-enhancing measures should be provided by both families and educators. In addition, studies or intervention projects focused on increasing self-control should be further evaluated and implemented to prevent and address substance use among adolescents.

In addition, the findings of this study provide valuable insights for psychology counselors (especially school psychology counselors) and substance abuse specialists. The psychological constructs of hope and self-control, which are the mediating variables of this study, may be added to school-based preventive intervention studies conducted during adolescence. Studies on the management of ostracism may emphasize school-based interventions. To prevent the development of positive attitudes toward substance abuse, family- and community-based curriculum programs are also implemented in many countries. The findings of this study can also be added to family- and community-based curricula. In these programs, components such as managing ostracism and promoting hope and self-control can be added.

On the other hand, the current study has several limitations. First, since a cross-sectional design was used, it is difficult to draw causal inferences between variables. Future studies could design a controlled laboratory study to further confirm the results of the current study. Second, the sample of this study included only adolescents who continued their education in one region of Turkey, which may limit the generalizability of the results; therefore, future studies can use students from different regions of Turkey or other countries to validate the current results. Finally, the results of this study were tested with a correlational model. Future studies can test the current variables by establishing experimental models to support the results of this study.

Author Contributions: Conceptualization, S.C. and M.E.T.; methodology, M.E.T. and E.Ç.; S.C., M.E.T. and E.Ç.; validation, S.C., M.E.T. and E.Ç.; formal analysis, S.C., M.E.T. and E.Ç.; investigation, M.E.T., S.C. and E.Ç.; resources, M.E.T., S.C. and E.Ç.; data curation, M.E.T., S.C. and E.Ç.; writing—original draft preparation, S.C., M.E.T. and E.Ç.; writing—review and editing, S.C., M.E.T. and E.Ç.; visualization, M.E.T., S.C. and E.Ç.; supervision, S.C., M.E.T. and E.Ç.; project administration, M.E.T. and S.C.; funding acquisition, E.Ç. All authors have read and agreed to the published version of the manuscript.

Funding: This research received no external funding.

Institutional Review Board Statement: The study was conducted by the Declaration of Helsinki and approved by the Ethics Committee Ethics of the Ağrı İbrahim Çeçen University Scientific Research Ethics Committee (Date: 23.08.2023; Decision: 193; Number: E-95531838-050.99-80732).

Informed Consent Statement: Informed consent was obtained from all subjects involved in the study.

Data Availability Statement: The data presented in this study are available on request from the corresponding author.

Conflicts of Interest: The authors declare no conflicts of interest.

References

1. Nawi, A.M.; Ismail, R.; Ibrahim, F.; Hassan, M.R.; Manaf, M.R.A.; Amit, N.; Ibrahim, N.; Shafurdin, N.S. Risk and protective factors of drug abuse among adolescents: A systematic review. *BMC Public Health* **2021**, *21*, 2088. [CrossRef] [PubMed]
2. Degenhardt, L.; Stockings, E.; Patton, G.; Hall, W.D.; Lynskey, M. The increasing global health priority of substance use in young people. *Lancet Psychiatry* **2016**, *3*, 251–264. [CrossRef] [PubMed]
3. Substance Abuse and Mental Health Services Administration. Key Substance Use and Mental Health Indicators in the United States: Results from the 2018 National Survey on Drug Use and Health. Available online: https://www.samhsa.gov/data/ (accessed on 20 March 2023).
4. Ogundipe, O.; Amoo, E.O.; Adeloye, D.; Olawole-Isaac, A. Substance use among adolescents in sub-Saharan Africa: A systematic review and meta-analysis. *S. Afr. J. Child Health* **2018**, *2018*, 79–84. Available online: https://hdl.handle.net/10520/EJC-10deb396ce (accessed on 20 March 2023).
5. Henneberger, A.K.; Mushonga, D.R.; Preston, A.M. Peer influence and adolescent substance use: A systematic review of dynamic social network research. *Adolesc. Res. Rev.* **2021**, *6*, 57–73. [CrossRef]
6. Kraus, L.; Seitz, N.N.; Piontek, D.; Molinaro, S.; Siciliano, V.; Guttormsson, U.; Arpa, S.; Monshouwer, K.; Leifman, H.; Vicente, J.; et al. 'Are the times A-Changin'? Trends in adolescent substance use in Europe. *Addiction* **2018**, *113*, 1317–1332. [CrossRef]
7. Gocet Tekin, E.; Yilmaz, F.B.; Satici, S.A. Impulsivity and substance misuse among Turkish people: Serial mediating effect of emotion dysregulation and general anxiety disorder. *J. Ethn. Subst. Abus.* **2023**, 1–18. [CrossRef]
8. Uncu, B.; Doğan, E.; Duman, R. Common health risks and problems in adolescence. *Sak. Univ. J. Holist. Health* **2023**, *6*, 338–352. [CrossRef]
9. Çelik, Ö.; Kadakal, F.; Sarar, E.; Özdemir, E.; Sarac, S. Smoking habits, related factors and knowledge levels of vocational school students about smoking. *Sak. Med. J.* **2021**, *11*, 542–553. [CrossRef]
10. Sönmez, M.B.; Cakir, D.; Cinar, R.K.; Gorgulu, Y.; Vardar, E. Substance use and parent characteristics among high school students: Edirne sample in Turkey. *J. Child Adolesc. Subst. Abus.* **2016**, *25*, 260–267. [CrossRef]
11. Volkow, N.D.; Poznyak, V.; Saxena, S.; Gerra, G.; UNODC-WHO Informal International Scientific Network. Drug use disorders: Impact of a public health rather than a criminal justice approach. *World Psychiatry* **2016**, *16*, 213–214. [CrossRef]
12. Wilchek-Aviad, Y.; Ne'eman-Haviv, V. Do meaning in life, ideological commitment, and level of religiosity, related adolescent substance abuse and attitude? *Child Indic. Res.* **2016**, *9*, 261–276. [CrossRef]
13. Kiuru, N.; Salmela-Aro, K.; Laursen, B.; Vasalampi, K.; Beattie, M.; Tunkkari, M.; Junttila, N. Profiles of Loneliness and Ostracism During Adolescence: Consequences, Antecedents, and Protective Factors. *Child Psychiatry Hum. Dev.* **2024**, 1–21. [CrossRef] [PubMed]
14. Wölfer, R.; Scheithauer, H. Ostracism in childhood and adolescence: Emotional, cognitive, and behavioral effects of social exclusion. *Soc. Influ.* **2013**, *8*, 217–236. [CrossRef]
15. Rabiul, M.K.; Al Karim, R.; Ahmed, S.U.M. Task performance of hotel employees: Role of ostracism, meaningfulness, and emotional exhaustion. *J. Hosp. Tour. Manag.* **2023**, *56*, 314–321. [CrossRef]
16. Rudert, S.C.; Janke, S.; Greifeneder, R. Ostracism breeds depression: Longitudinal associations between ostracism and depression over a three-year-period. *J. Affect. Disord. Rep.* **2021**, *4*, 100118. [CrossRef]
17. Ali, H.; Hameed, M.; Abbasi, M.A.; Ali, A.; Abbas, Z.; Valiyakath, C.R.; Abbasi, G.A.; Qureshi, A.U.; Kainaat, M.; Amer, A. Ostracism predicting suicidal behavior and risk of relapse in substance use disorders. *Cureus* **2024**, *16*, e61519. [CrossRef]
18. Sprunger, J.G.; Hales, A.; Maloney, M.; Williams, K.; Eckhardt, C.I. Alcohol, affect, and aggression: An investigation of alcohol's effects following ostracism. *Psychol. Violence* **2020**, *10*, 585–593. [CrossRef]
19. Levine, S.A. *The Effects of Social Support and Sensitivity to Ostracism on Smoking Outcomes in College Students*; University of Maryland: College Park, MD, USA, 2006.
20. Fosnocht, A.Q.; Lucerne, K.E.; Ellis, A.S.; Olimpo, N.A.; Briand, L.A. Adolescent social isolation increases vulnerability to cocaine. *BioRxiv* **2018**, 320648. [CrossRef]
21. Williams, K.D. Ostracism: A temporal need-threat model. *Adv. Exp. Soc. Psychol.* **2009**, *41*, 275–314. [CrossRef]

22. Snyder, C.R.; Lopez, S.J.; Edwards, L.M.; Marques, S.C. *The Oxford Handbook of Positive Psychology*; Oxford University Press: Oxford, UK, 2020.
23. D'Souza, J.M.; Zvolensky, M.J.; Smith, B.H.; Gallagher, M.W. The unique effects of hope, optimism, and self-efficacy on subjective well-being and depression in German adults. *J. Well-Being Assess.* **2020**, *4*, 331–345. [CrossRef]
24. Çelebi, C.; Yılmaz, F.; Doğan, M. A research on metaphors for the "future" created by high school students. *Sak. Univ. J. Educ.* **2022**, *12*, 367–389. [CrossRef]
25. Gutierrez, D. Spiritus contra spiritum: Addiction, hope, and the search for meaning. *Spiritual. Clin. Pract.* **2019**, *6*, 229–239. [CrossRef]
26. Sethi, N.; Moulds, M.L.; Richardson, R. The role of focus of attention and reappraisal in prolonging the negative effects of ostracism. *Group Dyn. Theory Res. Pract.* **2013**, *17*, 110–123. [CrossRef]
27. Vazsonyi, A.T.; Huang, L. Where self-control comes from: On the development of self-control and its relationship to deviance over time. *Dev. Psychol.* **2010**, *46*, 245–257. [CrossRef] [PubMed]
28. Yöyen, E.; Bal, F.; Barış, T.G.; Arslan, M.S.; Çokluk, G.F. Mediator role of dissociative experiences in the effect of childhood traumas on emotion regulation difficulty and parental child-containing function. *Children* **2024**, *11*, 618. [CrossRef]
29. Büyükşakar, S.; Çelik, E. Attachment styles and loneliness as predictors of phubbing amongst university students. *Sak. Univ. J. Educ.* **2024**, *14*, 18–32. [CrossRef]
30. Li, C.; Dang, J.; Zhang, X.; Zhang, Q.; Guo, J. Internet addiction among Chinese adolescents: The effect of parental behavior and self-control. *Comput. Hum. Behav.* **2014**, *41*, 1–7. [CrossRef]
31. DeWall, C.N.; Gilman, R.; Sharif, V.; Carboni, I.; Rice, K.G. Left out, sluggardly, and blue: Low self-control mediates the relationship between ostracism and depression. *Personal. Individ. Differ.* **2012**, *53*, 832–837. [CrossRef]
32. Gottfredson, M.R.; Hirschi, T. A general theory of crime. In *A General Theory of Crime*; Stanford University Press: Redwood City, CA, USA, 1990.
33. Gowan, T.; Whetstone, S.; Andic, T. Addiction, agency, and the politics of self-control: Doing harm reduction in a heroin users' group. *Soc. Sci. Med.* **2012**, *74*, 1251–1260. [CrossRef]
34. Schaefer, B.P.; Vito, A.G.; Marcum, C.D.; Higgins, G.E.; Ricketts, M.L. Examining adolescent cocaine use with social learning and self-control theories. *Deviant Behav.* **2015**, *36*, 823–833. [CrossRef]
35. Harman, J.P.; Hansen, C.E.; Cochran, M.E.; Lindsey, C.R. Liar, liar: Internet faking but not frequency of use affects social skills, self-esteem, social anxiety, and aggression. *CyberPsychology Behav.* **2005**, *8*, 1–6. [CrossRef]
36. Iranmanesh, M.; Foroughi, B.; Nikbin, D.; Hyun, S.S. Shyness, self-esteem, and loneliness as causes of FA: The moderating effect of low self-control. *Curr. Psychol.* **2021**, *40*, 5358–5369. [CrossRef]
37. Zhang, M.; Pan, J.; Shi, W.; Qin, Y.; Guo, B. The more self-control, the more anxious?—A network analysis study of the relationship between self-control and psychological anxiety among Chinese university students. *BMC Psychol.* **2024**, *12*, 648. [CrossRef]
38. Botvin, G.J.; Griffin, K.W. School-based programmes to prevent alcohol, tobacco and other drug use. *Int. Rev. Psychiatry* **2007**, *19*, 607–615. [CrossRef]
39. Throuvala, M.A.; Griffiths, M.D.; Rennoldson, M.; Kuss, D.J. School-based prevention for adolescent internet addiction: Prevention is the key. A systematic literature review. *Curr. Neuropharmacol.* **2019**, *17*, 507–525. [CrossRef] [PubMed]
40. Walcott, C.M.; Meyers, A.B.; Landau, S. Adolescent sexual risk behaviors and school-based sexually transmitted infection/HIV prevention. *Psychol. Sch.* **2008**, *45*, 39–51. [CrossRef]
41. Gilman, R.; Carter-Sowell, A.; DeWall, C.N.; Adams, R.E.; Carboni, I. Validation of the Ostracism Experience Scale for Adolescents. *Psychol. Assess.* **2013**, *25*, 319–330. [CrossRef] [PubMed]
42. Akın, A.; Uysal, R.; Akın, Ü. The validity and reliability of Turkish version of the ostracism experience scale for adolescents. *Kastamonu Educ. J.* **2016**, *24*, 895–904.
43. Steger, M.F.; Samman, E. Assessing meaning in life on an international scale: Psychometric evidence for the meaning in life questionnaire-short form among Chilean households. *Int. J. Wellbeing* **2012**, *2*, 182–195. [CrossRef]
44. Eroğlu, A. The Mediating Role of Self-Control in the Relationship Between Internet Addiction and Religiosity in Adolescents (Karaman Sample). Master's Thesis, Marmara University, Istanbul, Türkiye, 2022.
45. Snyder, C.R.; Harris, C.; Anderson, J.R.; Holleran, S.A.; Irving, L.M.; Sigmon, S.T.; Yoshinobu, L.; Gibb, J.; Langelle, C.; Harney, P. The will and the ways: Development and validation of an individual differences measure of hope. *J. Personal. Soc. Psychol.* **1991**, *60*, 570–585. [CrossRef]
46. Tarhan, S.; Bacanlı, H. Adaptation of dispositional hope scale into Turkish: Validity and reliability study. *J. Happiness Well-Being* **2015**, *3*, 1–14.
47. Aksoy, K. Attitudes of High School Students Towards Addictive Substances and Examination of Variables Affecting These Attitudes (Malatya Province Example). Master's Thesis, Inonu University, Malatya, Türkiye, 1996. Unpublished.
48. Hayes, A.F.; Preacher, K.J. Statistical mediation analysis with a multicategorical independent variable. *British J. Math. Stat. Psychol.* **2014**, *67*, 451–470. [CrossRef]

49. Preacher, K.J.; Kelley, K. Effect size measures for mediation models: Quantitative strategies for communicating indirect effects. *Psychol. Methods* **2011**, *16*, 93–115. [CrossRef] [PubMed]
50. Curran, P.J.; West, S.G.; Finch, J.F. The robustness of test statistics to nonnormality and specification error in confirmatory factor analysis. *Psychol. Methods* **1996**, *1*, 16. [CrossRef]
51. Beard, S.J.; Hastings, P.D.; Ferrer, E.; Robins, R.W.; Guyer, A.E. Neural response to social exclusion moderates the link between adolescent anxiety symptoms and substance use. *Biol. Psychiatry Cogn. Neurosci. Neuroimaging* **2022**, *7*, 180–191. [CrossRef]
52. Pharo, H.H. The Behavioural and Psychological Effects of Ostracism in Adolescence and Emerging-Adulthood. Ph.D. Thesis, University of Otago, Dunedin, New Zealand, 2012.
53. Bacon, A.K.; Engerman, B. Excluded, then inebriated: A preliminary investigation into the role of ostracism on alcohol consumption. *Addict. Behav. Rep.* **2018**, *8*, 25–32. [CrossRef]
54. Haribhakti, P. Ostracism, Belongingness, and Alcohol Use: Comparing Different Racial/Ethnic Groups. Ph.D. Thesis, Texas A&M University, College Station, TX, USA, 2020.
55. Laws, H.B.; Ellerbeck, N.E.; Rodrigues, A.S.; Simmons, J.A.; Ansell, E.B. Social rejection and alcohol use in daily life. *Alcohol. Clin. Exp. Res.* **2017**, *41*, 820–827. [CrossRef]
56. Ruggieri, S.; Bendixen, M.; Gabriel, U.; Alsaker, F. The impact of ostracism on the well-being of early adolescents. *Swiss J. Psychol.* **2013**, *72*, 103–109. [CrossRef]
57. Quancai, L.; Meng, C.; Kunjie, C. Social control and self-control: Factors linking exposure to domestic violence and adolescents' Internet gaming addiction. *Front. Psychiatry* **2023**, *14*, 1245563. [CrossRef]
58. Forgas, J.P.; Harmon-Jones, E. It is better to give than to receive: The role of motivation and self-control in determining the consequences of ostracism for targets and sources. In *Motivation and Its Regulation*; Psychology Press: London, UK, 2014; pp. 369–384.
59. Warburton, W.A.; Williams, K.D.; Cairns, D.R. When ostracism leads to aggression: The moderating effects of control deprivation. *J. Exp. Soc. Psychol.* **2006**, *42*, 213–220. [CrossRef]
60. Bhatt, B.; Rana, N. The relationship between workplace ostracism and adaptive performance: Moderating role of hope. *Int. J. Res. Manag.* **2022**, 38–43.
61. Johnson, C.B. *Personality and Ostracism: Do Hope, Optimism, and Forgiveness Moderate the Effects of Social Exclusion?* Purdue University: West Lafayette, IN, USA, 2010.
62. Russo, C.; Barni, D.; Zagrean, I.; Lulli, M.A.; Vecchi, G.; Danioni, F. The resilient recovery from substance addiction: The role of self-transcendence values and hope. *Mediterr. J. Clin. Psychol.* **2021**, *9*, 1–20. [CrossRef]
63. Güngör, H.; Erçetin, Ş.Ş. Factors affecting future expectations of 12. grade students' preparation for higher education in schools. *Sak. Univ. J. Educ.* **2021**, *11*, 220–246. [CrossRef]
64. Marlatt, G.A.; Larimer, M.E.; Witkiewitz, K. *Harm Reduction: Pragmatic Strategies for Managing High-Risk Behaviors*; Guilford Press: New York, NY, USA, 2011.
65. Mathis, G.M.; Ferrari, J.R.; Groh, D.R.; Jason, L.A. Hope and substance abuse recovery: The impact of agency and pathways within an abstinent communal-living setting. *J. Groups Addict. Recovery* **2009**, *4*, 42–50. [CrossRef] [PubMed]
66. Koehn, C.; Cutcliffe, J.R. The inspiration of hope in substance abuse counseling. *J. Humanist. Couns.* **2012**, *51*, 78–98. [CrossRef]
67. Çiftci, N.; Yıldız, M.; Çiftci, K. The mediating role of social ostracism in the effect of social media addiction on loneliness in adolescents. *J. Pediatr. Nurs.* **2023**, *73*, 177–183. [CrossRef]
68. Taş, İ. The relationship between social ignore and social media addiction among adolescents: Mediator effect of satisfaction with family life. *Youth Soc.* **2021**, *55*, 708–729. [CrossRef]
69. Erdoğan Kaya, A.; Yazici, A.B.; Kaya, M.; Yazici, E. The relationship between expressed emotion, personality traits and prognosis of alcohol and substance addiction: 6-month follow-up study. *Nord. J. Psychiatry* **2021**, *75*, 596–606. [CrossRef]

children

MDPI

Article

Parents' Educational Background and Child's Learned Skills Are More Predictive for a Positive School Career than Earlier Parenting Behavior or Child's Mental Health—Results from an 18-Year Longitudinal Observation Study

Beate Muschalla [1,*], Ann-Katrin Job [2] and Wolfgang Schulz [1]

[1] Psychotherapy and Diagnostics, Technische Universität Braunschweig, 38106 Braunschweig, Germany; wolfgang.schulz@tu-braunschweig.de
[2] Institute of Psychology, University of Kassel, 34127 Kassel, Germany; a-k.job@uni-kassel.de
* Correspondence: b.muschalla@tu-braunschweig.de

Abstract: Background/Objectives: Developmental research has shown that mental health and functioning is determined by social background and child and family characteristics. Until now, there have been few longitudinal studies which considered several aspects at the same time and observed children's development over ten or more years. **Methods**: The aim of this 18-year-longitudinal study is to find out to which degree different child, family, and socioeconomic factors during early childhood (4 years of age) are associated with educational and professional outcomes in young adulthood (22 years of age). Of the initial sample of 280 participating families, 225 could again be investigated with standardized interviews and questionnaires at the 18 years follow-up (retention rate: 80%). **Results**: Educational degree of the parents was predictive of the child's school success ($\beta = -0.267$, $p < 0.001$, in regression analysis). Maternal mental health ($\beta = -0.005$, $p = 0.953$), parenting behavior ($\beta = -021$, $p = 0.782$), and early child mental health problems ($\beta = 0.071$, $p = 0.551$) only had a low impact. The child's sex did not predict school success. Better early learned skills (i.e., crystalline intelligence), but not cognitive skills, as measured by the child-specific intelligence test K-ABC, made children more likely to achieve good school-leaving grades ($\beta = -0.240$, $p = 0.008$). Children's early mental health problems had no relevant impact on school degree ($d = 0.00$, $p = 0.934/d = 0.02$, $p = 0.52$ 3) or professional status ($d = 0.04$, $p = 0.157/d = -0.02$, $p = 0.299$) at age 22. **Conclusions**: Besides the not-changeable parental education level, (learnable) competency aspects may be more predictive of a child's educational success until young adulthood than earlier mental health problems in parents and children. This is good news as it supports the idea that mental health deficits can be compensated for through learning and competency training.

Keywords: educational and professional degree; young adults; capacities; mental health; prediction; longitudinal study

1. Introduction

1.1. What Predicts School and Professional Performance?

Many social, emotional, and cognitive school-relevant capacities are developed in early childhood [1,2]. In addition, various individual child, family, and socioeconomic factors during early childhood are associated with later academic performance, school completion, and career prospects [3–5]. The strongest influence on an individual's school performance is exerted by cognitive and metacognitive capacities and prior knowledge [5], as well as social–emotional competencies [6]. On the side of non-cognitive characteristics student's motivational [7] and classroom characteristics [8] as well as family conditions [9] are considered predictive. Sociodemographic, school, and educational factors seem to have somewhat weaker effects [8]; however, in some countries, the socioeconomic family background is highly related to children's school success [10,11], and of course the quality of school impacts on students competency development [12].

Research so far has often focused on specific predictors for healthy development [13] or specific achievements [14,15]. Thus, there is still a need for evidence of broader developmental prediction perspectives which include aspects of family characteristics as well as aspects of child and parental mental health and behavior, to find out which aspects are more or less important for broader school success in young adults.

Accordingly, the aim of this 18-year-longitudinal study was to examine differentiated aspects of family characteristics, mental health, and behavior in parents and their young (4 years old) children, to find out which of them are predictive of children's school and professional success at 22 years of age.

1.2. *State of Research on Predictors for School and Professional Performance*

In the following, we summarize the empirical knowledge on the core predictors for school performance and professional performance in adolescence and young adulthood. These person and context factors have been assessed in this present longitudinal study, in order to examine their predictive value for school and professional performance outcomes in young adulthood.

1.2.1. Socioeconomic Status (SES) of the Family

School performance studies such as PISA [11], TIMSS [16], and LOGIK [17] consistently show that SES and school performance are directly related. For over 80 years, international results have also pointed to the relationship between SES and school performance [18,19]. A key finding of the PISA studies is that educational success is strongly related to SES in some countries [11]. Although the influence of socioeconomic factors on school success has decreased from 2003 to 2012, it still plays a crucial role [11]. It can thus be expected that children from families with high SES have better school achievements [20–25]. In the present study, we assessed the monthly household income of the family and the educational level of the parents at the first assessment (Pre) as indicators for SES.

1.2.2. Parenting Behavior and Parental Mental Health

The quality of the early family environment is particularly formative for intellectual and psychosocial development [3]. For children, the family not only represents a developmental and living space but also an important learning environment. In this context, the importance of parenting behaviors such as warmth, praise, responsiveness, and parental school engagement for positive school-related behavior in children has repeatedly been discussed [23,26]. Dysfunctional parenting behaviors during early childhood, in turn, have been shown to be associated with worse school performance in children at about 6 years of age [27,28].

Parental mental health problems also seem relevant in the sense that they—due to genetic reasons, or model learning, or parents' problems in socio emotional childcare—can affect child's mental health and result in problems that are relevant for children's school achievement [29–35].

1.2.3. Positive Parenting Programs (e.g., Triple P)

The Triple P is a well-established evidence-based preventive parenting program that trains parents how to positively interact as a family and with their very young children. The aim of such parent training is to strengthen the parental relationship and parenting skills to promote the healthy development of children. Several self-reflection exercises are used to train positive parental behavior [36,37].

According to these empirical findings, parental (maternal) mental health problems, dysfunctional parenting behavior, and participation in preventive parent training were assessed as potential predictors for child's school and professional outcomes.

1.2.4. Child's Sex

The sex difference in academic performance is most salient in language learning. In almost all European countries, girls usually perform better than boys of the same age in language subjects [11,38,39]. In contrast, boys' academic performance in mathematics is usually better than girls' [11,38]. Corresponding results are provided by a five-year longitudinal study of over 70,530 English children [40].

In the present study, we consider the sex of the child as a control variable in the prediction of later school success. As girls might achieve better grades in language subjects, but boys might achieve better grades in mathematics, the overall school success should not be dependent on the sex of the child.

1.2.5. Cognitive Capacities and Learned Skills

Cognitive functioning is a main aspect of health over the life span and is often determined by high education levels in youth [11]. Cognitive skills such as intelligence and attention are cited as relevant cross-domain competencies for school success [40,41]. A longitudinal study of 101 children demonstrated that cross-domain precursor skills such as intelligence and working memory performance in preschool age are related to children's performance in early school years [2]. In intelligence research, fluid intelligence and crystalline intelligence are distinguished. Fluid intelligence (capacities), on the one hand, encompasses basic processes of thinking and is largely independent of experience; it is very strongly genetically determined. Crystalline intelligence (learned skills), on the other hand, comprises the ability to apply acquired knowledge; it is considered to be predominantly culture-dependent [42].

In the present study, we assessed fluid capacities and learned skills as two dimensions of cognitive capacities in early childhood, and both are investigated as potential predictors for school and professional success in young adulthood.

Behavioral Problems, Mental Health, and Self Control

It has often been observed that self-control and behavioral or emotional problems during early childhood are related to later achievement [30,43–46]. Children's socio-emotional competencies and psychological behavioral problems are related to preschool competencies and later school performance [47–51]. For example, in one study, children with externalizing behavior problems during early childhood showed deficits in cognitive and preschool skills at age three [49]. The impact of psychopathology-related behavior problems on school performance was also investigated [47]: An initial survey of 1514 children assessed anxiety and emotional disturbance, depressive symptoms, and obsessive–compulsive disorders. The following year, 563 children were found to comprise an at-risk group and underwent a diagnostic interview to assess behavioral problems. Two years later, school performance could significantly be predicted by earlier mental health symptoms and behavioral problems. Especially, ADHD symptoms had a negative influence on school performance, as well as depressive symptoms and persistent anxiety. Social anxiety and generalized worrying, in turn, positively predicted school performance. The regression model explained a total of 27% of language achievement and 19% of math achievement.

In the present study, we dimensionally assessed child mental health problems by using observer reports from the mothers.

1.2.6. Adverse Childhood Events (ACEs) and Bullying

Adverse childhood events (ACEs) and bullying in youth may have a negative impact on children's school success and professional career. Until know, longitudinal research suggests that ACEs may influence children's behavioral and academic outcomes early in development [51]. Bullying is a frequent problem and reaction to the behavioral problems of children with observable neurocognitive or mental health problems [52]. Empirical findings show that bullying often occurs repeatedly, at school and later at work [53]. Therefore, in the present study, bullying in youth and ACEs were investigated as potential predictors for later school and professional problems in young adulthood.

1.3. Excursus: The German School System

In Germany, school attendance is obligatory for children and young people from the age of 6 until the end of the 9th school year. Attending state school is generally free for children and young people. Private schools, e.g., those run by church organizations, are only attended by very few children, even though there has been an increase in the last 5 to 10 years. The German school system is divided into primary, lower secondary, and upper secondary school depending on age and learning progress. The primary level is attended by all children regardless of their performance and lasts four or six years. In contrast to the school systems in many other countries, where all children, regardless of their performance, attend the same type of school at lower secondary level, most children in Germany attend a three-form school system with different school-leaving certificates. Depending on their performance level in primary school, children attend either Hauptschule (up to grade 9), Realschule (up to grade 10), or Gymnasium (up to grade 10 or 13; the last 3 years are also known as upper secondary level). There is a certain degree of mobility between the individual school types and, therefore, the possibility to switch between them. In addition, there have been more Integrative Gesamtschulen (inclusive comprehensive schools) in recent years, which can be attended by all children regardless of their performance in primary school, where all types of school qualifications are possible. With very few exceptions, there is no correlation between school quality and parental income [54].

1.4. Research Question

This aim of the present 18-year-longitudinal prediction study is to find out to which degree individual child-, family-, and socioeconomic factors during early childhood (4 years of age) as well as adverse childhood experiences (ACEs, up to age 18) and bullying in adolescence (at 14 years) are associated with educational and professional achievement in young adulthood (22 years of age). Because part of the families participated in the universal preventive Triple P Positive Parenting Program at the beginning of this study (for details, see Hahlweg and Schulz [55]), we also investigate the impact of program participation on school and professional success.

Although there is a large number of cross-sectional studies on the importance of family background for children's school and professional success, there is still a lack of longitudinal studies demonstrating the long-term effects over a long period of time. Particularly in Germany, with its three-form school system that differs from that of most other countries, there is a lack of longitudinal studies. The present study aims to close this research gap.

Based on the reported state of research, it will be explored to which degree school and professional success of young adults is determined by

- Educational level of parents and household income;
- Parenting behavior and approximate health;
- Parental participation in a preventive parenting program (Triple P [36]) 18 years ago;
- Cognitive capacities, self-control, and early mental health problems in the child;
- Problems with ACEs and bullying in the child.

2. Materials and Methods

A large longitudinal observation study was conducted with families from a German city over 18 years. This study repeatedly assessed child and family characteristics as well as child behavioral problems from early childhood at the age of 4 years (Pre) over adolescence (10-year follow-up, FU10) to young adulthood (18-year follow-up, FU18). Risk and protective factors were assessed in early childhood (Pre), bullying was assessed in youth, and mental health problems, ACEs, and school achievement were assessed in young adulthood (FU18).

2.1. Recruitment

Since most children at 4 years of age attend day care centers ("kindergarten") in Germany, recruitment was conducted via day care centers in the city. In the year 2001/02, all 33 day care centers (kindergarten) in the city of Braunschweig were informed about the research project, and 23 expressed their interest in participating. Out of the interested, 17 (i.e., 51.5% out of all the 33 day care centers) were randomly selected for family recruitment. The final eligible population from these 17 participating day care institutions included 915 families, of whom 280 families agreed to participate. The recruitment rate of 30.6% can be rated as very good for a universal prevention study. However, during the successive recruitment process, we observed that in areas of the city with lower socioeconomic level, the recruitment rate was lower than in socioeconomically higher-level areas. The non-participating parents were younger and more likely to receive state financial support. Parents who declined to participate usually feared an intrusion into their private lives, e.g., they expected the interview to be too personal, they did not want to be analyzed, or video recorded, or simply stated that they did not have time to participate in this study. Detailed information on the recruitment process and reasons for non-participation are reported by Bertram et al. [56].

Since participation of the families was conducted free-willingly, we expect that the participating families were interested in the research topic and somehow open for new experience. Families with a higher education background were over-represented (about 60% of parents had A-Levels) as compared to what would normally be expected in the general population. Due to these reasons, the sample represents a rather prototypically representative population, i.e., families with potentially better resources (socioeconomic background and education level). This limitation will be considered when interpreting the data.

At the Pre stage, each family received EUR 50 for their study participation. During the follow ups, the interviewed parent and the young adult each received EUR 40 (FU10) or EUR 50 (FU18) for participating in the approximately 2.5 h survey.

2.2. Instruments

Data were collected by using a combination of interviews and standardized questionnaires for children and parents (Table 1). The interviewers were prepared for the interviews with the families in advance through intensive training (12 to 15 h for each interviewer) by the project management. The training included role playing according to case vignettes, dealing with answers which are difficult to code, and assuring a private atmosphere, in order to keep the interviewed person motivated to answer all questions. The training's aim was to make sure all interviewers adhere to the interview manual, in order to collect reliable data. The questionnaires were completed with paper and pencil or at FU18 online via SurveyMonkey (www.surveymonkey.de, 4 April 2025).

Table 1. Instruments used in the first assessment (Pre), the 10-year follow-up (FU10), and in the 18-year follow-up (FU18).

Predictors and Characteristics	Type of Assessment and Psychometrics	Instruments Name and Content
Socio-demographics (Pre, FU10, FU18)	The sociodemographic interview checklist contains no psychometric contents	Categorical interview checklist exploring: age (childhood and young adulthood), biological sex (child), parenting status (2-parent family vs. single parent), highest school education (mother and father), monthly household income, and migration background
Intelligence—child (Pre)	Intelligence test conducted with child Cronbach's α for abilities 0.94; Cronbach's α for skills 0.98	Kaufman Assessment Battery for Children (K-ABC [42]), scales: intellectual abilities and intellectual skills
Self-control problems—child (Pre)	Psychometric questionnaire filled out by mother, each item scaled: 0–2 Retest reliability: 0.80 Split-half reliability: 0.90 Cronbach's α: 0.93	Child Self-Control Scale [57], 26 items from the domains of lack of control (e.g., "child gets angry quickly"), aggressiveness (e.g., "child gets into scuffles, fights easily"), and hyperactivity (e.g., "child cannot sit still, is restless or overactive")
Mental health problems—child (Pre)	Psychometric questionnaire filled out by mother, each item scaled: 0–2 Cronbach's α: 0.94 (mother)	Child Behavior Check List (CBCL 1.5–5 [58]), mother's report; higher scores = more child behavior problems
Dysfunctional parenting behavior—mother (Pre)	Psychometric questionnaire filled out by mother, each item scaled: 1–7 Retest reliability: 0.84 (mother) Cronbach's α: 0.80 (mother)	German version of the Parenting Scale (EFB [59]), mother's report, higher scores = more dysfunctional parenting behavior
Mental health problems—mother (Pre)	Psychometric questionnaire filled out by mother, each item scaled: 1–4 Cronbach's α: 0.96 (mother)	Depression–Anxiety–Stress Scale (DASS) [60], higher values = more symptom severity
Bullying—adolescent (FU10)	Psychometric questionnaire filled out by child, each item scaled: 1–5 Cronbach's α: 0.68–0.83	Bully–Victim Questionnaire (BVQ [61]); bullying yes or no

Table 1. *Cont.*

Predictors and Characteristics	Type of Assessment and Psychometrics	Instruments Name and Content
ACE—child (FU18)	Psychometric questionnaire filled out by child, each item scaled: 0–1 Cronbach's α: 0.76	German version of the Adverse Childhood Experiences Questionnaire (ACE-D [62]), sum score from 10 items (e.g., "Before your 18th birthday: Did a parent or another adult in your household often or very often push you, grab you, hit you or throw something at you?"); higher score = more ACE
School-related data—young adult (FU18)	The sociodemographic interview checklist contains no psychometric contents	Type of school (FU10), school-leaving grades (overall grade, 1.0 = top grade; FU18), school-leaving certificate (FU18), professional certificate (FU18)—explored in interview

At baseline (Pre), when children were on average 4 years old, socio-demographics of the family were assessed by personal interviews (for details see Table 1). Child's characteristics in terms of self-control problems, mental health, and intelligence, as well as parenting behavior and mothers' self-reported mental health problems, were assessed by standardized tests and questionnaires (Table 1).

At FU10, when the children were on average 14 years old, family socio-demographics, the children's school achievements, and whether the child was involved in bullying was assessed (Table 1).

At FU18, when the children were on average 22 years old, again, family socio-demographics were assessed, as well as the children's ACEs, school-leaving achievements, and professional status (Table 1).

2.3. Statistical Analysis

First, for a basic overview of the descriptive data, means and percentages on all sample characteristics are reported (Table 2). Second, for a basic view on associations between predictors (family's characteristics) and outcomes (school-leaving degree, professional degree, and overall school grade), correlations were calculated (Table 3).

Third, hierarchical regression analyses (Tables 4–6) were conducted, to estimate the relative predictive value of each predictor by including all relevant predictors according to the research question. Depending on the level of the outcome variable, either multiple linear regression (for continuous outcome variable, Table 6), or multinomial logistic regression (for categorial outcome variable, Tables 4 and 5) were calculated. Five models were calculated for each of the hierarchical regressions, with additional variables added at each level (see Tables 4–6).

Our hierarchical structure is based on the following logic:

Level 1: socio-demographic data (Pre);
Level 2: psychological characteristics of the child (Pre);
Level 3: characteristics of the mothers (Pre);
Level 4: Triple P intervention (Pre);
Level 5: psychological characteristics of the child (FU10 and across the lifespan).

Table 2. Sample characteristics from Pre to the 18-year follow-up (FU18). N = 225.

Characteristics	M	SD
Age child in years (Pre)	4.00	1.0
Age adolescent in years (FU10)	14.4	1.1
Age young adult in years (FU18)	22.6	1.1
Overall school grade (FU18)Lower grades indicate better school achievements	2.54	0.65
School-leaving degree parents [1] (Pre)	2.51	0.63
Household income [2] (Pre)	8.74	2.81
IQ fluid capacities (Pre)	103.47	12.11
IQ learned skills (Pre)	102.56	13.76
Self-control problems [3] (Pre)	13.89	9.74
Early mental health problems (child) [4] (Pre)	48.63	10.24
Dysfunctional parenting (Pre)	3.22	0.56
Parental mental health problems (mother) (Pre)	22.80	16.02
ACE adverse childhood experiences (FU18)	1.03	1.58
	N	%
Sex of the child (Pre)		
- girl	111	49.3
- boy	114	50.7
Parent status (Pre)		
- two-parent family	184	81.8
- mother only	40	17.8
- father only	1	0.4
Education level mother (Pre)		
- without school-leaving certificate. 9 classes	16	7.1
- 10 classes	78	34.8
- A-Levels/High school	130	58.0
Education level father (Pre)		
- without school-leaving certificate. 9 classes	21	11.4
- 10 classes	47	25.5
- A-Levels/High school	116	63.0
Monthly household income (EUR/USD) (Pre)		
- <1.000	1	0.5
- 1.000 to <1.500	5	2.3
- 1.500 to <2.000	4	1.8
- 2.000 to <2.500	19	8.7
- 2.500 to <3.000	6	2.7
- 3.000 to <3.500	14	6.4
- 3.500 to <4.000	15	6.8
- 4.000 to <4.500	20	9.1
- 4.500 to <5.000	18	8.2
- 5.000 to <6.000	44	20.1
- 6.000 to <8.000	44	20.1
- 8.000 to <10.000	26	11.9
- ≥10.000	3	1.4

Table 2. *Cont.*

Characteristics	M	SD
Migration background (Pre)		
- with	24	10.7
- without	201	89.3
Bullying (FU10)		
- bullying	47	22.2
- no bullying	165	77.8
School-leaving certificate (young adult. FU18)		
- no school-leaving degree	3	1.3
- special school-leaving degree	1	0.4
- 9 classes school-leaving degree	11	4.9
- 10 classes school-leaving degree	30	13.4
- 12/13 classes A-Levels/high school	179	79.9
Professional certificate (young adult. FU18)		
- no professional certificate, not in any professional education	31	14.0
- currently in professional education	19	8.6
- professional certificate	39	17.6
- college/university studies	101	45.5
- college/university certificate	32	14.4

Note. [1] 3-stepped scale: 1 = no school-leaving degree, 9 classes, 2 = 10 classes school-leaving degree, and 3 = 12/13 classes A-Levels; mean of mother (and if available father) school-leaving degree; [2] 13-stepped scale: 1 < 1.000 DM to 13 > 10.000 DM); [3] high values = low self-control; [4] t-values.

Table 3. Means, standard deviations, and correlations of study variables (Pre, FU10, and FU18).

Characteristics	N	N	%	School-Leaving Degree [5]	Professional Degree [5]	Overall School Grade [6]
School-leaving degree (FU18) - no school-leaving degree. 9 classes - 10 classes school-leaving degree - 12/13 classes A-Levels/high school	224	15 30 179	6.7 14.4 79.9	-	0.675 ***	−0.169 **
Professional degree (FU18) - without professional education - in professional education - in college/university studies	222	31 58 133	14.0 26.1 59.9	0.675 ***	-	−0.270 ***
Biological sex - female - male	225	111 114	49.3 50.7	0.098	0.088	0.111
Parenting status (Pre) - 2-parent family - single parent	225	184 41	81.8 18.2	0.128	0.103	0.095
Parental training Triple P (Pre) - no participation - participation	225	104 121	46.2 53.8	0.085	0.094	−0.072
Bullying (FU10) - bullying - no bullying	212	165 47	77.8 22.2	0.365 ***	0.211 **	−0.192 **

Table 3. *Cont.*

Characteristics	N	M	SD	School-leaving degree [6]	Professional degree [6]	Overall school grade [7]
Overall school grade (FU18) Lower grades indicate better school achievements	215	2.54	0.65	−0.169 **	−0.270 ***	-
School-leaving degree parents [1] (Pre)	224	2.51	0.63	0.363 ***	0.291 ***	−0.288 ***
Household income [2] (Pre)	219	8.74	2.81	0.183 ***	0.223 ***	−0.216 **
IQ fluid capacities (Pre)	218	103.47	12.11	0.253 ***	0.211 ***	−0.290 ***
IQ learned skills (Pre)	220	102.56	13.76	0.257 ***	0.237 ***	−0.292 ***
Self-control problems [3] (Pre)	223	13.89	9.74	−0.169 **	−0.155 **	0.072
Early mental health problems (child) [4] (Pre)	223	48.63	10.24	−0.161 **	−0.150 **	0.138 *
Dysfunctional parenting (Pre)	223	3.22	0.56	−0.106	−0.083	0.105
Parental mental health problems (mother) (Pre)	223	22.80	16.02	−0.058	−0.107 *	0.115
ACE	211	1.03	1.58	−0.164 **	−0.161 **	0.067

Note. *** $p < 0.001$, ** $p < 0.05$, * $p < 0.01$; all tests were one sided, test for sex was 2-sided; [1] 3-stepped scale: 1 = no school-leaving degree, 9 classes, 2 = 10 classes school-leaving degree, and 3 = 12/13 classes A-Levels; mean of mother (and if available father) school-leaving degree; [2] 13-stepped scale: 1 < 1.000 DM to 13 > 10.000 DM); [3] high values = low self-control; [4] t-values; [5] φ coefficient; [6] Kendall τ; [7] Spearman r_s.

The multiple coefficients of determination R^2 were interpreted according to Cohen [63]: $R^2 > 0.02$ is interpreted as low variance clarification, $R^2 > 0.13$ is interpreted as moderate variance clarification, and $R^2 > 0.26$ is interpreted as high variance clarification. Interpretation of the effect sizes (Cohen's d) and ß values is as follows: A Cohen's d/ß value of 0.20–0.50/0.10–0.30 is interpreted as a small effect, a value of 0.50–0.80/0.30–0.50 is interpreted as a medium effect, and a value of >0.80/>0.50 is interpreted as a large effect; r > 0.10 is interpreted as a small effect, r > 0.30 is interpreted as a medium effect, and r > 0.50 is interpreted as a large effect 0.57.

Almost all multinomial logistic regressions showed sufficient model quality (LQ-Test p significant; Goodness of Fit (except the first model for professional degree which was not significant)). For the dependent variable school degree >82.5% of the young adults were correctly assigned by the model, and for professional degree, the rate was >62.8%. Nagelkerkes R^2 was acceptable or good for all models concerning school degree (>0.297), and acceptable for professional degree (>0.245; except the first model therein). To verify multicollinearity, on the one hand, correlations between the twelve predictors were calculated and, on the other hand, the VIF values were determined [64]. None of the 66 correlations are >0.80; the VIF values fluctuate between 1.01 and 3.09 (<10). It can, therefore, be assumed that there is no multicollinearity between the predictors. Variance clarification (R^2) was moderate; all models were significant.

Table 4. Prediction of school-leaving degree (FU18): multinomial logistic regression (inclusion method, hierarchical).

Dependent Variable: Without School-Leaving Degree or 9 Classes Versus 12/13 Classes															
Predictor	**Model 1**			**Model 2**			**Model 3**			**Model 4**			**Model 5**		
	B	*p*	**d**	**B**	*p*	**d**	**B**	*p*	**d**	**B**	*p*	**d**	**B**	*p*	**d**
School-leaving degree parents [1] (Pre)	−2.068	<0.001 ***	−1.14 ###	−1.416	0.032 *	−0.78 ###	−1.585	0.031 *	−0.87 ###	−1.625	0.027 *	−0.90 ###	−3.001	0.096	−1.65 ###
Household income [2] (Pre)	−0.257	0.023 *	−0.14	−0.304	0.051	−0.17	−0.364	0.033 *	−0.20 #	−0.323	0.073	−0.18	0.077	0.807	0.04
Sex of the child	0.071	0.910	0.04	−0.303	0.718	−0.17	−0.373	0.675	−0.21 #	−0.417	0.643	−0.23 #	0.498	0.781	0.27 #
IQ Fluid capacities (Pre)				−0.096	0.042 *	−0.05	−0.093	0.057	−0.05	−0.089	0.069	−0.05	−0.149	0.140	−0.08
IQ Learned skills (Pre)				−0.026	0.490	−0.13	−0.041	0.290	−0.02	−0.043	0.275	−0.02	−0.098	0.297	−0.05
Self-control problems [3] (Pre)				0.075	0.205	−0.04	0.092	0.152	0.05	0.090	0.164	0.05	0.138	0.253	0.08
Mental health problems (child) [4] (Pre)				−0.013	0.832	−0.01	−0.018	0.792	−0.01	−0.010	0.884	−0.01	0.008	0.934	0.00
Dysfunctional parenting (Pre)							0.395	0.654	0.22 #	0.475	0.610	0.26	0.177	0.898	0.10
Parental mental health problems (mother) (Pre)							−0.036	0.085	−0.02	−0.037	0.088	−0.02	−0.062	0.292	−0.03
Parental training (Triple P) participation (Pre)										−0.740	0.428	−0.41 #	1.723	0.356	−0.95 ###
ACE adverse childhood experiences (FU18)													1.006	0.016 *	0.55 ##
Bullying (FU10)													−2.230	0.037 *	−1.23 ###
Dependent variable: School-leaving degree after 10 classes versus after 12/13 classes															
Predictor	**Model 1**			**Model 2**			**Model 3**			**Model 4**			**Model 5**		
	B	*p*	**d**	**B**	*p*	**d**	**B**	*p*	**d**	**B**	*p*	**d**	**B**	*p*	**d**
School-leaving degree parents [1] (Pre)	−1.408	<0.001 ***	−0.78 ##	−1.515	<0.001 ***	−0.83 ###	−1.546	<0.001 ***	−0.85 ###	−1.610	<0.001 ***	−0.89 ###	−1.837	<0.001 ***	−1.01 ###
Household income [2] (Pre)	0.019	0.820	0.01	0.066	0.515	0.04	0.050	0.628	0.03	0.079	0.457	0.04	0.120	0.350	0.07
Sex of the child	0.771	0.080	0.43 #	0.672	0.167	0.37 #	0.682	0.165	0.38 #	0.636	0.200	0.35 #	0.822	0.187	0.45 #
IQ Fluid capacities (Pre)				0.005	0.846	0.00	0.006	0.802	0.00	0.008	0.771	0.00	−0.019	0.537	−0.01
IQ Learned skills (Pre)				−0.032	0.165	−0.02	−0.034	0.135	−0.02	−0.035	0.133	−0.02	−0.013	0.617	−0.01
Self-control problems [3] (Pre)				0.000	0.997	0.000	0.006	0.878	0.00	0.010	0.806	0.01	0.036	0.441	0.02
Mental health problems (child) [4] (Pre)				0.011	0.782	0.01	0.015	0.711	0.01	0.022	0.581	0.01	0.030	0.523	0.02
Dysfunctional parenting (Pre)							−0.199	0.685	−0.11	−0.278	0.581	−0.15	−0.353	0.541	−0.19
Parental mental health problems (mother) (Pre)							−0.008	0.579	−0.00	−0.009	0.575	−0.01	−0.014	0.389	−0.01

Table 4. *Cont.*

Dependent variable: School-leaving degree after 10 classes versus after 12/13 classes															
Predictor	**Model 1**			**Model 2**			**Model 3**			**Model 4**			**Model 5**		
	B	***p***	**d**	**B**	***p***	**d**	**B**	***p***	**d**	**B**	***p***	**d**	**B**	***p***	**d**
Parental training (Triple P) participation (Pre)										−0.791	0.106	−0.44 $^{\#}$	−10.260	0.037 *	−0.69 $^{\#\#}$
ACE adverse childhood experiences (FU18)													0.300	0.167	0.17
Bullying (FU10)													−0.133	0.545	−0.07
LQ-Test	$\chi^2 = 52.1, p < 0.001$			$\chi^2 = 73.5, p < 0.001$			$\chi^2 = 77.2, p < 0.001$			$\chi^2 = 80.1, p < 0.001$			$\chi^2 = 76.6, p < 0.001$		
Goodness of Fit	$\chi^2 = 77.4, p = 0.918$			$\chi^2 = 176.4, p = 1.000$			$\chi^2 = 173.2, p = 1.000$			$\chi^2 = 170.3, p = 1.000$			$\chi^2 = 117.9, p = 1.000$		
Nagelkerkes R^2	$R^2 = 0.297$			$R^2 = 0.426$			$R^2 = 0.443$			$R^2 = 0.457$			$R^2 = 0.552$		
Correct prediction	82.5%			86.5%			87.0%			86.5%			87.5%		

Note. *** $p < 0.001$, * $p < 0.01$; $^{\#}$ > 0.20, <−0.20 small effect, $^{\#\#}$ > 0.50, <−0.50 medium effect, $^{\#\#\#}$ > 0.80, <−0.80 large effect; [1] 3-stepped scale: 1 = no school-leaving degree, 9 classes, 2 = 10 classes school-leaving degree, and 3 = 12/13 classes A-Levels; mean of mother (and if available father) school-leaving degree; [2] 13-stepped scale: 1 < 1.000 DM to 13 > 10.000 DM; [3] high values = low self-control; [4] t-values.

Table 5. Prediction of professional degree (FU18): multinomial logistic regression (inclusion method, hierarchical).

Dependent Variable: Without Professional Education Versus College/University															
Predictor	**Model 1**			**Model 2**			**Model 3**			**Model 4**			**Model 5**		
	B	***p***	***d***	***B***	***p***	***d***	***B***	***p***	***d***	***B***	***p***	***d***	***B***	***p***	***d***
School-leaving degree parents [1] (Pre)	−1.041	0.002 **	−0.57 $^{\#\#}$	−0.965	0.013 *	−0.53 $^{\#\#\#}$	−1.081	0.007 **	−0.60 $^{\#\#}$	−1.164	0.004 **	−0.64 $^{\#\#}$	−1.356	0.009 **	−0.758 $^{\#\#}$
Household income [2] (Pre)	−0.169	0.030 *	−0.09	−0.171	0.050	−0.09	−0.199	0.027 *	0.11	−0.169	0.069	−0.09	0.034	0.784	0.02
Sex of the child	0.644	0.138	0.36 $^{\#}$	0.667	0.165	0.37 $^{\#}$	0.672	0.168	0.37 $^{\#}$	0.639	0.201	0.35 $^{\#}$	20.043	0.011 *	10.13 $^{\#\#\#}$
IQ Fluid capacities (Pre)				−0.012	0.620	−0.01	−0.008	0.768	−0.00	−0.005	0.849	−0.00	0.016	0.603	0.01
IQ Learned skills (Pre)				−0.023	0.308	−0.01	−0.029	0.197	−0.02	−0.029	0.199	−0.02	−0.010	0.721	−0.01
Self-control problems [3] (Pre)				0.028	0.458	0.02	0.043	0.274	0.02	0.050	0.217	0.03	0.012	0.805	0.01
Mental health problems (child) [4] (Pre)				0.010	0.789	0.01	0.019	0.636	0.01	0.023	0.562	0.01	0.074	0.157	0.04
Dysfunctional parenting (Pre)							−0.409	0.387	−0.23	−0.495	0.309	−0.27 $^{\#}$	−0.588	0.319	−0.32 $^{\#}$
Parental mental health problems (mother) (Pre)							−0.024	0.181	−0.01	−0.024	0.184	−0.01	−0.025	0.288	−0.01
Parental training (Triple P) participation (Pre)										−0.913	0.067	−0.50 $^{\#\#}$	−0.813	0.174	−0.45 $^{\#}$
ACE adverse childhood experiences (FU18)													0.804	<0.001 ***	0.45 $^{\#}$
Bullying (FU10)													−0.291	0.157	−0.16

Table 5. *Cont.*

Dependent variable: professional education versus college/university															
Predictor	**Model 1**			**Model 2**			**Model 3**			**Model 4**			**Model 5**		
	B	*p*	*d*	*B*	*p*	*d*	*B*	*p*	*d*	*B*	*p*	*d*	*B*	*p*	*d*
School-leaving degree parents [1] (Pre)	−0.939	0.001 ***	−0.52 ##	−0.702	0.027 *	−0.39 #	−0.708	0.030 *	−0.39 #	−0.719	0.028 *	−0.40 #	−0.569	0.119	−0.32 #
Household income [2] (Pre)	−0.109	0.090	−0.06	−0.091	0.199	−0.05	−0.096	0.183	−0.05	−0.092	0.211	−0.05	−0.141	0.096	−0.08
Sex	0.207	0.540	0.11	0.090	0.806	0.05	0.076	0.837	0.04	0.044	0.905	0.02	−0.062	0.877	−0.03
IQ Fluid capacities (Pre)				−0.011	0.573	−0.01	−0.011	0.569	−0.01	−0.011	0.581	−0.01	−0.013	0.525	−0.01
IQ Learned skills (Pre)				−0.037	0.032 *	−0.02	−0.037	0.035 *	−0.02	−0.038	0.033 *	−0.02	−0.046	0.027	−0.03
Self-control problems [3] (Pre)				0.046	0.137	0.03	0.046	0.143	0.03	0.048	0.131	0.03	0.062	0.069	0.03
Mental health problems (child) [4] (Pre)				−0.028	0.347	−0.02	−0.026	0.393	−0.01	−0.025	0.413	−0.01	−0.036	0.299	−0.02
Dysfunctional parenting (Pre)							−0.113	0.752	−0.06	−0.132	0.712	−0.07	−0.058	0.881	−0.03
Parental mental health problems (mother) (Pre)							−0.001	0.937	−0.00	−0.001	0.920	−0.00	−0.009	0.520	−0.01
Parental training (Triple P) participation (Pre)										−0.178	0.631	−0.10	−0.067	0.872	−0.04
ACE adverse childhood experiences (FU18)													−0.222	0.259	−0.12
Bullying (FU10)													−0.016	0.926	−0.01
LQ-Test	$\chi^2 = 31.4, p < 0.001$			$\chi^2 = 47.6, p < 0.001$			$\chi^2 = 51.9, p < 0.001$			$\chi^2 = 54.9, p < 0.001$			$\chi^2 = 74.4, p < 0.001$		
Goodness of Fit	$\chi^2 = 128.6, p = 0.015$			$\chi^2 = 333.0, p <= 0.991$			$\chi^2 = 329.1, p = 0.991$			$\chi^2 = 325.6$, $p = 0.9$[illegible]2			$\chi^2 = 260.0, p = 1.000$		
Nagelkerkes R^2	$R^2 = 0.161$			$R^2 = 0.245$			$R^2 = 0.262$			$R^2 = 0.278$			$R^2 = 0.397$		
Correct prediction	62.8%			65.0%			66.5%			65.0%			68.5%		

Note. *** $p < 0.001$, ** $p < 0.05$, * $p < 0.01$; # > 0.10 small effect, ## > 0.30 medium effect, ### > 0.50 large effect; [1] 3-stepped scale: 1 = no school-leaving degree, 9 classes, 2 = 10 classes school-leaving degree, and 3 = 12/13 classes A-Levels; mean of mother (and if available father) school-leaving degree; [2] 13-stepped scale: 1 < 1.000 DM to 13 > 10.000 DM); [3] high values = low self-control; [4] t-values.

Table 6. Prediction of school grade (FU18): multiple linear regression (inclusion method. hierarchical).

	Model 1		**Model 2**		**Model 3**		**Model 4**		**Model 5**	
Predictors	β	*p*	β	*p*	β	*p*	β	*p*	β	*p*
School-leaving degree parents [1] (Pre)	−0.329 ##	<0.001 ***	−0.251 #	0.001 ***	−0.252 #	0.001 ***	−0.254 #	0.001 ***	−0.267 #	<0.001 ***
Household income [2] (Pre)	−0.118 #	0.107	−0.062	0.411	−0.060	0.433	−0.054	0.495	−0.077	0.335
Sex of the child	0.109 #	0.120	0.113 #	0.108	0.113 #	0.111	0.110 #	0.[illegible]27	0.077	0.286

Table 6. *Cont.*

	Model 1		Model 2		Model 3		Model 4		Model 5	
Predictors	β	p	β	p	β	p	β	p	β	p
IQ Fluid capacities (Pre)			−0.009	0.915	−0.011 #	0.903	−0.011 #	0.904	−0.011	0.895
IQ Learned skills (Pre)			−0.236 #	0.008 **	−0.235 #	0.009 **	−0.236 #	0.009 **	−0.240 #	0.008 **
Self-control problems [3] (Pre)			−0.075	0.507	−0.074	0.517	−0.071	0.537	−0.065	0.568
Mental health problems (child) [4] (Pre)			0.088	0.447	0.087	0.466	0.092	0.445	0.071	0.551
Dysfunctional parenting (Pre)					−0.023	0.767	−0.025	0.743	−0.021	0.782
Parental mental health problems (mother) (Pre)					0.019	0.814	0.017	0.831	−0.005	0.953
Parenting training (Triple P) participation (Pre)							−0.029	0.687	−0.025	0.736
ACE adverse childhood experiences (FU18)									−0.117 #	0.121
Bullying (FU10)									−0.118 #	0.102
	R^2	0.151	R^2	0.203	R^2	0.203	R^2	0.204	R^2	0.228
	corrected R^2	0.137	*corrected* R^2	0.170	*corrected* R^2	0.161	*corrected* R^2	0.157	*corrected* R^2	0.173
	p	<0.001 ***	p	<0.001 ***	p	<0.001 ***	p	<0.001 ***	p	<0.001 ***
	Change in R^2	0.151	*Change in* R^2	0.052	*Change in* R^2	0.001	*Change in* R^2	0.001	*Change in* R^2	0.024
	Change in p	<0.001 ***	*Change in p*	0.028 *	*Change in p*	0.939	*Change in p*	0.687	*Change in p*	0.076
	Durbin-Watson-Statistik	2.015	Durbin-Watson-Statistik	2.105	Durbin-Watson-Statistik	2.105	Durbin-Watson-Statistik	2.105	Durbin-Watson-Statistik	2.105
	VIF	1.01–1.101	VIF	1.06–2.88	VIF	1.07–3.03	VIF	1.09–3.06	VIF	1.12–3.09

Note. *** $p < 0.001$, ** $p < 0.05$, * $p < 0.01$; # > 0.10 small effect, ## > 0.30 medium effect; VIF = variance-inflation factor; [1] 3-stepped scale: 1 = no school-leaving degree, 9 classes, 2 = 10 classes school-leaving degree, and 3 = 12/13 classes A-Levels; mean of mother (and if available father) school-leaving degree; [2] 13-stepped scale: 1 < 1.000 DM to 13 > 10.000 DM); [3] high values = low self-control; [4] t-values.

3. Results

3.1. Sample Characteristics

The initial sample consisted of 280 families. Based on a randomized assignment, nearly half (48.6%) of the families received a brief parenting intervention (Triple P, [36]) after baseline assessment as part of the experimental condition (for details, see Hahlweg and Schulz [55]). Parents allocated to the control group were not provided with any training. In both groups, changes were observed over the time of data collection. At the first assessment point (Pre), the children were on average 4.1 years old (SD = 1.0). For the 10-year follow-up (FU10), 249 families could still be recruited (retention rate: 89%). At this time, the adolescents were on average 14.4 years old (SD = 1.2). In the 18-year follow-up (FU18), 225 families still participated (retention rate: 80%). The reasons for dropout were as follows: only about 5% of families refused to participate after being contacted by email or telephone, 10% could not be contacted in person, although contact details seemed to be up to date, and 5% could not be located at all.

The following analysis has been conducted with the FU18 sample.

The FU18 sample of young adults consists of 49.3% women and 50.7% men. The mean age was 22.6 years (SD = 1.1). The educational level of the parents was slightly higher than in the general population: in our sample, about 60% of parents (Pre) had the highest possible school degree (A-Levels/high school, 12 years completed; Table 1), but there were also about 10% without a school-leaving certificate. At FU18, 79.9% of the young adults had a school-leaving degree with 12 or 13 completed school years (high school level). Moreover, 59.9% had already finished a college degree or were in a study program at college. Thus, in our sample, there is enough variance of persons with the highest and lowest education, but the distribution is slightly different as compared to the general population. Further details on sample characteristics are displayed in Table 2.

There were some differences in sociodemographic data between families who participated in FU18 and those who did not (dropouts): the dropouts were more likely to be single parents ($p = 0.003$), the parents were more likely to have a lower high school diploma ($p < 0.001$), the household income was slightly lower ($p = 0.014$), and the mothers were younger ($p = 0.029$). These differences limit the representativeness compared to the initial sample.

3.2. Which Factors Are Associated with Young Adults School and Professional Performance at Age 22? Results from Correlation and Regression Models

3.2.1. Bivariate Correlative Analysis

All correlations were in the expected directions (see Table 3). The school-leaving degree of the parents showed a comparatively high correlation with the school degree, overall grade, and professional degree of the young adults. Similarly, household income was significantly associated with the young adults' school and professional achievements.

The school and professional degree of the young adults at age 22 and the overall school-leaving grade were also significantly associated with the child's early cognitive capacities and skills (IQ) as well as with the child's mental health problems at preschool age. Children's early self-control was also significantly associated with their later school-leaving and professional degree. In contrast, there were no significant associations with maternal dysfunctional parenting or maternal mental health problems in early childhood. Significant correlations, however, were found for adverse childhood events (ACEs), on the one hand, and bullying, on the other hand: young adults with fewer ACEs and no experiences of bullying in childhood or youth reported higher school and professional degrees.

The results of the bivariate analysis can be summarized as follows: a low socioeconomic family background, low child cognitive capacities and skills (IQ), early child mental health problems, adverse childhood experiences, and bullying experiences correspond with lower school and professional success until the age of 22 years.

3.2.2. Regression Analysis

Concerning school and professional degrees, the lowest qualification status was compared with the highest qualification (e.g., no school-leaving certificate or lower secondary school-leaving certificate compared with 12/13 classes, i.e., high school and A-Levels; Table 4), and the intermediate qualification was compared with the highest qualification (e.g., intermediate school-leaving certificate of 10 classes compared with 12/13 classes, i.e., high school and A-Levels; Table 4).

The results of the multinomial logistic hierarchical regression analysis (school-leaving certificate and professional qualification status) and the multiple linear hierarchical regression analysis (overall school-leaving grade) can be summarized as follows (see Tables 4–6): as expected, the predictive power of the models improves with the number of variables included. The improvements across the five models are particularly evident for school-leaving degree as well as professional degree and less so for the overall school-leaving grade. Improvements in the model fit appear with the inclusion of early childhood characteristics (Model 1 to Model 2) as well as ACEs and bullying (Model 4 to Model 5). The school-leaving degree was slightly better predicted than the professional degree (QL test, Goodness of Fit, Nagelkerke's R2, and correct prediction).

The parents' school-leaving degree proved to be an important predictor, particularly for the prediction of children's school-leaving degree (Tables 4 and 5). In contrast to the bivariate comparison, household income had no significant influence. Early learned skills of children rather than fluid intelligence capacities significantly predicted school grades. Children's sex, early self-control, and early mental health problems as well as early dysfunctional parenting and early mental health problems of the mothers had no significant impact on the young adults' school or professional success.

In the multinomial comparison between the lowest and the highest school degree (Table 4), adverse childhood experiences (ACEs) and bullying were both identified as significant predictors. At the same time, the parents' school-leaving degree was no longer significant. This means that ACEs and bullying experiences were more predictive for the young adults' highest school degree than the parents' school-leaving degree. This effect was no longer found when comparing the middle and highest school-leaving degree (Table 4, lower part).

In the multinomial comparison between the lowest and the highest professional degree Table 5), ACEs, but not bullying, proved to be significant predictors. At the same time, the influence of the parents' school-leaving degree remained significant. This means that both ACEs and the parents' school-leaving degree significantly predicted the young adult's professional degree. This effect was no longer found in the comparison between the middle and highest professional degree (Table 5, lower part).

In the prediction for overall school-leaving grade (Table 6), besides parents' school degree, only children's early learned skills (IQ) appeared to be of additional importance. All other predictors did not make a significant contribution to the prediction model. In addition, young women achieved slightly better grades than young men (small effect-size in models 1 to 4); however, the effect of the young adult's sex was not significant.

Parental participation in the Triple P parenting intervention at child's preschool age had no significant effect on the young adults' professional degree and overall school-leaving grade. Young adults of parents who participated in the Triple P at the beginning of the longitudinal study, however, were a bit more likely to have a high school degree (12/13 classes completed) than a 10 classes school degree (ß = 0.037 **, Table 4).

4. Discussion

4.1. Predictors for School and Professional Performance in Young Adulthood: Findings from the Longitudinal Study

This 18-year longitudinal study aimed to predict school and professional achievement in young adults by using various context, parental, and child characteristics that were collected in childhood. The results from this investigation on children from age 4 to 22 years old and their families support some findings from earlier research but also bring about some unexpected new findings regarding the prediction of children's school and professional success.

It was initially assumed that socioeconomic and family characteristics would have a significant impact on children's school development. The first robust finding of the current investigation is that parents' educational level significantly predicted their children's school and professional success 18 years later. This aligns with U.S. findings showing that parents' educational level when the child was 8 years old significantly predicted the child's educational and occupational success 40 years later [65]. It is widely known that more educated people are generally healthier than lower educated people (e.g., Wang et al. [66]). More educated parents may thus have better resources for educating their children about coping with life problems, knowledge, and health behavior (e.g., nutrition and mobility) and to support them to learn skills and academic contents at school, which form the basis for starting a successful life. In addition, these parents usually place more value on academic education and, therefore, try to create a modern and adaptable academic environment for their children [67].

Besides the parents' educational level, other family variables did not have great impact on children's school and professional achievements until the age of 22 years, i.e., maternal parenting behavior and maternal mental health problems. This may be partly astonishing, since it is well known that mental disorders have a relevant genetic component, and that parental mental health problems significantly predict child mental health (e.g., [68,69]). Mental health problems and school achievements, however, are different things, and apparently children's school achievement can develop positively even if a parent (here: the mother) has some own mental health problems. Socioeconomic background (assessed by household income) turned out to be only partially predictive. Considering the well-known narrow association between a family's socioeconomic background and their children's academic achievements, our finding is partly unexpected. The results illustrate the importance of examining family factors (e.g., parents' educational level, parenting behavior, and parental mental health) and contextual factors (e.g., household income, ACEs, and bullying experiences) in a very differentiated way. Thus, there is hope that not only context and economic aspects determine school and professional success, but that there are degrees of freedom for positive child developments. A starting point, e.g., could be the child's learning history outside the core family. Although the core family is of great importance in young childhood, children's later school performance can also benefit from skills learning in other contexts, such as kindergartens or preschools [70], school environments in urban location with health policies [71], practice-oriented school activities [72], and peer-support [73].

Children's learned skills—thus behavioral and therefore modifiable aspects of intelligence—turned out to be important cognitive capacities in the children themselves which may be helpful on the way to school and professional achievements. In contrast, children's early mental health problems (symptoms severity) did not significantly impact school and professional long-term outcome. This finding demonstrates the importance of distinguishing between behavioral skills and learned capacities (what a person can do and activities), on the one hand, and mental health problems (i.e., symptoms and behavioral problems due to mental disorders), on the other hand. (Recurrent) Mental health *symptoms* cannot be prevented by means of environment and parenting [68,69], because they are chronic due to their (partly biologically determined) nature (e.g., [67,68,74–76]). *Behavioral and participation problems* (which are often byproducts of mental health symptomatology), however, can be reduced by training and skills learning. For example, a person with a chronic affect dysregulation symptomatology can learn to notice when he or she becomes affectively tense and at risk to react impulsively. He or she can learn to leave the situation in good time before the emotional outburst or learn to cool down by using self-regulation skills. However, this will not prevent him or her from recurring affective tension as such. Our findings indicate that learned skills, on the one hand, and mental health symptomatology, on the other hand, differentially impact child development even in a longitudinal study over 18 years. Mental health symptomatology is often chronic, and skills can be learned and enable people to cope with recurring symptoms.

The multinomial comparisons furthermore showed that adverse childhood experiences (ACEs) in particular, but also bullying experiences in adolescence, significantly predicted school and professional success. These findings are consistent with other results that found significant associations for ACEs and bullying experiences with mental health problems [77–79]. However, there are few studies that have investigated the association between ACEs or bullying experiences and school and professional success [79]. In the current investigation, ACEs and bullying experiences were even more important for the prediction of the school-leaving degree than the parents' school education and socioeconomic background. Individual stressful experiences in childhood and adolescence may thus be important for school achievements. Because there is a wide variety of possible stressful events in childhood and youth, in and out of the core family or at school, it can be assumed that there is hardly one common way for how stressful events may impact child's school career. Peer conflicts or family trouble at a young age, in some cases, can lead to problematic family communication, the induction of irritation in the child, and resulting problems with learning and school participation. Preventive activities aiming to support coping with unavoidable stress and conflict management may focus, e.g., on functional parenting behavior and resilience training for children: through targeted support, resilience can be strengthened as early as kindergarten age. This can be realized, e.g., by child-centered support programs [80] or parent training with low-threshold access for families with increased risk exposure. Cognitive-behavioral parent training has already been proven to be effective in this context [36].

Longitudinal studies offer a great opportunity to identify long-term effects. However, the results should be interpreted with caution. Even in longitudinal studies, significant influences can actually be due to other variables, especially if there is a longer period of time between surveys. Another problem lies in the generalizability of the results to the present situation. The first assessment (Pre) was conducted in 2001−2003. More than 20 years have passed since then, raising the question to what extent the living conditions of families with young children and the distribution of children in kindergartens have changed. For example, demographic change has led to an increase in the proportion of children with a migration background, technological change has led to new learning methods, e.g., at school, and new academic programs and professions as well as improved childcare options have emerged over the last 20 years. The independent variables we analyzed, however, are fairly universal, and the assessment methods used are likely to remain reliable and valid over time. It would be highly speculative to assume different processes and mechanisms of influence today; nevertheless, social changes and new challenges call for caution and far-reaching conclusions.

4.2. Implications for Research

Our aim was to analyze which variables best predict school and professional success, i.e., to find the 'best' predictors. Future studies should conduct mediator analyses to examine how parental background affects child factors (e.g., intelligence and mental health) and how this in turn affects school and professional success.

As the study sample is not representative, particularly with regard to socioeconomic status, and the variance is therefore lower than in a representative sample, it can be assumed that the results would certainly be more significant in a representative sample. This would, of course, have to be verified in samples with a larger number of children with a low socioeconomic background.

In addition to maternal variables, future studies should also consider variables from fathers or other caregivers to provide a complete picture of family influences on child school and professional success.

4.3. Strengths and Limitations

We analyzed data of a longitudinal study that repeatedly and prospectively assessed family, parental, and individual characteristics of children over 18 years from early childhood to young adulthood. The high retention rate of 80% even after 18 years is a major strength of the present investigation. One reason for the high response rate is the maintenance of intensive contact with the participating families over the whole study period, i.e., reporting results to the families and in the local media, and regular contact with the families, e.g., in terms of Christmas greetings and informational letters. The families furthermore obtained some financial compensation for their effort to participate in the interviews. A lot of families were interested in the longitudinal research themselves, many of them were higher educated and thus may have a sense for the importance of continuing their participation in a longitudinal study. Until FU10, the interviews were conducted in person which may also increase commitment for continued participation. Finally, the families were recruited in the city of research, which may foster the perception of being part of a common project. School success was not only operationalized by the young adults' school-leaving degree but also by the overall school-leaving grade, and we also considered the current professional degree at age 22 years as another outcome variable for educational success.

Limitations of this study are a rather small sample size of families with a low socioeconomic background (low household income and low highest school-leaving qualification of parents) and a small sample size of families with a migration background; therefore, the representativeness of the current sample is somewhat limited. Furthermore, almost 80% of the young adults had reached a high school degree (12/13 school years completed), and almost 60% had already completed a college degree or were in college. This high level of education may somewhat limit the significance of the results, because obviously less well-educated young adults are underrepresented in the sample, too.

Another limitation is that about half of the families participated in a parent training after the baseline assessment. However, since 18 years have passed, there are multiple other developmental impact factors, which were broadly included in the prediction models; moreover, participation in the parent training was also included in the analysis to control for potential intervention effects.

5. Conclusions

Parents' educational level explains a large part of variance in children's school and professional success. There are, however, some other aspects of interest: skills and competency aspects may be more predictive for young adults' school and professional success than early life economic and health conditions of parents and children. This is good news as it supports the idea that health deficits can be partly compensated for by learning and skills training. For children's development and educational achievements, the findings imply that education, preventive interventions, and treatment should also focus on strengthening behavioral skills rather than just focusing on reducing or even fully erasing mental health symptoms.

Aside from the implications already mentioned, the present results confirm that children from families with low-educated parents in particular deserve special support. It might furthermore be useful to conduct performance tests with all children at an early age to assess their early learned skills. This would allow children with special needs to be identified at an early stage and supported with indicated prevention measures.

As adverse childhood experiences and bullying experiences in childhood and youth may also have a negative impact, but are not always avoidable, preventive interventions should also address coping and resilience and thus support child development with regard to positive school and career achievements.

Author Contributions: Conceptualization, B.M. and W.S.; methodology, W.S.; software, W.S.; validation, B.M. and A.-K.J.; formal analysis, W.S.; investigation, A.-K.J.; resources, B.M.; data curation, W.S.; writing—original draft preparation, B.M.; writing—review and editing, W.S., A.-K.J. and B.M.; funding acquisition, W.S. and A.-K.J. All authors have read and agreed to the published version of the manuscript.

Funding: This study was carried out within the framework of the German Research Foundation project (DFG; HA 1400/14-1, 2, 3/17-1, 2, JO 1632/1-1).

Institutional Review Board Statement: The Human Subjects Protection Board of the German Association of Psychology and the ethic committee of the Faculty of Life Sciences of the Technische Universität Braunschweig approved all procedures (DGPs; FF-III identification number: WS 12_2010, 20 January 2011; FF-IV identification number: D-2019-01; 11 February 2019, Faculty of Life Sciences). Informed written consent was obtained from all individual participants included in this study. All methods were performed in accordance with the relevant BioMed Central guidelines and regulations.

Informed Consent Statement: Informed consent was obtained from all subjects included in this study.

Data Availability Statement: The datasets generated and/or analyzed during the current study are not publicly available as they contain sensitive material. Furthermore, it is a longitudinal study with several assessment points, so that the data could possibly be used to draw conclusions about individuals. The questionnaires used can be found in the corresponding references.

Acknowledgments: We thank all the families for their continuous participation over 18 years and M.W. for his pilot work.

Conflicts of Interest: The authors declare no conflicts of interest.

References

1. Mähler, C.; Cloos, P.; Koch, K. Forschung zur Entwicklung und Förderung in der frühen Kindheit. In *Entwicklung und Förderung in der Frühen Kindheit*; Mähler, C., Cloos, P., Koch, K., Eds.; Beltz Juventa: Bad Langensalza, Germany, 2015; pp. 13–24. Available online: https://download.e-bookshelf.de/download/0003/5344/32/L-G-0003534432-0006898040.pdf (accessed on 13 March 2025).
2. Mähler, C.; Piekny, J.; von Goldammer, A.; Balke-Melcher, C.; Schuchardt, K.; Grube, D. Kognitive Kompetenzen als Prädiktoren im Grundschulalter. In *Entwicklung und Förderung in der Frühen Kindheit*; Cloos, P., Koch, K., Mähler, C., Eds.; Beltz Juventa: Bad Langensalza, Germany, 2015; pp. 60–77.
3. Neuenschwander, M.P. *Schule und Familie: Was sie zum Schulerfolg Beitragen*; Haupt: Bern, Switzerland, 2005. Available online: https://www.researchgate.net/profile/Markus-Neuenschwander/publication/304704676_Schule_und_Familie_-_Was_sie_zum_Schulerfolg_beitragen/links/5e42e60992851c7f7f2f8cb7/Schule-und-Familie-Was-sie-zum-Schulerfolg-beitragen.pdf (accessed on 13 March 2025).

4. Vollmar, M.; Klaukien, A. *Berufsbildung auf Einen Blick*; Statistisches Bundesamt: Wiesbaden, Germany, 2013. Available online: https://www.statistischebibliothek.de/mir/servlets/MCRFileNodeServlet/DEMonografie_derivate_00001580/BerufsbildungBlick0110019129004[1].pdf (accessed on 13 March 2025).
5. Roos, J.; Schöler, H. (Eds.) *Entwicklung des Schriftspracherwerbs in der Grundschule*; Verlag für Sozialwissenschaften: Wiesbaden, Germany, 2009.
6. O'Connor, E.E.; Cappella, E.; McCormick, M.P.; McClowry, S. An examination of the efficacy of INSIGHTS in enhancing the academic and behavioral development of children in early grades. *J. Educ. Psychol.* **2014**, *106*, 1156–1169. [CrossRef]
7. Sauer, J.; Gamsjäger, E. *Ist Schulerfolg Vorhersagbar?* Hogrefe: Göttingen, Germany, 1996.
8. Jerusalem, M. Schulklasseneffekte. In *Enzyklopädie der Psychologie, Themenbereich D Praxisgebiete, Serie I Pädagogische Psychologie, Bd. 3 Psychologie des Unterrichts und der Schule*; Weinert, F.E., Ed.; Hogrefe: Göttingen, Germany, 1997; pp. 253–278.
9. Heller, K.A. Individuelle Bedingungsfaktoren der Schulleistung—Literaturüberblick. In *Entwicklung im Grundschulalter*; Weinert, F.E., Helmke, A., Eds.; Beltz: Weinheim, Germany, 1997; pp. 183–201.
10. Maaz, K.; Neumann, M.; Baumert, J. (Eds.) *Herkunft und Bildungserfolg von der Frühen Kindheit bis ins Erwachsenenalter: Forschungsstand und Interventionsmöglichkeiten aus Interdisziplinärer Perspektive*; Springer VS: Wiesbaden, Germany, 2014.
11. OECD. *Education at a Glance 2021: OECD Indicators*; OECD Publishing: Paris, France, 2021. [CrossRef]
12. Ansari, A.; Pianta, R.C. Variation in the long-term benefits of child care: The role of classroom quality in elementary school. *Dev. Psychol.* **2018**, *54*, 1854–1867. [CrossRef] [PubMed]
13. Lövdén, M.; Fratiglioni, L.; Glymour, M.M.; Lindenberger, U.; Tucker-Drob, E.M. Education and Cognitive Functioning Across the Life Span. *Psychol. Sci. Public Interest* **2020**, *21*, 6–41. [CrossRef] [PubMed]
14. Park, S.K.; Philips, J.; Pavuluri, N. Systematic Review of Predictors of Success for the North American Pharmacist Licensure Examination. *Am. J. Pharm. Educ.* **2021**, *85*, 8591. [CrossRef]
15. Madigan, S.; Prime, H.; Graham, S.A.; Rodrigues, M.; Anderson, N.; Khoury, J.; Jenkins, J.M. Parenting Behavior and Child Language: A Meta-analysis. *Pediatrics* **2019**, *144*, e20183556. [CrossRef]
16. Schwippert, K.; Kasper, D.; Köller, O.; McElvany, N.; Selter, C.; Steffensky, M.; Wendt, H. (Eds.) *TIMSS 2019. Mathematische und Naturwissenschaftliche Kompetenzen von Grundschulkindern in Deutschland im Internationalen Vergleich*; Waxmann: Münster, Germany, 2020. [CrossRef]
17. Schneider, W. (Ed.) *Entwicklung von der Kindheit bis zum Erwachsenenalter: Befunde der Münchner Längsschnittstudie LOGIK*; Beltz PVU: Weinheim, Germany, 2008.
18. Bradley, R.H.; Corwyn, R.F. Socioeconomic status and child development. *Annu. Rev. Psychol.* **2002**, *53*, 371–399. [CrossRef]
19. Davis-Kean, P.E. The influence of parent education and family income on child achievement: The indirect role of parental expectations and the home environment. *J. Fam. Psychol.* **2005**, *19*, 294–304. [CrossRef]
20. Early, E.; Miler, S.; Dunne, L.; Thurston, A.; Filiz, M. The influence of socio-economic background and gender on school attainment in the United Kingdom: A systematic review. *Rev. Educ.* **2020**, *8*, 120–152. [CrossRef]
21. Halle, T.G.; Kurtz-Costes, B.; Mahoney, J.L.; Clarke, A.; Fletcher, A.; Hearne, S.; Parker, B. Family Influences on School Achievement in Low-Income, African American Children. *J. Educ. Psychol.* **1997**, *89*, 527–537. [CrossRef]
22. Schlemmer, E. *Familienbiografien und Schulkarrieren von Kindern: Theorie und Empirie*; VS Verlag für Sozialwissenschaften: Wiesbaden, Germany, 2004.
23. Schmitt, M. *Soziale Beziehungen und Schulerfolg: Die Bedeutung Sozialer Beziehungen für Schulerfolg im Primar- und Sekundarbereich*; University of Bamberg Press: Bamberg, Germany, 2012.
24. Schneider, T. Der Einfluss des Einkommens der Eltern auf die Schulwahl. *Z. Soziol.* **2004**, *33*, 471–492. [CrossRef]
25. Vukojevic, M.; Zovko, A.; Talic, I.; Tanovic, M.; Resic, B.; Vrdoljak, I.; Splavski, B. Parental Socioeconomic Status as a Predictor of Physical and Mental Health Outcomes in Children—Literature Review. *Acta Clin. Croat.* **2017**, *56*, 742–748. [CrossRef]
26. Horner, R.H.; Sugai, G.; Anderson, C.M. Examining the evidence base for schoolwide positive behavior support. *Focus Except. Child.* **2010**, *42*, 1–14. [CrossRef]
27. Janius, N.; Bin Amdan, M.A.; Bin Kasdiah, M.A.H.; Harifin, N.I.B.; Bhari, F.A.N.B.S. Safety practices and injury prevention strategies in recreational facilities catering (RFC) for children. *Int. J. Sci. Res. Arch.* **2024**, *12*, 2182–2192. [CrossRef]
28. Tsela, D.; Tsela, R.D.; López, I.G. Relations between Parenting Style and Parenting Practices and Children's School Achievement. *Soc. Sci.* **2023**, *12*, 5. [CrossRef]
29. Woodcock, R.W.; Bonner, M. *Woodcock-Johnson III Tests of Achievement–Revised*; Riverside: Itasca, IL, USA, 1989.
30. Brennan, L.M.; Shaw, D.S.; Dishion, T.J.; Wilson, M.N. Longitudinal Predictors of School-Age Academic Achievement: Unique Contributions of Toddler-Age Aggression, Oppositionality, Inattention, and Hyperactivity. *J. Abnorm. Child Psychol.* **2012**, *40*, 1289–1300. [CrossRef]

31. Dougherty, L.R.; Tolep, M.R.; Smith, V.C.; Rose, S. Early Exposure to Parental Depression and Parenting: Associations with Young Offspring's Stress Physiology and Oppositional Behavior. *J. Abnorm. Child Psychol.* **2013**, *41*, 1299–1310. [CrossRef]
32. Brophy, S.; Todd, C.; Rahman, M.A.; Kennedy, N.; Rice, F. Timing of parental depression on risk of child depression and poor educational outcomes: A population based routine data cohort study from Born in Wales, UK. *PLoS ONE* **2021**, *16*, e0258966. [CrossRef]
33. Ranning, A.; Laursen, T.; Agerbo, E.; Thorup, A.; Hjorthøj, C.; Jepsen, J.R.M.; Nordentoft, M. School performance from primary education in the adolescent offspring of parents with schizophrenia and bipolar disorder- a national, register-based study. *Psychol. Med.* **2018**, *48*, 1993–2000. [CrossRef]
34. Weissman, M.M.; Wickramaratne, P.; Nomura, Y.; Warner, V.; Pilowsky, D.; Verdeli, H. Offspring of Depressed Parents: 20 Years Later. *Am. J. Psychiatry* **2006**, *163*, 1001–1008. [CrossRef]
35. Wright, C.A.; George, T.P.; Burke, R.; Gelfand, D.M.; Teti, D.M. Early Maternal Depression and Children's Adjustment to School. *Child Study J.* **2000**, *30*, 153–169.
36. Sanders, M.R.; Kirby, J.N.; Tellegen, C.L.; Day, J.J. The Triple P-Positive Parenting Program: A systematic review and meta-analysis of a multi-level system of parenting support. *Clin. Psychol. Rev.* **2014**, *34*, 337–357. [CrossRef] [PubMed]
37. Sanders, M.R. Development, evaluation, and multinational dissemination of the Triple P Positive Parenting Program. *Annu. Rev. Clin. Psychol.* **2012**, *8*, 345–379. [CrossRef] [PubMed]
38. Driessen, G.; van Langen, A. Gender differences in primary and secondary education: Are girls really outperforming boys? *Int. Rev. Educ.* **2013**, *59*, 67–86. [CrossRef]
39. Eurydice. *Gender Differences in Educational Outcomes*; European Commission: Brussels, Belgium, 2010.
40. Deary, I.J.; Strand, S.; Smith, P.; Fernandes, C. Intelligence and educational achievement. *Intelligence* **2007**, *35*, 13–21. [CrossRef]
41. Gut, J.; Reimann, G.; Grob, A. Kognitive, sprachliche, mathematische und sozialemotionale Kompetenzen als Prädiktoren späterer schulischer Leistungen. *Z. Pädagog. Psychol.* **2012**, *26*, 213–220. [CrossRef]
42. Melchers, P.; Preuß, U. *Kaufman-Assessment Battery for Children. German Version K-ABC*, 6th ed.; PITS: Frankfurt, Germany, 2001.
43. Frick, P.J.; Kamphaus, R.W.; Lahey, B.B.; Loeber, R.; Christ, M.A.; Hart, E.L.; Tannenbaum, L.E. Academic Underachievement and the Disruptive Behavior Disorders. *J. Consult. Clin. Psychol.* **1991**, *59*, 289–294. [CrossRef]
44. Malinauskiene, O.; Vosylis, R.; Zukauskiene, R. Longitudinal Examination of Relationships between Problem Behaviors and Academic Achievement in Young Adolescents. *Procedia Soc. Behav. Sci.* **2011**, *15*, 3415–3421. [CrossRef]
45. Plück, J.; Beiling, M.; Hautmann, C.; Kuschel, A.; Heinrichs, N.; Schmeck, K.; Döpfner, M. Die Erfassung von Verhaltensauffälligkeiten im Vorschulalter mit dem Elternfragebogen für Klein- und Vorschulkinder (CBCL 1 ½ -5). *Diagnostica* **2013**, *59*, 155–166. [CrossRef]
46. Robson, D.A.; Allen, M.S.; Howard, S.J. Self-regulation in childhood as a Predictor of future outcomes: A meta-analytic review. *Psychol. Bull.* **2020**, *146*, 324–354. [CrossRef]
47. Voltas, N.; Hernández-Martínez, C.; Aparicio, E.; Arija, V.; Canals, J. Psychopathological factors that can influence academic achievement in early adolescence: A three-year prospective study. *Span. J. Psychol.* **2014**, *17*, e100. [CrossRef]
48. Hasselhorn, M.; Schneider, W. Trends und Desiderate der Frühprognose schulischer Kompetenzen: Eine Einführung. In *Frühprognose Schulischer Kompetenzen*; Hasselhorn, M., Schneider, W., Eds.; Hogrefe: Göttingen, Germany, 2011; pp. 1–12.
49. Friedman-Weieneth, J.L.; Harvey, E.A.; Youngwirth, S.D.; Goldstein, L.H. The relation between 3-year-old children's skills and their hyperactivity, inattention, and aggression. *J. Educ. Psychol.* **2007**, *99*, 671–681. [CrossRef]
50. Brennan, L.M.; Shelleby, E.C.; Shaw, D.S.; Gardner, F.; Dishion, T.J.; Wilson, M.N. Indirect effects of the Family Check-Up on school-age academic achievement through improvements in parenting in early childhood. *J. Educ. Psychol.* **2013**, *105*, 762. [CrossRef] [PubMed]
51. McKelvey, L.M.; Edge, N.C.; Mesman, G.R.; Whiteside-Mansell, L.; Bradley, R.H. Adverse experiences in infancy and toddlerhood: Relations to adaptive behavior and academic status in middle childhood. *Child Abuse Negl.* **2018**, *82*, 168–177. [CrossRef] [PubMed]
52. Abregú-Crespo, R.; Garriz-Luis, A.; Ayora, M.; Martín-Martínez, N.; Cavone, V.; Carrasco, M.Á.; Fraguas, D.; Martín-Babarro, J.; Arango, C.; Díaz-Caneja, C.M. School bullying in children and adolescents with neurodevelopmental and psychiatric conditions: A systematic review and meta-analysis. *Lancet Child Adolesc. Health* **2023**, *15*, 122–134. [CrossRef]
53. Brendgen, M.; Poulin, F. Continued Bullying Victimization from Childhood to Young Adulthood: A Longitudinal Study of Mediating and Protective Factors. *J. Abnorm. Child Psychol.* **2018**, *46*, 27–39. [CrossRef]
54. Köller, O.; Hasselhorn, M.; Hesse, F.W.; Maaz, K.; Schrader, J.; Solga, H.; Spieß, C.K.; Zimmer, K. *Das Bildungswesen in Deutschland. Bestand und Potenziale*; Julius Klinkhardt: Bad Heilbrunn, Germany, 2019.

55. Hahlweg, K.; Schulz, W. Universelle Prävention kindlicher Verhaltensstörungen durch Elterntrainings. *Z. Klin. Psychol. Psychother.* **2018**, *47*, 1–15. [CrossRef]
56. Bertram, H.; Heinrichs, N.; Kuschel, A.; Kessemeier, Y.; Saßmann, H.; Hahlweg, K. Projekt "Zukunft Familie". Erste Ergebnisse der Rekrutierung. *Verhaltensther. Verhaltensmed.* **2003**, *2*, 187–204.
57. Nickel, A.-K. Die Skala kindlicher Selbstkontrolle (SKS). Entwicklung und Evaluation einer Skala zur Erfassung Kindlicher Selbstkontrolle im Rahmen des Projekts Zukunft Familie. Unpublished Bachelor Thesis, Technische Universität Braunschweig, Braunschweig, Germany, 2012.
58. Plück, J.; Scholz, K.-K.; Döpfner, M. Für die Arbeitsgruppe Deutsche Child Child Behavior Checklist. In *CBCL/1½ -5, C-TRF/1½ -5: Deutsche Kleinkind- und Vorschulalter-Formen der Child Behavior Checklist von Thomas M. Achenbach und Leslie A. Rescorla*; Hogrefe: Göttingen, Germany, 2022.
59. Naumann, S.; Bertram, H.; Kuschel, A.; Heinrichs, N.; Hahlweg, K.; Döpfner, M. Der Erziehungsfragebogen (EFB). Ein Fragebogen zur Erfassung elterlicher Verhaltenstendenzen in schwierigen Erziehungssituationen. *Diagnostica* **2010**, *56*, 144–157. [CrossRef]
60. Köppe, E. Glückliche Eltern, Liebe Kinder: Auswirkungen von Partnerschaft und Psychischer Symptomatik der Eltern auf das Verhalten ihrer Kinder. Unpublished Doctoral Thesis, Technische Universität Braunschweig, Braunschweig, Germany, 2001.
61. Lösel, F.; Averbeck, M.; Bliesener, T. Gewalt zwischen Schülern der Sekundarstufe: Eine Untersuchung zur Prävalenz und Beziehung zu allgemeiner Aggressivität und Delinquenz. *Empir. Pädagog.* **1997**, *11*, 327–349.
62. Wingenfeld, K.; Schäfer, I.; Terfehr, K.; Grabski, H.; Driessen, M.; Grabe, H.; Löwe, B.; Spitzer, C. The reliable, valid, and economic assessment of early traumatization: First psychometric characteristics of the German version of the Adverse Childhood Experiences Questionnaire (ACE). *Psychother. Psychosom. Med. Psychol.* **2011**, *61*, e10–e14. [CrossRef]
63. Cohen, J. *Statistical Power Analysis for the Behavioral Sciences*, 2nd ed.; Erlbaum: Hillsdale, NJ, USA, 1988.
64. Field, A. *Discovering Statistics Using IBM SPSS Statistics*, 5th ed.; Sage: London, UK, 2018.
65. Dubow, E.; Boxer, P.; Huesmann, L.R. Long-term Effects of Parents' Education on Children's Educational and Occupational Success: Mediation by Family Interactions, Child Aggression, and Teenage Aspirations. *Merrill-Palmer Q.* **2009**, *55*, 224–249. [CrossRef] [PubMed]
66. Wang, T.; Li, Y.; Zheng, X. Association of socioeconomic status with cardiovascular disease and cardiovascular risk factors: A systematic review and meta-analysis. *J. Public Health* **2023**, *21*, 385–399. [CrossRef] [PubMed]
67. Hanafi, Z. The relationship between aspects of socio-economic factors and academic achievement. Aspects of Socio-Economic Factors. *J. Pendidik.* **2008**, *33*, 95–105.
68. Lynch, S.J.; Sunderland, M.; Newton, N.C.; Chapman, C. A systematic review of transdiagnostic risk and protective factors for general and specific psychopathology in young people. *Clin. Psychol. Rev.* **2021**, *87*, 102036. [CrossRef]
69. Schulz, W.; Muschalla, B. What Predicts internal and external mental disorders in adolescent boys and girls? Results from a 10-year longitudinal study. *Eur. J. Dev. Psychol.* **2021**, *19*, 234–250. [CrossRef]
70. Zhu, Y.T.; Li, X.; Jiao, D.D.; Tanaka, E.; Tomisaki, E.; Watanabe, T.; Sawada, Y.; Zhu, Z.; Ajmal, A.; Matsumoto, A.; et al. Development of Social Skills in Kindergarten: A Latent Class Growth Modeling Approach. *Children* **2021**, *8*, 870. [CrossRef]
71. Sellström, E.; Bremberg, S. Is there a "school effect" on pupil outcomes? A review of multilevel studies. *J. Epidemiol. Community Health* **2006**, *60*, 149–155. [CrossRef]
72. Berezowitz, C.K.; Bontrager, A.B.; Schoeller, D.A. School Gardens Enhance Academic Performance and Dietary Outcomes in Children. *J. Sch. Health* **2015**, *85*, 508–518. [CrossRef]
73. Butler, N.; Quigg, Z.; Bates, R.; Jones, L.; Ashworth, E.; Growland, S.; Jones, M. The Contributing Role of Family, School, and Peer Supportive Relationships in Protecting the Mental Wellbeing of Children and Adolescents. *Sch. Ment. Health* **2022**, *14*, 776–788. [CrossRef]
74. Stansfeld, S.A.; Clark, C.; Caldwell, T.; Canner, R.; North, F.; Marmot, M. Psychosocial characteristics and anxiety and depressive disorders in midlife: The effect of prior psychological distress. *Occup. Environ. Med.* **2008**, *65*, 634–642. [CrossRef]
75. Linden, M.; Deck, R.; Muschalla, B. Rate and spectrum of participation impairment in patients with chronic mental disorders: Comparison of self- and expert ratings. *Contemp. Behav. Health Care* **2018**, *3*, 1–5. [CrossRef]
76. Caspi, A.; Moffitt, T.E.; Newman, D.L.; Silva, P.A. Behavioral observations at age 3 years predict adult psychiatric disorders. Longitudinal evidence from a birth cohort. *Arch. Gen. Psychiatry* **1996**, *53*, 1033–1039. [CrossRef] [PubMed]
77. Hughes, K.; Bellis, M.A.; Hardcastle, K.A.; Sethi, D.; Butchart, A.; Mikton, C.; Jones, L.; Dunne, M.P. The effect of multiple adverse childhood experience on health: A systematic review and meta-analysis. *Lancet Public Health* **2017**, *2*, e356–e366. [CrossRef] [PubMed]
78. Moore, S.E.; Norman, R.E.; Suetani, S.; Thomas, H.J.; Sly, P.D.; Scott, J.G. Consequences of bullying victimization in childhood and adolescence: A systematic review and meta-analysis. *World J. Psychiatry* **2017**, *7*, 60–76. [CrossRef]

79. Tyrone, R.S.; Fletcher, L.M.; Walker, C.S.; Compretta, C.; Burns, P.; Reneker, J.C. Adverse Childhood Experiences and Academic Performance Among U.S. Students: A Systematic Review and Meta-Analysis. *J. Educ.* **2023**, *204*, 748–773. [CrossRef]
80. Fröhlich-Gildhoff, K.; Dörner, T.; Rönnau-Böse, M. *Prävention und Resilienzförderung in Kindertageseinrichtungen—PriK*; Ernst Reinhardt Verlag: München, Germany, 2019.

children

MDPI

Article

Promoting Peer Interaction and Acceptance Among Students with Special Needs Through an Experiential Learning Program

Hsiu-Ming Lin [1], Szu-Yin Chu [1,*], Wen-Hsuan Chang [2], I-Hsuan Lo [1] and Hsin-Ting Peng [1]

[1] Department of Special Education, National Tsing Hua University, Hsinchu 300044, Taiwan; emely21481@tmail.hc.edu.tw (H.-M.L.); lihsuan20058@gapp.nthu.edu.tw (I.-H.L.); saskia12tw@gapp.nthu.edu.tw (H.-T.P.)

[2] Department of Educational Psychology, Texas A& M University, College Station, TX 77840, USA; wenhsuan.chang@tamu.edu

* Correspondence: chusy@mx.nthu.edu.tw

Abstract: Background/Objectives: Inclusive education emphasizes positive interactions between students with and without special needs to foster mutual understanding and acceptance. This study explored the effect of an experiential learning program (ExL Prog) on interaction and acceptance between students with and without special needs. Based on Kolb's ExL theory, this study explores how the ExL Prog fosters experiential learning, reflection, and mutual growth through activities that enhance interpersonal skills, promote empathy, and create an inclusive classroom environment where students with and without special needs deepen their understanding and acceptance of one another. Methods: The study used a mixed-methods approach with 2 students with special needs and 16 students without special needs from the same sixth-grade class. Researchers divided participants into two groups: one intervention group that underwent the 8-activity ExL Prog and one comparison group that participated in regular activities. Data collection methods included questionnaires, interviews, and feedback forms, which enabled qualitative and quantitative analysis. Results: The results indicated the implementation of the ExL Prog facilitated increased opportunities for positive interactions between students with and without special needs. Regarding attitudes of acceptance toward students with special needs, students without special needs in the EXL group demonstrated lower scores than those in the control group in the cognitive dimension, higher scores in the affective dimension, and no significant difference in the behavioral dimension. The program fostered mutual listening, respect, and understanding, particularly among the intervention group, which promoted empathy and supportive relationships among participants. Conclusions: The students in the ExL Program developed a greater understanding of others and reflected on improving their relationship-building approaches. This transformation fostered increased openness, goodwill, and mutual reciprocity, promoting growth in interpersonal relationships and communication skills.

Keywords: experiential learning; peer interaction; acceptance; students with special needs

1. Introduction

Interpersonal interaction is crucial for developing social skills, communication abilities, understanding of others, peer emotional connections, and acceptance of peers with different traits among school-age children [1–3]. The current trend in inclusive education policies is the integration of students with special needs into general education classrooms alongside students without special needs. This practice aims to achieve educational equity and

https://doi.org/10.3390/children12050543

foster broad understanding and interaction between students with special needs and their peers. They promote shared learning, raise awareness of the difficulties of others, enhance understanding of different perspectives, and increase empathy, all contributing to a positive cycle of interpersonal interaction for both parties [4–6]. However, integrating students with special needs into general education classrooms often presents challenges in peer interaction and acceptance [6,7]. Even when provided with opportunities for peer relationships, students with special needs may encounter obstacles such as negative experiences and biases related to their disability categories or severity of their disability [8,9]. Therefore, during this integrating process, addressing the negative experiences and biases and identifying positive interpersonal relationships that mutually benefit students with special needs and students without special needs is essential.

Drawing on empirical research and theories of interpersonal development, scholars advocate for experiential learning (ExL) as a potent approach for mitigating negative peer interactions and promoting acceptance [10]. This study is based on Kolb's [11] ExL theory, where learners engage in experiential activities to gain experiences, then reflect on their feelings and actions from those experiences to generate new ideas. ExL refers to generating reflections through experiences while integrating students' prior knowledge, enabling them to become active participants in life [12]. ExL promotes direct engagement in activities, empowering individuals to cultivate crucial interpersonal skills through hands-on experiences. Through the ExL program (ExL Prog), individuals reflect on their interactions with others, prompting synthesis and reinterpretation of these experiences. This process enables them to develop interpersonal sensitivity, nurture empathy, and forge deeper, more meaningful connections with others [11,13–15]. In the ExL Prog, students with special needs and their peers jointly engage in activities [16]. It promotes mutual growth and creates an inclusive classroom environment in which all students feel accepted and valued. Consequently, it nurtures richer interpersonal connections, encourages positive interactions, and deepens understanding and acceptance between students without special needs and those with special needs.

1.1. Peer Interaction and Acceptance

Experiences of recognition and acceptance by peers are vital for both students with and without special needs. A harmonious social integration network fosters a positive peer atmosphere, broadens individual interpersonal resources, and supports the development of mature interpersonal skills and a strong social self-concept [17,18]. Positive peer interaction involves establishing confident and constructive relationships that enrich interpersonal experiences and promote harmony [3]. Inclusive education aims to create a mutually supportive community between students without special needs and those with special needs [5], which benefits the psychological well-being and social development of both groups, breaks down barriers, and promotes mutual growth.

Peer acceptance is a type of attitude that varies in the degree to which someone accepts individual differences among their peers, including different behaviors, traits, and backgrounds. In interpersonal interactions, everyone holds certain attitudes and standards towards other members of their peer group. Students with special needs, characterized by unique behavioral expressions or cognitive–emotional traits [7,19,20] may face challenges in forming stable friendships [21] and may experience peer rejection or social isolation in inclusive education settings [22–24].

In brief, positive interactions and acceptance, exemplified by experiential and friendly engagement, are crucial for nurturing mutual peer relationships between students without special needs and those with special needs. Favorable peer relationships aid in resolving interpersonal problems along with empathy and sharing values. In inclusive education settings, interpersonal issues often arise from a lack of understanding. Therefore, ExL Progs are designed to help individuals understand the significance of teamwork and enhance their comprehension of others. These activities also encourage individuals to embrace everyone's uniqueness with an open mind [25–27]. This, in turn, enables them to engage actively and effectively in various social and interpersonal settings, contributing positively to their connections and affairs.

1.2. Theoretical Foundations of ExL Cycle

The core philosophy of ExL, 'learning by doing', posits that transforming life experiences through active engagement is key to successful learning [14,28,29]. The ExL theory introduces a cycle (the ExL cycle; Figure 1) that comprises four phases of experience and understanding, starting as individuals participate in activities, thus generating 'concrete experiences (referred to as experiencing)'. They then observe and reflect on the activity process, a phase known as reflective observation (referred to as reflecting). Next, individuals deepen their understanding or reconstruct what they have learned, a phase known as abstract conceptualization (applying). Finally, they apply insights from these experiences to practical situations and adjust their behavior for greater adaptability in a phase known as active experimentation (referred to as generalizing; [11,13–15]). The ExL theory asserts that this cycle is a dynamic progression, where individuals continuously advance through these four phases in a spiral manner, thereby gaining a more comprehensive understanding of their experiences and enhancing their ability to apply what they have learned practically.

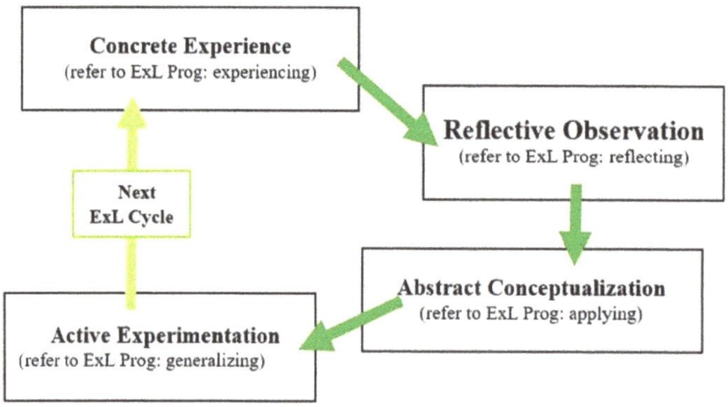

Figure 1. ExL Prog experiential learning cycle.

Some scholars suggest that applying the ExL framework to interpersonal interaction programs (referred to as the ExL Prog in this study) in inclusive settings can yield a wide range of profound collaborative experiences [4,5]. By reflecting on interpersonal feelings and behaviors and adopting new interaction patterns during the ExL cycle, individuals enhance their interpersonal skills [14,30]. Essentially, ExL Progs, through structured activities, enrich the self-awareness, empathy, and cooperation of individuals. Individuals can establish more adaptive and open-minded interpersonal interaction patterns.

1.3. The ExL Prog to Boost Peer Interaction and Acceptance

Relevant studies explore the ExL approach as a comprehensive framework for intergroup contact, aimed at comprehending the learning process and developing skills through reflection and action [14,15]. ExL Prog focus on understanding and applying the effects of interactions and collaborative activities [17,31], prioritizing reflection on real-life interpersonal interactions to enhance social skills through various hands-on experiences [15,29]. Furthermore, educational and developmental researchers apply the ExL Prog in inclusive settings to enhance educational outcomes. These intervention activities encompass peer tutoring and acceptance programs [32,33], social relationship maps and peer network interventions [17], and picture book teaching [34,35], each contributing to enhanced interpersonal interactions and acceptance. They discovered that implementing an ExL Prog through collaborative activities in inclusive settings benefits both students with special needs and their peers.

Accordingly, the ExL Prog promotes initial steps in peer interpersonal interactions in inclusive environments, demonstrating that such programs and related activities effectively initiate interactions between students without special needs and those with special needs. The ExL Prog also contributes to the subsequent co-occurrence of positive interaction and acceptance by gaining insight from reflection or applying these understandings to improve the quality of relationships between both groups [6,16,36]. Overall, the ExL Prog highlights how individuals can shape their perceptions of those with disabilities. Both parties learn from interacting with each other and become more understanding and accepting.

While the studies above demonstrate the effectiveness of the ExL Prog in inclusive settings for students with and without special needs, research on the application of the ExL Prog concerning peer interaction and acceptance is scarce, particularly among senior-grade elementary school students [17,31]. Considering that children actively reflect on interpersonal interactions, they often form a second- or third-person perspective [37,38]. This study investigated the effectiveness of the ExL Prog in promoting interaction relationships and acceptance attitudes in an inclusive environment for senior-grade elementary school students. The study anticipates that the ExL Prog will encourage understanding among students without special needs towards their peers with special needs and foster mutual assistance and acceptance during activities. It also expects the program to boost overall positive experiences of compassion and friendship relationships in both directions.

The study's research questions were as follows: (1) What changes in 'interaction relationships' and 'acceptance attitudes' between students without special needs and students with special needs result from the ExL Prog (quantitative analysis)? (2) What are the experiences of students without special needs and students with special needs during the ExL Prog (qualitative analysis)? (3) After the ExL Prog, what are the experiences of students without special needs regarding 'interaction relationships' and 'acceptance attitudes' towards students with special needs (qualitative analysis)? (4) What are the feelings and thoughts of the classroom teachers of the participating students regarding the intervention's effects after the ExL Prog (qualitative analysis)? The study investigated the practical effects of the ExL Prog on peer interaction and acceptance among students, as well as the evaluations of participating students and teachers regarding this intervention method.

2. Method

2.1. Study Design

To address the four research questions outlined above, we employed a mixed-methods approach that combined surveys and interviews with both quantitative and qualitative analyses. Quantitative data were derived from two questionnaires, and qualitative analysis was gleaned from feedback and interviews.

2.2. Procedures

We employed a quasi-experimental design without randomization research and divided students into two groups: an intervention group and a comparison group during the COVID-19 period. Each group comprised eight students without special needs and one student with special needs. The intervention group participated in the ExL Prog, whereas the comparison group continued with their regular activities. Quantitative data were collected through a questionnaire administered four weeks after the experiential activity intervention, and students' responses were analyzed based on their scores. Qualitative data were collected through interviews conducted after the intervention. Furthermore, the qualitative data from the interviews were compared with the quantitative data gathered from the completed questionnaires.

2.3. Participants and the Setting

In total, 18 sixth-grade elementary school students aged 11–12 years in Taiwan were recruited, including 2 students with special needs (Table 1). The students with special needs (1) were enrolled in an inclusive classroom, (2) shared the same disability category (both had autism spectrum disorder), and (3) did not experience academic learning difficulties but had special needs in interpersonal interactions. The students without special needs (1) were in the same class as the students with special needs, (2) did not have academic learning difficulties, and (3) did not exhibit overtly friendly or unfriendly behavior in their interactions with the students with special needs. A teacher from the same school ensured the proper execution of the intervention activities within the ExL Prog. The researchers interviewed three classroom teachers to see if the students maintained the effects of the intervention after returning to their original classrooms. The first author, who has special education training, implemented the ExL Prog.

Table 1. Comparison of Peer Interaction in Intervention and Comparison Groups in the Same Class.

Condition	Category	Peer Interaction
ExL Prog	ASD (boy, $n = 1$)	1. Often experiences conflicts and quarrels with classmates. 2. When reminded by classmates, the student often does not respond and continues behaviors that lead to further conflicts. After multiple conflicts, peer relationships deteriorate. 3. Is perceived by peers as intentionally uncooperative due to an invisible disability.
	General (boy, $n = 5$; girl, $n = 3$)	Exhibits subdued participation in class, rarely provides suggestions, and generally assumes a more passive role.
Non-ExL Prog	ASD (girl, $n = 1$)	1. Few conflicts with peers, though experiences a history of rejection and frustration in forming friendships. 2. Often engages in solitary activities, such as walking or reading after class. 3. Peer interactions mainly revolve around academic discussions, with less engagement in playful or casual interactions with this student, due to an invisible disability.
	General (boy, $n = 4$; girl, $n = 4$)	Actively participates in class, is proactive, willing to provide suggestions, and is considered a more active participant in the class.

The schools participating in this study are located in suburban areas, with a total of 25 classes (including one resource class) for grades 1 to 6, and are considered small public schools. Among the participants, the students with special needs are all Taiwanese, with one indigenous student in both ExL Prog. and non-ExL Prog. groups. The students with special needs rank in the bottom 3% of academic performance, while their peers' academic performance range between the top 3% and 10%. However, all participants speak Mandarin. The two students with disabilities in this study come from lower-middle socioeconomic backgrounds. In addition, there are four students from low socioeconomic backgrounds and four from lower-middle socioeconomic backgrounds in both ExL Prog. and non-ExL Prog. groups.

2.4. The ExL Prog

The ExL Prog was conducted over 4 days during the summer, consisting of two activities each day, culminating in a total of eight intervention activities (Table S1 presents Supplementary Information). The researchers divided all students into two groups: those participating in the ExL Prog, which involved intervention activities during a regular 40 min summer course, and those who did not receive any intervention, engaging solely in regular summer 40 min course activities.

The program is modelled after the ExL cycle, as proposed by Kolb [11,13], and further developed by Morris [14]. It guides students through a series of activities aimed at promoting interactions with peers. The process begins with interactive activities, which leads students to recall and reflect on these interactions and experiences, with the goal of distilling key insights and lessons learned. Subsequently, students engage in discussions to strategize adjustments and improvements for future interactions, with the overarching aim of fostering positive relationships and enhancing attitudes of acceptance.

A total of eight thematic activities within the program guided the students through four distinct phases of the ExL cycle. In Activity 1, students initially immersed themselves in the activity (Table S1). After concluding, children progressed to the second to fourth phases (experiencing, reflecting, applying, and generalizing), engaging in reflective review and extended thinking. They explored improvements in interpersonal skills and potential positive changes for the future, and sought sustainable methods for improvement.

To confirm the efficacy of the ExL Prog, the researchers recorded all eight activities. A teacher from the same school selected three of the eight activities to assess adherence to the 12 elements of the four phases within the ExL cycle. The percentage was calculated by dividing the number of items that matched the assessor's selections by the total number of items, then multiplied the result by 100%. This calculation indicates a high level of compliance, with a degree of conformity of 92%.

2.5. Instruments

Interaction Relationship and Acceptance Attitude Questionnaires. After reviewing the literature on children's interpersonal interactions and peer acceptance, the researchers developed a two-part questionnaire covering interaction relationships and acceptance attitudes (Table S2) that employs a four-point Likert-type scale, where higher cumulative scores indicate better interaction relationships or more favorable acceptance attitudes. The researchers asked five experts to review the content and wording of the draft to establish expert validity. The 'Interaction Relationship Questionnaire' had 22 items, and the 'Acceptance Attitude Questionnaire' had 20 items. After the content and wording were reviewed by five experts (with expertise in the well-being of individuals with disabilities, peer interaction and acceptance, and elementary education and counselling), the researchers eliminated inappropriate items. The final version of the 'Interaction Relationship Questionnaire' had 21 items, categorized into 'Affective Experiences' and 'Interaction Performance', comprising 7 and 14 items, respectively. The 'Acceptance Attitude Questionnaire' had 17 items, categorized into 'Cognitive', 'Affective', and 'Behavioral' aspects, comprising four, seven, and six items, respectively. Due to the limited reading comprehension ability of the student with special needs, the researchers administered the questionnaire only to the students without special needs after the completion of the ExL Prog.

Feedback Form and Interviews for The ExL Prog with Activities. To gather feedback from the students, one week after the completion of all eight activities of the ExL Prog, researchers conducted a semi-structured interview using the 'Experiential Activity Feedback Form' to gather reflections from all nine participants, including one with special needs, following each ExL activity. This feedback aims to capture the participants' insights into the activities, providing information about what they have learned. It also serves as a basis for adjusting the content of subsequent activities. In addition, the researchers employed additional semi-structured interviews using the 'Student and Teacher Interview Form'. The interviews focused on two aspects: interaction relationships (involving both students without special needs and students with special needs, totaling nine interviewees) and acceptance attitudes (specifically from students without special needs towards students with special needs, totaling eight interviewees). Moreover, interviews were conducted with the homeroom teacher and two subject teachers after the completion of the ExL Prog. The interviews aimed to compare the evaluations of interaction outcomes and peer acceptance between students and teachers, ensuring consistency. The first author (who was also a special education teacher at the school) conducted one-on-one interviews to ensure that their perspectives and ideas would not influence each other.

2.6. Data Collection and Analysis

Descriptive statistics were used to present the quantitative data from the Interaction Relationship and the Acceptance Attitude Questionnaires. Further statistical comparison of the differences in positive changes among the students without special needs with and without the ExL Prog was conducted. Qualitative data consist of feedback forms from all students who participated in the ExL Prog and interviews from the students without special needs who participated in the ExL Prog, as well as their homeroom teachers and two subject teachers. Qualitative data were employed to complement the limitations of quantitative findings. A thematic analysis approach [23] was utilized to identify recurring concepts among participants through in-depth examination of interview content, thereby enhancing the interpretation and presentation of results. After the first author completed the transcription, the interview content was validated with the participants to ensure accuracy. An initial analysis was then conducted, followed by a cross-verification of the qualitative data with the corresponding author to ensure the accuracy of the coding. Consensus on the results of the analysis was achieved, with an agreement rate exceeding 90%.The organized descriptive information is coded with T1 to T3, representing teacher codes; students without special needs are coded as S1 to S8, and the student with special needs is coded as S9.

2.7. Ethics Declarations

The study received approval from the university's thesis review committee and was supported by a grant that had undergone review by the university's Institutional Review Board. All participants provided written informed consent before participation. The authors declare no competing interests. The data that support the findings of this study are available from the corresponding author upon reasonable request.

3. Results

3.1. Group Comparison on Peer Interaction and Acceptance

To address the first research question, Tables 2 and 3 present descriptive statistics from the Interaction Relationship and Acceptance Attitude Questionnaires. The total score of positive interactions in the intervention group, as well as the average values for the two dimensions (affective experience and interaction performance), were both lower than those of the control group. However, after analyzing the median, it was found that the total score of positive interactions and the scores for the two dimensions (affective experience and interaction performance) in the intervention group was higher than those of the control group. It is speculated that this discrepancy may be due to the small sample size of only eight students in both the intervention and control groups, where the influence of extreme values might be more pronounced.

Table 2. Descriptive statistics of general education students' Interaction Relationship Questionnaire.

Statistics	Intervention (n = 8)			Comparison (n = 8)		
	Total	Affective Experiences	Interaction Performance	Total	Affective Experiences	Interaction Performance
Mean	51.75	15.50	36.25	53.75	16.75	37.00
SD	11.20	4.11	8.14	12.20	4.17	8.37
Median	51.00	16.50	37.50	50.50	15.50	34.00
Minimum	37.00	9.00	28.00	40.00	12.00	28.00
Maximum	69.00	22.00	47.00	77.00	25.00	52.00

Table 3. Descriptive statistics of general education students' Acceptance Attitude Questionnaire.

Statistics	Intervention (n = 8)				Comparison (n = 8)			
	Total	Cognitive	Affective	Behavioral	Total	Cognitive	Affective	Behavioral
Mean	55.00	13.75	22.13	19.13	55.38	14.38	21.13	19.88
SD	8.73	1.17	4.32	3.72	7.09	1.85	3.64	2.75
Median	54.00	14.00	21.00	19.50	55.0	15.00	20.00	19.50
Minimum	44.00	12.00	17.00	14.00	45.00	11.00	18.00	16.00
Maximum	66.00	16.00	28.00	24.00	68.00	16.00	28.00	24.00

The "cognitive" dimension of students without disabilities' acceptance attitude toward students with special needs was lower than that of the control group, while the "affective" dimension was higher than that of the control group. The "behavioral" dimension was the same as that of the control group. Overall results indicated an equal distribution of high scorers between the two groups, suggesting no difference in population distribution. Notably, Figure 2 highlights a significant index that, compared with the comparison group (interaction relationships and acceptance attitudes: range = 23 and 12, SD = 11.50 and 6.00), the intervention group's scores exhibit more central tendency (interaction relationships and acceptance attitudes: range = 14 and 10, SD = 5.91 and 4.79). This suggests that the ExL Prog may enable students without special needs to consistently improve in their interaction relationships and acceptance attitudes.

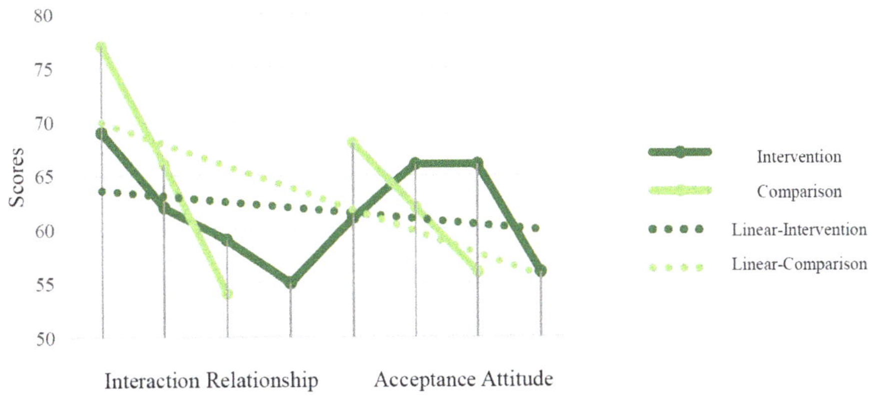

Figure 2. Trends in score distribution of above-average students.

3.2. The Experiences of Cultivating Relationships and Acceptance During ExL Prog

Table S3 presents examples of the feedback from participating students who participated in the ExL Prog after each activity. The students' feedback illustrates considerable development in experience, interactive relationships, and acceptance attitudes throughout the eight activity units. Students preliminarily encountered and reflected on their interpersonal reactions during the initial ExL Prog. They advanced towards more profound experiential reflections and the assimilation of diverse perspectives in the latter stages of ExL Prog. Quotes such as 'Sometimes the advice we give may not be what the other person needs; we should try to understand their needs first and then offer advice to help them' (S3) and 'I learned to accept others and observe them with care' (S2, S7, S9) highlight transformative experiences. This awareness suggests that students have shifted their viewpoints and undergone substantial transformations through repeated practices, leading to the refinement of their relationship concepts and increased consideration of others.

3.3. The Experiences of Navigating Positive Interaction and Promoting Peer Acceptance After the ExL Prog

Students without special needs participating in the ExL Prog reported positive experiences and enjoyed the activities. Many students gained insight into the significance of observing the requirements of students with special needs during these activities. In addition, they demonstrated compassion along with empathy towards the student with special needs by understanding his challenges from his perspective. For instance, one student shared, 'When engaging with him [the student with special needs], I make a conscious effort not to overstep boundaries. I take into his limits and try hard to not annoying him intentionally' (S5). Another student echoed, 'When he [the student with special needs] refused to cooperate with the activity, I felt very angry… If a teacher reminds me to be mindful of his needs, I will speak to him appropriately, but I might still be accustomed to speaking loudly, as I did before' (S6).

Previously, students without special needs who participated in the ExL Prog exhibited lower acceptance towards their classmates with special needs. However, their acceptance of these students noticeably transformed through participation in the ExL Prog. For example, one student remarked, 'I would think he [the student with special needs] was intentionally causing trouble before, but now I try to think about why he would do that' (S5). Another student also shared, 'I might have thought that it's his [the student with special needs] business in the past, but I understand that it's just a matter of differences between us' (S4). Another student commented, 'Now, I'll engage with him [the student with special needs] in a new way, aiming to discover and learn more about him [the student with special needs]' (S7).

The student with special needs (S9) felt relaxed and less pressured in the group interactions. He learned the importance of valuing different perspectives, which led him to shift from previous reactions of anger and unwillingness to adopt the suggestions and opinions of classmates. The student (S9) shared: 'When my peers are trying to be friend with me, I feel comfortable and enjoy being with them' and 'I learned to be more cooperative with others, and I realized that I should take others' thoughts and feelings into considerations'.

3.4. Teacher Interviews on Positive Class Dynamics and Peer Support

The ExL Prog influenced class dynamics, enabling a shift from passive to proactive assistance among students without special needs towards their peers with special needs. A teacher noticed, 'After the ExL Prog, the students without special needs began using a softer tone to address issues caused by the special needs student' (T1). Another teacher commented, 'In the class, conflicts involving the student with special needs were common prior to the intervention. Yet, I've observed increased maturity among the students without special needs. They demonstrated more initiative in assisting the student with special needs when they see him not following classroom rules or team rules' (T2 and T3). Generally, disruptive relationships and rejection among students decreased, leading to greater patience and cooperation in peer interactions. Conflicts were replaced with mutual understanding and acceptance.

4. Discussion

The quantitative data show that the median scores of intervention group's positive interaction scores between students with special needs and peers without special needs were higher than those of the control group. However, the intervention group's acceptance scores were lower than those of the control group, meaning that the effect of the ExL Prog on improving peer acceptance was less significant, except for the "Affective" dimension, which was higher than that of the control group. Based on the results shown in Figure 2, the scores of the intervention group demonstrate a more central tendency than those of the control group, indicating reduced polarization and greater consistency in participants' perceptions. This more balanced distribution may help explain the relatively lower acceptance scores, as increased exposure to the ExL Prog could have fostered more reflective attitudes among students. The qualitative data show that students without special needs in the intervention group reported a change in how they viewed peers with special needs through the ExL Prog. Their perspective shifted from negative tolerance to positive understanding, and they also learned to observe the needs of others before interacting. Students with special needs in the intervention group expressed that they learned to respect different opinions and were happy to have more opportunities to play with their classmates. The interviews predominantly reflected positive feelings and interaction styles.

This study found that the ExL Prog can enhance positive interaction between students without special needs and students with special needs. Throughout the ExL Prog, students without special needs reported their own attitudes toward their peers with special needs shifted from impatience to positive understanding and compassion. The students without special needs learned to observe each other's needs and cooperate consciously. The student with special needs not only was pleased to have more opportunities to play with his peers through these constructive interactive experiences but also developed consideration for others' perspectives. Regarding the effects on peer acceptance attitudes, the students without special needs indicated positive changes in their views toward the student with special needs after the ExL Prog. They learned to be respectful of the unique characteristics and difficulties for students with special needs in case of misunderstandings. In addition, both the homeroom teacher and subject teachers held positive views on the ExL Prog. Through intensive and comprehensive engagement in the ExL Prog, both students without special needs and students with special needs reacquainted themselves. Then, they became willing to listen, understand, and assist each other. This added value of change benefits teachers in class management by alleviating the burden of handling peer interaction and acceptance issues while enhancing cohesion among classmates.

The overall findings of this study demonstrate the effectiveness of the ExL Prog in enhancing positive interactions and acceptance between students without special needs and students with special needs. The program is consistent with the ExL theory [11,13,14] and previous related research [6,16,36]. The ExL Prog promotes structured participation in students across four distinct phases within the ExL cycle. Starting with immersion in the activity, students then transition to the subsequent phases, which involve reflective reviews, and engage in extended cognitive deliberation. This process enables the exploration of advancements in interpersonal aptitudes and the anticipation of prospective positive transformations. Ultimately, it creates a sustainable avenue for fostering a cohesive and inclusive atmosphere. More importantly, this study further emphasizes the critical role of senior-grade elementary school children in the bidirectional perspective of ExL [15,17,31], presenting more age-specific and comprehensive intervention effectiveness.

4.1. Practical Implications

4.1.1. Advocating for Empathy and Respect Towards Differences

The sixth-grade students without special needs and students with special needs participating in this study's ExL Prog fostered an appreciation for the uniqueness of each individual. The ExL Prog meaningfully transformed their peer interactions, enabling students to reconnect and reshape their interpersonal dynamics. Inclusive classrooms must promote students without special needs' awareness and understanding of the challenges faced by students with special needs [4–6]. This enhanced awareness encourages students without special needs to develop an empathetic and respectful mindset that motivates them to provide support and compassion to those with visible physical or sensory impairments, as well as hidden cognitive or emotional disabilities. Likewise, students with special needs profit from increased peer resources and opportunities for positive outcomes. Hence, inclusive classrooms should prioritize refining a culture of understanding and acceptance through programs like ExL, rather than mere compliance.

4.1.2. Enhancing Positive Dynamics in Inclusive Classrooms with the ExL Prog

Based on our findings and positive feedback across students with and without special needs, and their teachers, the ExL Prog could be used in inclusive education. The ExL Prog prompted the students to provide students with special needs with time to adapt, to kindly acknowledge differences, and to constructively balance mutual respect. A designed ExL Prog can promote peer interactions and acceptance among both students with special needs and students with special needs. By encouraging the recognition and understanding of differences, these activities lead to increased mutual assistance [4,5,39]. Additionally, using group cooperative work allows students to engage in experiencing, reflecting, applying, and generalizing [14,15]. To ensure effective program implementation, instructors should have a basic understanding of students with special needs and the dynamics between students without special needs and students with special needs.

4.2. Limitations and Future Research

The focus of this study on interpersonal interactions meant that participants' interaction relationships could not be randomly assigned based on their inherent characteristics. As students with special needs experienced difficulties in comprehending the questionnaire items, their quantitative data were not included in the current study. This limitation should be addressed in future research. Moreover, the absence of a pretest for interaction relationships and the sole reliance on the statements of class teachers as references indicate that rigorous control of variables was not implemented. It is possible that the intervention group started with lower baseline acceptance levels, which could have influenced post-intervention outcomes. This suggests that researchers should interpret the research results with caution to account for potential interference or covariate factors. Since this research was conducted during the COVID-19 pandemic, it was not possible to carry out a pilot study in advance to assess the feasibility of the program. It is recommended that future studies include a pilot phase to better evaluate and refine the program design before full implementation. Additionally, the relatively small sample size and limited diversity in cultural backgrounds may have reduced statistical power, making it more difficult to detect subtle changes and potentially contributing to the central tendency observed in the score distribution. As a result, the interpretation and application of the research findings should be approached with caution, and further studies are needed to provide supporting evidence. Furthermore, the intervention timeframe of the ExL Prog was short, and the sustainability of its effectiveness still requires further confirmation in future research. Lastly, although our activity design in the program accounted for various aspects of ExL, it was limited to only eight activities, serving as instructional references. Future research could incorporate a variety of activities to apply the ExL Prog to enhance the interpersonal relationships and acceptance attitudes among students with and without special needs.

5. Conclusions

These findings are consistent with Kolb's ExL theory [11,13,14], which emphasizes the importance of concrete experiences and reflective observation in shaping learning. The students involved in the ExL Prog recognize the importance of understanding others and have reflected on how their previous approaches might be ineffective in fostering relationships. Their consideration for others has been cultivated, but the transition from knowing to implementing these newfound skills sometimes demands ongoing support and reinforcement. These changes led to a newfound openness for interactions and goodwill from their peers, highlighting a growing sense of mutual reciprocity. Overall, the ExL Prog promoted transformative growth in interpersonal relationships and communication skills for the students. Future research should consider both sample representativeness and inferential validity to more thoroughly investigate the potential correlation between students' positive interactions and their attitudes toward peer acceptance, as well as the extent to which these factors may mutually influence one another.

Supplementary Materials: The following supporting information can be downloaded at: https://www.mdpi.com/article/10.3390/children12050543/s1, Table S1: The ExL Prog Activities and Core Objectives; Table S2: The Interaction Relationship and The Acceptance Attitude Questionnaires; Table S3: Feedback Summary of General Education Students in the ExL Prog Intervention Group.

Author Contributions: Conceptualization, H.-M.L. and S.-Y.C.; materials and methods, H.-M.L. and S.-Y.C.; results, H.-M.L., S.-Y.C. and I.-H.L.; discussion and recommendations for future research, S.-Y.C. and W.-H.C.; limitations, S.-Y.C. and I.-H.L.; conclusions, S.-Y.C. and I.-H.L.; formal analysis, H.-M.L. and S.-Y.C.; writing—original draft preparation, S.-Y.C. and H.-T.P.; writing—review and editing, I.-H.L. and W.-H.C.; supervision, S.-Y.C.; funding acquisition, S.-Y.C. All authors have read and agreed to the published version of the manuscript.

Funding: This research reported here was supported by the National Science and Technology Council, Taiwan, under [Grant 111-2628-H-007-004-MY3] and [Grant 113-2627-M-008-001] to the principal investigator, Szu-Yin Chu.

Institutional Review Board Statement: This research was approved by the thesis committee and received informed consent from the families of the participating children. The study was supported by a grant that was reviewed and approved by the Institutional Review Board (IRB) of National Tsing Hua University, Taiwan, (protocol code 11010HT113 and date of approval 5 November 2021).

Informed Consent Statement: All participants provided written informed consent before participation.

Data Availability Statement: The original contributions presented in the study are included in the article, further inquiries can be directed to the corresponding author.

Conflicts of Interest: The authors declare no conflicts of interest.

References

1. Adams, D.; Hussain, S.; Tan, K.L. Inclusive leadership for schools: Practices, challenges, and future directions. In *Educational Leadership: Contemporary Theories, Principles, and Practices*; Adams, D., Ed.; Springer Nature: Singapore, 2023; pp. 85–99. [CrossRef]
2. Beazidou, E.; Botsoglou, K. Peer acceptance and friendship in early childhood: The conceptual distinctions between them. *Early Child Dev. Care* **2016**, *186*, 1615–1631. [CrossRef]
3. Osher, D.; Cantor, P.; Berg, J.; Steyer, L.; Rose, T. Drivers of human development: How relationships and context shape learning and development. *Appl. Dev. Sci.* **2020**, *24*, 6–36. [CrossRef]
4. Esposito, M.K.; Tang, K.; Kulkarni, S.S. Ensuring inclusive environments for students with disabilities: School leaders play a linchpin role. *J. Educ. Adm. Hist.* **2019**, *51*, 43–52. [CrossRef]
5. Pazey, B.; Combes, B. Principals' and school leaders' roles in inclusive education. *Oxf. Res. Encycl. Educ.* **2020**. [CrossRef]
6. Petry, K. The relationship between class attitudes towards peers with a disability and peer acceptance, friendships and peer interactions of students with a disability in regular secondary schools. *Eur. J. Spec. Needs Educ.* **2020**, *33*, 254–268. [CrossRef]
7. de Boer, A.; Pijl, S.J. The acceptance and rejection of peers with ADHD and ASD in general secondary education. *J. Educ. Res.* **2016**, *109*, 325–332. [CrossRef]
8. Schwab, S. Social dimensions of inclusion in education of 4th and 7th grade pupils in inclusive and regular classes: Outcomes from Austria. *Res. Dev. Disabil.* **2015**, *43*, 72–79. [CrossRef]
9. Schwab, S.; Gebhardt, M.; Krammer, M.; Gasteiger-Klicpera, B. Linking self-rated social inclusion to social behaviour: An empirical study of students with and without special education needs in secondary schools. *Eur. J. Spec. Needs Educ.* **2015**, *30*, 1–14. [CrossRef]
10. Chen, L.-J. Incorporating experiential learning in tour planning and design: Practice and reflection. *J. Teach. Pract. Pedagog.* **2023**, *6*, 83–122. [CrossRef]
11. Kolb, D.A. *Experiential Learning: Experience as the Source of Learning and Development*, 1st ed.; Prentice-Hall: Hoboken, NJ, USA, 1984.
12. Kolb, A.; Kolb, D. Experiential Learning Theory: A Dynamic, Holistic Approach to Management Learning, Education and Development. In *Handbook of Management Learning, Education and Development*; Armstrong, S.J., Fukami, C., Eds.; SAGE: Los Angeles, CA, USA, 2011. [CrossRef]
13. Kolb, D.A. *Experiential Learning: Experience as the Source of Learning and Development*, 2nd ed.; FT Press: Upper Saddle River, NJ, USA, 2014.
14. Morris, T.H. Experiential learning—A systematic review and revision of Kolb's model. *Interact. Learn. Environ.* **2020**, *28*, 1064–1077. [CrossRef]
15. Seaman, J.; Brown, M.; Quay, J. The evolution of experiential learning theory: Tracing lines of research in the JEE. *J. Exp. Educ.* **2017**, *40*, NP1–NP21. [CrossRef]
16. Wozencroft, A.J.; Pate, J.R.; Griffiths, H.K. Experiential learning and its impact on students' attitudes toward youth with disabilities. *J. Exp. Educ.* **2015**, *38*, 129–143. [CrossRef]
17. Kamps, D.; Thiemann-Bourque, K.; Heitzman-Powell, L.; Schwartz, I.; Rosenberg, N.; Mason, R.; Cox, S. A comprehensive peer network intervention to improve social communication of children with autism spectrum disorders: A randomized trial in kindergarten and first grade. *J. Autism Dev. Disord.* **2015**, *45*, 1809–1824. [CrossRef]
18. Pijl, S.J.; Frostad, P. Peer acceptance and self-concept of students with disabilities in regular education. *Eur. J. Spec. Needs Educ.* **2010**, *25*, 93–105. [CrossRef]
19. Bakopoulou, I.; Dockrell, J.E. The role of social cognition and prosocial behaviour in relation to the socio-emotional functioning of primary aged children with specific language impairment. *Res. Dev. Disabil.* **2016**, *49*, 354–370. [CrossRef] [PubMed]
20. Calder, L.; Hill, V.; Pellicano, E. Sometimes I want to play by myself: Understanding what friendship means to children with autism in mainstream primary schools. *Autism* **2013**, *17*, 296–316. [CrossRef]
21. Avramidis, E.; Strogilos, V.; Aroni, K.; Kantaraki, C.T. Using sociometric techniques to assess the social impacts of inclusion: Some methodological considerations. *Educ. Res. Rev.* **2017**, *20*, 68–80. [CrossRef]
22. Bossaert, G.; Colpin, H.; Pijl, S.J.; Petry, K. Truly included? A literature study focusing on the social dimension of inclusion in education. *Int. J. Incl. Educ.* **2013**, *17*, 60–79. [CrossRef]
23. Braun, V.; Clarke, V. Using thematic analysis in psychology. *Qual. Res. Psychol.* **2006**, *3*, 77–101. [CrossRef]
24. Pinto, C.; Baines, E.; Bakopoulou, I. The peer relations of pupils with special educational needs in mainstream primary schools: The mportance of meaningful contact and interaction with peers. *Br. J. Educ. Psychol.* **2019**, *89*, 818–837. [CrossRef]
25. Bialka, C.S.; Havlik, S.A. Partners in learning: Exploring two transformative university and high school service-learning partnerships. *J. Exp. Educ.* **2016**, *39*, 220–237. [CrossRef]
26. Fifolt, M.; Morgan, A.F.; Burgess, Z.R. Promoting school connectedness among minority youth through experience-based urban farming. *J. Exp. Educ.* **2018**, *41*, 187–203. [CrossRef]
27. Isaak, J.; Devine, M.; Gervich, C.; Gottschall, R. Are we experienced? Reflections on the SUNY experiential learning mandate. *J. Exp. Educ.* **2018**, *41*, 23–38. [CrossRef]

28. Collins, R.H.; Sibthorp, J.; Gookin, J. Developing ill-structured problem-solving skills through wilderness education. *J. Exp. Educ.* **2016**, *39*, 179–195. [CrossRef]
29. Deringer, S.A. Mindful place-based education: Mapping the literature. *J. Exp. Educ.* **2017**, *40*, 333–348. [CrossRef]
30. Asfeldt, M.; Hvenegaard, G.; Purc-Stephenson, R. Group writing, reflection, and discovery: A model for enhancing learning on wilderness educational expeditions. *J. Exp. Educ.* **2018**, *41*, 241–260. [CrossRef]
31. Slininger, D.; Sherrill, C.; Jankowski, C.M. Children's attitudes toward peers with severe disabilities: Revisiting contact theory. *Adapt. Phys. Act. Q.* **2000**, *17*, 176–196. [CrossRef]
32. Fırat, T. An exploration of the effects of learning through 'Interaction Activities' on eighth-graders' social acceptance of students with special needs in Turkey. *Education* **2021**, *49*, 792–808. [CrossRef]
33. Sardohan Yildirim, A.E.; Atbaşi, Z.; Erol, E. The effect of peer-mediated skill generalisation activities on the social acceptance of individuals with special needs in Turkey. *Education* **2022**, *52*, 227–239. [CrossRef]
34. Hayden, H.E.; Prince, A.M. Disrupting ableism: Strengths-based representations of disability in children's picture books. *J. Early Child. Lit.* **2023**, *23*, 236–261. [CrossRef]
35. Kale, M.; Demir, S. Determining the effects of interactive book reading implementations on the social acceptance of students with special needs. *Read. Writ. Q.* **2023**, *39*, 36–53. [CrossRef]
36. Schwab, S. The impact of contact on students' attitudes towards peers with disabilities. *Res. Dev. Disabil.* **2017**, *62*, 160–165. [CrossRef] [PubMed]
37. Denham, S.A. *The Development of Emotional Competence in Young Children*; Guilford Publications: New York, NY, USA, 2023.
38. Glen, C.; Taylor, L.K.; Dautel, J.B. Promoting prosocial behavior toward refugees: Exploring the empathy-attitude-action model in middle childhood. In *Children and Peace: From Research to Action*; Bavlin, N., Christie, D., Eds.; Psychology Book Series; Springer: Cham, Switzerland, 2020; pp. 71–87. [CrossRef]
39. Mégret, F. The disabilities convention: Human rights of persons with disabilities or disability rights? *Hum. Rights Q.* **2008**, *30*, 494–516. [CrossRef]

children

MDPI

Article

When Parent–Teacher Collaboration Turns Violent: Corporal Punishment in American Schools and Subsequent (Secondary) Trauma

Da'Shay Templeton [1,*], Ruslan Korchagin [1], Bree Valla [1] and Jesse R. Ford [2]

[1] Educational Leadership, California Lutheran University, Thousand Oaks, CA 61360, USA; rkorchag@callutheran.edu (R.K.); bvalla@callutheran.edu (B.V.)
[2] Teacher Education and Higher Education, University of North Carolina at Greensboro, Greensboro, NC 27412, USA; jrfordjr@uncg.edu
* Correspondence: dtempleton@callutheran.edu; Tel.: +1-661-305-3502

Abstract: Methods. Through the lens of childhood trauma theory, a qualitative phenomenological study was conducted using purposive and snowball sampling methods to gain a deeper understanding of the experiences of former students with corporal punishment and how those experiences have shaped their academic and psychological outcomes. Interviews were conducted via Zoom with 19 men and women of different ages and races who attended schools in Mississippi. **Results/Conclusions.** The study revealed that parents and school personnel collaborated to punish the student corporally both on campus and at home. Related, beaten students did not share their punishment with their parents/caregivers, and if their families did find out, they received another beating at home. There was a general lack of consistency in how and who administered corporal punishment. In addition to the well-documented ways that corporal punishment is administered in school, we also found that students were made to hold painful positions or perform painful tasks. There were also peer effects of trauma, with students experiencing fear or anger following a friend or classmate being beaten in front of them. Race was an influence if the abused students felt that their punishment was racist, with Black American participants feeling there were racial undertones regardless of the perpetrator's race. The study's findings align with those of previously conducted research, but also extend them and can be used to create policy to allow schools to address trauma and create instructional practices that eliminate the fear and racial disparities that have been proven to exist in schools with corporal punishment.

Keywords: corporal punishment; trauma; trauma-informed policy; childhood trauma theory

1. When Parent–Teacher Collaboration Turns Violent: Corporal Punishment in American Schools and Subsequent (Secondary) Trauma

When does collaboration between teachers and parents turn violent? When does someone else's trauma become your own? In several states, corporal punishment in the home results in a visit from Child Protection Services and, in some cases, incarceration; yet, select school personnel are exempt from child abuse charges for corporal punishment in school (CPS) [1]. In the U.S., twenty-three states do not expressly prohibit the use of CPS, making it a form of state-sanctioned violence [2]. School personnel use brutal tactics and techniques to dole out CPS via hands, feet, or objects such as canes, rulers, paddles, yardsticks, and belts. The assault takes various forms: choking, kicking, punching, pinching, slapping, and shaking as well as requiring the child to hold painful positions for extended periods of time [3,4].

CPS has deleterious consequences for the youth on whom the pain is inflicted; however, the extent to which these consequences extend to peer effects has yet to be explored in the literature and is investigated in-depth in this study. CPS is associated with negative life outcomes, including mental (e.g., increased aggressive behaviors, maladaptive behaviors, depression, and anxiety) [5,6], physical (increased bodily injury) [1], academic (increased dropout rates and chronic absenteeism and decreased GPA) [7,8], and socio-emotional effects (decreased sense of belonging and trust in authority figures) [9].

While the legality and administration of CPS have declined in America, about 600 students are still struck each day [1]. Instances of CPS are often underreported, so these estimates could be greater [5]. Whether a child is beaten at school is random, but in Mississippi—a state with the highest rates of CPS in America—the probability is increased [1], making it an ideal location for a case study. Using in-depth interviews of 19 former Mississippi public school students, we sought to answer this question: How has CPS shaped the academic and psychological outcomes of Mississippi public school students? This study contributes to a long line of research studies on CPS but provides an in-depth and contemporary analysis of a state with the highest instances of corporal punishment in schools, particularly regarding how parents and teachers work together to administer corporal punishment as well as the secondary effects of trauma on peers.

We found that students experienced primary, compounded, and secondary trauma as well as secrecy and shame for fear of telling their guardians and receiving an additional corporal punishment. Generally, there were a perceived lack of consistency and increased racial biases. Lastly, we recorded their recommendations for change, which align well with previous research. The findings underscore the critical role school personnel and parents play in creating traumatic conditions for vulnerable youth and their peers. The study concludes with practical suggestions that the state, parents, and school personnel can implement to protect our students and increase their success. The following section outlines the theory used to anchor and guide this study.

2. Childhood Trauma Theory

In order to investigate the long-term effects of CPS on Mississippi public school students, this study leverages childhood trauma theory. Childhood trauma theory has no single founder; instead, it has been developed over time by scholars in the fields of psychology, psychiatry, and psychoanalysis. Traumatic events are experienced by many children, and their psychological and developmental consequences are often severe [10]. The term childhood trauma refers to the harm, potential harm, or threat of harm caused by the actions of a child's caregiver [11]. As defined by the American Psychiatric Association, traumatic exposure occurs when an individual is confronted with death, serious injury, or other threats to physical integrity [12]. Men and women report physical abuse, physical neglect, and emotional abuse as the most common forms of trauma [13]. The effects of interpersonal trauma often manifest in a greater number of global and profound changes in children than they do in adults, who are conceivably more resistant to stress and possess more cognitive resources to mitigate risks and promote resilience. Children who experience such events are likely to lose their sense of self-esteem, their sense of lovability, their sense of vulnerability, and their faith in family, friends, and a higher power as a result [9].

In children, posttraumatic stress and its pathological manifestation, posttraumatic stress disorder, have been the most extensively studied psychological consequences of traumatic exposure [12]. As a result of prolonged exposure to trauma, changes in brain structure and function may also occur, particularly in areas associated with emotional regulation and fear processing [13]. In accordance with the findings of neuroscientific researchers, trauma can adversely affect a child's academic health in a number of ways, including impaired brain development related to language and communication, impaired self-esteem, impaired learning, compromised ability to pay attention in class, diminished memory, difficulty following instructions, poor organizational skills, and difficulty grasping cause-and-effect relationships. Researchers have demonstrated that protective and compensatory experiences are critical to the healing and improvement of those who have suffered adverse childhood experiences [14–18]. The sooner these protective measures are implemented, the sooner the vicious cycle that leads to failure or social and personal disadvantage will end. The next section reviews the extant literature.

3. Literature Review

Secondary Trauma

We first review the literature on secondary trauma, which we propose researchers leverage in addition to childhood trauma theory. Hearing about or witnessing another person's traumatic experiences may cause secondary trauma, also known as secondary traumatic stress, vicarious traumatization, or compassion fatigue [19]. Figley [20] conceptualizes secondary traumatic stress as the natural, subsequent feelings and behaviors associated with knowing about a traumatizing event experienced by a significant other as well as the stress caused by helping or wanting to assist someone in distress. People who witness traumatic events or care for trauma survivors suffer secondary trauma. It occurs when a person is exposed to a traumatic event experienced by another person [21]. Experiencing trauma situations and identifying with those in them can also cause secondary trauma reactions, especially when these experiences evoke fear reactions in the witness [22,23].

As a result of secondary traumatic stress, individuals may experience cognitive difficulties, such as intrusive thoughts and difficulty concentrating, as well as physical changes, such as insomnia or fatigue [24]. A secondary traumatic stress disorder is characterized by intrusive imagery, avoidant reactions, physiological arousal, distressing emotions, and functional impairment [25]. As a result of secondary trauma, a variety of symptoms may appear, including anger, anxiety, depression, low self-esteem, emotional exhaustion, difficulty concentrating, body aches, sleep problems, changes in eating habits, startle reactions, and an increase in addictive behaviors, as well as withdrawal from others [26].

Typically, secondary trauma of childhood refers to negative psychological experiences caused by a child's close relationship with a traumatized individual. An emotional bond may exist between a child and a parent, guardian, relative, or anyone else with whom the child has a close relationship [26]. A child's secondary trauma can have a significant impact on their cognitive ability, emotional health, behavior, physical health, and personal relationships [27]. In order to heal secondary trauma, children should be provided with a secure nonthreatening environment where safety and the establishment of trust are prioritized [26]. A relatively limited amount of research has been conducted on the measurement of secondary trauma, and the majority of the assessment devices that exist are designed for therapists and not for the general public or for children [26]. There are relatively few empirical studies on secondary trauma in children, and systematic, controlled research is lacking. Secondary trauma is a field that is in its infancy and relatively lacking in empirical studies.

4. Impacts of Corporal Punishment on Students

Corporal punishment uses a punishing stimulus after a student has exhibited an undesirable behavior with the intent that the negative experience will deter the child from repeating the offensive behavior [4,7,28]—though research supporting that notion is limited and controversial [1]. Corporal punishment is often administered using an object to inflict pain, such as a paddle or cane, which routinely leads to physical injury to the student, ranging from bruises and cuts to broken bones [4]. School personnel administer corporal punishment; they are the individuals hurting the child. The same individuals who are responsible for motivating children on campus are physically injuring them. This dichotomy is difficult for students to understand and conflicts with their sense of self-efficacy and safety in schools.

The act of hitting a child does not teach nor explain why their behavior was offensive, thereby not providing a learning opportunity for the student. For punishment to be effective in changing behavior, it must be administered immediately, consistently, and after every instance of the behavior [4]. When students cannot understand the "why" behind their punishment, coupled with the fact that it is violent punishment, their self-regulation and self-efficacy are negatively impacted. They cannot make sense of the reason for the violent punishment being inflicted on them by a school official who is supposed to protect them [1].

Students who experience corporal punishment are more likely to be depressed, suffer from anxiety, and report a disconnect from their schools [4,6], symptoms that are commonly seen in those who cannot exercise self-efficacy, resulting in an inability to recover from the violent, traumatic event [29]. Not surprisingly, students who were the victims of corporal punishment also had lower grade-point averages [4], higher dropout rates, and increased absenteeism [30–33]. Once again, these students cannot self-regulate and struggle to see the likelihood of attaining their future goals [29] because of the traumatic effect of corporal punishment. Students in southern states and Black American students have a higher chance of receiving CPS [1,34]; unfortunately, those same groups are disproportionally punished corporally at home.

5. Corporal Punishment in Black American Culture

As revealed in the study conducted by Patton et al. [35], Black American children are more likely to be injured or killed by their parents than by police because of white supremacy. White supremacy ensures that Black American parents and guardians beat their children to ensure that they are prepared for the expected social violence. Black American parents and guardians believe that corporal punishment is necessary to prevent the incarceration of their youth and prepare them for police violence. Patton et al. [35] argue that physical punishment is the legacy of slavery. This notion is supported by research that links slavery and lynching to increased CPS [34].

A qualitative study conducted by LeCuyer et al. [36] with southern Black American mothers of young children found that corporal punishment was considered normal in this population. Taylor et al. [37] found that Black Americans living in southern states believe that corporal punishment is a necessary component of effective parenting. Black American families use corporal punishment at higher rates than non-Latino White or Latino families, even after controlling for socioeconomic status [38]. Compared to other racial groups, Black American parents approve of corporal punishment at a higher rate [39]. At the same time, Klevens et al. [40] found that the majority of parents, regardless of their racial or ethnic affiliation, believe that most other parents hit their children.

A recent study conducted by Duong et al. [41] found some trends in the usage of corporal punishment by Black American parents. First, the change in the current social environment does not support child physical discipline, and it no longer works in favor of Black American parents. Second, as a result of feeling misunderstood and unfairly evaluated by society, Black American parents resisted social pressures not to use corporal punishment. Third, Black American parents believe corporal punishment is an effective and normal disciplinary method that worked well in their youth. Fourth, Black American parents believe that non-physical discipline leads to undesirable consequences.

6. Consistency in the Administration of School Discipline

For discipline to be effective, it must also be consistent [4]; however, research evidences that school discipline is inconsistent. Welsh [42] found that a substantial amount of language used in school-level training materials reflects interventionist disciplinary philosophies, such as "behavior cannot be shaped unless interventions are implemented consistently". Irby and Clough [43] emphasized that consistency is a guiding principal of school discipline culture. They identified three ways in which consistency functions across schools. First, consistency serves as a means of maintaining collegial relations. Second, teachers employ consistency to promote fairness and equality in the treatment of their students. Third, consistency is essential to ensuring that students are aware of rules and expectations at school and can comply with them. Furthermore, Williams III [44] found that Black American students are less likely to be suspended when school administrators are more consistent.

At the same time, a group of researchers highlight issues with consistency in the implementation of school discipline. Griffith and Tyner [45] discovered that school discipline protocols are inconsistently implemented. Smith and Hains [46] highlight that school discipline policies vary depending on the philosophies and beliefs of educators guiding disciplinary practices. Kennedy et al. [47] highlight a tension between consistency and individualization in school administrators' decisions to follow centralized school discipline guidelines. On the one hand, guidelines provide easy choices when applying school discipline. On the other hand, many administrators did not feel comfortable with the rigidity of the code and made compromises in their decisions based on numerous factors. Shabazian [48] examined how administrative perspectives shape the implementation of school discipline policy and determined that an administrator's decision to exclude students was influenced by five normative values: productive efficiency, equality versus equity, legal liability, prescribing a cultural deficit ideology, and the notion of strict surveillance. Discipline varies by state, districts, and even schools within the same district, but below, we provide information on the legality and administration of discipline in Mississippi public schools.

7. Administration of School Discipline in Mississippi

Mississippi is one of the states that allows corporal punishment for students as long as they do not have disabilities [49]. According to Education Code §49001 (a), corporal punishment is the "willful infliction of, or willfully causing the infliction of, physical pain on a pupil". Mississippi Code 37-11-57 (2) defines corporal punishment as "reasonable use of physical force or physical contact by a teacher, assistant teacher, principal or assistant principal, as may be necessary to maintain discipline, to enforce a school rule, for self-protection, or for the protection of other students from disruptive students". Furthermore, MI Code 37-11-52 (2) states that when a "public school teacher, assistant teacher, principal or assistant principal" administers corporal punishment in a "reasonable manner" or uses "any reasonable action to maintain control and discipline of a student", they cannot be found negligent or guilty of child abuse. In addition, they are shielded from any civil damages that could arise from a student who may suffer due to the application of corporal punishment.

Mississippi law explicitly gives the power to suspend or expel a student to the superintendent or school principal anytime their presence in the classroom disrupts the educational environment or if their presence is detrimental to the other students and the teacher (§37-9-71). If the suspension is more than 10 days, the student has the right to due process (§37-9-71). However, if a student receives corporal punishment, the student has no opportunity for due process. Based on the Mississippi Education Code and the restraints on suspension and expulsion, these forms of discipline are considered more extreme than corporal punishment. According to Mississippi governmental officials, physical infliction of pain is less injurious than having a student not attend school.

According to federal data, in 2017–2018, the most recent year with data, Mississippi had the highest rates of corporal punishment administration of any state, with nearly 30% of all incidents occurring in Mississippi [50]. In 2019, Mississippi restricted corporal punishment so that it could not be used on students with disabilities, which resulted in a decrease of over 23,000 instances of corporal punishment [51]. In 2019, Mississippi realized that the deleterious effects of corporal punishment were too extreme and inappropriate for students with disabilities. However, non-disabled students still receive corporal punishment.

School discipline, specifically corporal punishment, is applied inequitably. In 2020–2021, Mississippi students were 47.72% Black or African American, 43.13% White, 4.39% Hispanic or Latin*, 3.33% two or more races, 1.15% Asian, 0.22% American Indian or Alaskan Native, and 0.06% Native Hawaiian or Pacific Islander [52]. Comparatively, for the same school year, Black/African American students received 53.1% of the corporal punishment, disproportionately higher than that meted out to all other races. All other races (see Table 1 below) received corporal punishment less often in proportion to their racial representation in the population.

Table 1. National data on population and instances of corporal punishment by racial group.

	Black/African American	White American	Hispanic/Latin *	Two or More Races	Asian	American Indian/Alaskan Native	Native Hawaiian/Pacific Islander
Enrollment	47.74%	43.13%	4.39%	3.33%	1.15%	0.22%	0.06%
Corporal Punishment	53.1%	43.0%	1.9%	1.2%	<1.0%	<1.0%	0%
Teachers	22.6%	75.6%					
Principals	37.1%	62.9%					

[52]. The asterisk is used to indicate both genders or (Latin(a/o) and not to indicate a need for a notation.

This study will further explore if these disparities influence the disproportionate administration of corporal punishment to Black American students. These statistics are important since the Mississippi Education Code allows teachers and principals to administer corporal punishment.

8. Methodology

Using a qualitative phenomenological research design, we interviewed 19 former students who had experienced corporal punishment in primary and secondary school in Mississippi as recently as the 2022–2023 school year. We recruited participants through both purposive and snowball sampling by contacting the participants following a study administered through Prime Panels. We interviewed participants for up to 90 min in exchange for a USD 100 Amazon gift card. Interviews were carried out via Zoom, an online virtual platform, from 21 March 2024 to 28 March 2024. For more information on how each participant self-identified in the interview, see Table 2 below. Due to the subject matter of the interviews, participants were informed prior to the interview that they could stop at any time and did not need to answer any questions that they felt uncomfortable about. Throughout the interview participants were reminded of the opportunity to stop, take a break, skip questions, reschedule, or cancel the interviews. However, even with these prompts, the researchers recognize that they could have inadvertently caused secondary trauma to participants by asking them to retell their lived experiences. This limitation could be mitigated in the future by offering participants resources to assist them with navigating the secondary trauma, providing them with coping strategies and pausing the interview at regular intervals, and offering the participants time to apply the strategies before continuing to explore their experiences [53].

Table 2. Self-identified race, gender, and age of each participant along with their pseudonym.

Number	Name	Race	Gender	Age
1	Mark	Black American	Man	20
2	Rally	Black American	Man	21
3	Bella	Black American	Woman	25
4	LaShawna	Black American	Woman	38
5	Laila	Black American	Woman	22
6	Tony	Black American	Man	24
7	Jim	Black American	Man	25
8	Jason	Black American	Man	22
9	Jamal	Black American	Man	21
10	Felix	Black American	Man	18
11	Jazz	Black American	Man	20
12	Stanley	Black American	Man	21
13	Sammy	Black American	Woman	37
14	Mindy	Black American	Woman	23
15	Sarah	Black American	Woman	31
16	Christina	Black American	Woman	49
17	Adam	White American and American Indian	Man	58
18	Megan	White American	Woman	45
19	Janet	White American	Woman	53

Interviews were transcribed by Zoom and Rev first, and then by hand for accuracy. The process of data coding and analysis followed a three-stage framework outlined by Strauss [54].

Prior to the data coding process, the transcriptions were thoroughly examined to ensure their accuracy. Coding, as defined by Silverman and Marvasti [55], is the process of categorizing data according to predetermined theoretical categories for the purpose of analysis (p. 507). Then, we performed a second cycle, thematic analysis [56,57]. To enhance the research, trustworthiness was assessed using memoing, peer debriefing, and member checking. After each interview, we recorded feelings during the research process. We recognize the importance of memoing as a tool in the process. Keeping memos after interviews was crucial, as this enabled us to explore personal emotions and shared identities, reducing bias in data collection. In addition to memoing, our team used peer debriefing to enhance in-depth reflection [58]. This analysis illuminated consistent patterns in the data, which led to our overarching themes. We found the following overarching themes: primary trauma, compounded trauma, secrecy and shame, secondary trauma, lack of consistency, racial bias, and recommendations for change (see Figure 1 for a visual display of our findings). These themes are presented in this order in the next segment of this paper.

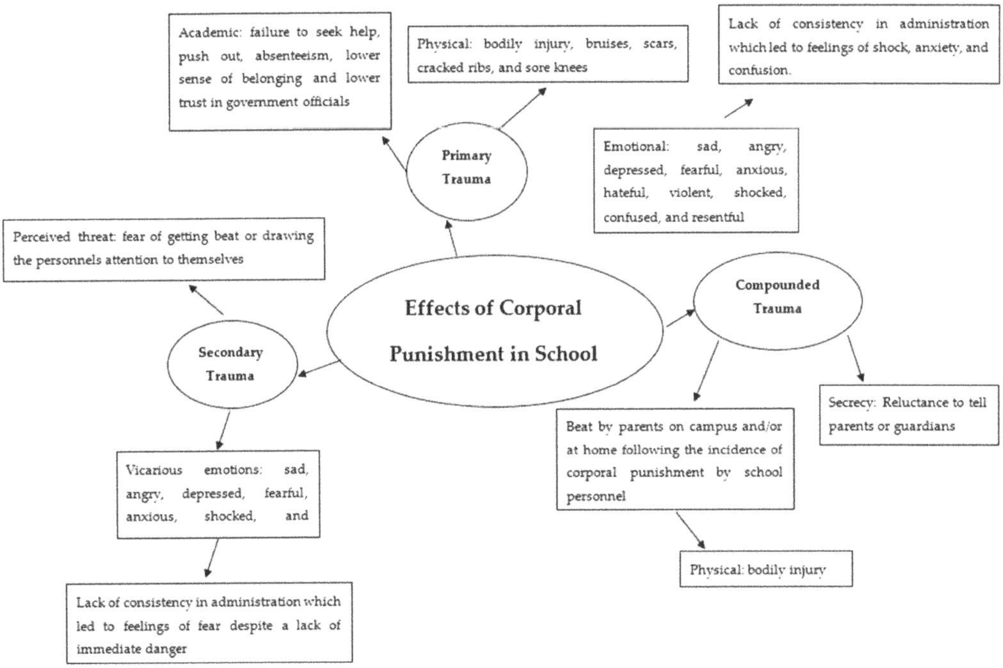

Figure 1. The Traumatic Effects of Corporal Punishment in Mississippi public schools. *Note:* We did not include recommendations for change, which include more government oversight and scholarly research on corporal punishment in schools as well as more humane treatment and individual therapy and counseling instead of corporal punishment in schools.

9. Primary Trauma

Every participant felt pain, with most additionally feeling aggression, anger, depression, sadness, and embarrassment. For pain, each former student felt pain that lasted days and even weeks. One student, Jazz, said "I received four strokes of the cane. I remember I would never forget it was counted, and it was in class in public, so it was very, very painful. I must say it was a painful experience". Another student recounts trying to run away from the pain of the caning: "Since the caning was very, very painful, I attempted to run, but I was held down, and to complete the strokes. So it was really, really a painful experience". Lastly, Jim, a 25-year-old Black American man, shared that "I was in pain for weeks, you know. It affected me psychologically. You know. I just I was just so down, and the feeling was not a good one. It was not a good one".

For aggression, some students felt aggressive toward the students and school personnel following the incident. Two students recount the aggression they felt after their corporal punishment: "it made me feel like, it made me feel like I'm fighting, fighting whoever that was paddling me there" and "I wanted to hit the lady myself". Another common and related feeling was anger: "I was mad before, and I was mad after. I was mad"; "I felt very betrayed and and and fed up"; and lastly, "It made me mad, I was angry. I was angry and I was emotional and in pain. I was emotional because the licks hurted, they hurt". For depression, most students felt very sad or even depressed after the incident: "I was also feeling bad and depressed because I could not feel happy again throughout my stay in school for the day. I was just so depressed because it was painful". And "I felt so bad like, I cried, even when I was kneeling down. So it was a very bad experience, like the worst experience I had". After having an argument with his teacher, Stanley, a 21-year-old Black

American man, recounts his traumatic experience: "Well, I still have the scar on my back. Yeah, I still have the scars on my back. . . . before he used the ruler on me, he! He actually slapped me on the face so, and then he he used the ruler to hit my back. . . . he actually cracked one of my ribs". Many former students had scars or bruises following the incident. One student recounts the depression and pain she felt following the incident: "I felt so depressed, and I felt pain all over my body because she flogged me all over my body. She even asked me to stretch out my hands".

For embarrassment, most students felt embarrassed, often because the punishment was carried out in public in front of the class. Sammy, a 37-year-old Black American woman, recounts the embarrassment she felt: "I felt like that should have been done at least privately because now I got to worry about the classmates who aren't my friends. Probably back there laughing. It was extremely embarrassing for me". Likewise, Megan, a 45-year-old White American woman, recounts how the embarrassment negatively affected her academic performance: "I definitely did not learn anything after I was embarrassed". Ultimately, these feelings and experiences were traumatic for the student—with most incidences negatively impacting their academic performance.

10. Compounded Trauma

Most participants received corporal punishment at home from their parents or guardians following the corporal punishment they received at school. They were also more likely to receive corporal punishment regularly in the home. This finding is supported by Taylor et al.'s [37] study, which revealed that Black Americans from southern states believe corporal punishment is a necessary component of effective parenting. One former student, Felix, an 18-year-old Black American man, recounts the following: "sometimes, they [school administration] would report me to my parent, and my dad is going to give me the beating of my life". Moreover, most participants whose parents were available during the school day (e.g., the parents left work early or did not work) received corporal punishment first by their teacher or principal and then by their parents on the school campus. Sarah, a 31-year-old Black American woman, recounts her mother beating her at school: "So I had got a paddling that day and then my mom came up that day as well and took me in the [school] bathroom and whooped me as well". Those parents who could not leave home beat their child once they returned home from school.

When rationalizing why his parents signed the school's consent form that permitted corporal punishment, former student Jason, a 22-year-old Black American man, believed that it was part of the Black American culture: "Yeah, I felt like they signed it because in the Black culture, corporal punishment is even adopted in homes in the Black culture. So, I felt like they had assigned it as a way of getting me disciplined". According to Jason, corporal punishment at home happened regularly, so it occurring at school was not unexpected or surprising. This statement of the participant is supported by the study conducted by Duong et al. [41], which indicates that Black American parents believe corporal punishment is an effective and normal method of disciplinary action that worked for them when they were children. Still, one student, who was not corporally punished at previous schools and was rarely beaten at home, felt shock; she said, "It was traumatic because like I said, I came from somewhere where that [school beatings] wasn't an option. I didn't know anything about it. It wasn't nothing that I was aware of it. Well, I'm not going to say kind of, it scarred me". Most students experienced compounded trauma at home and on campus which, in turn, led to subsequent secrecy and shame.

11. Secrecy and Shame

Students who experienced corporal punishment at school often did not tell their parents for fear of additional disciplining at home. Laila, a 22-year-old Black American woman, talks about having to keep this traumatic experience a secret: "I couldn't tell my parents about it, because I know they wouldn't stand with me. They might give me another punishment". In contrast, Tony, a 24-year-old Black American man, said he told his father, who just laughed at him. His father told him not to take the incident seriously and that students are always flogged in school. CPS is normal. As a result of his father laughing at him, he did not tell anyone else about the harsh beating. He felt like he was solely responsible for the traumatic experience. Mindy, a 23-year-old Black American woman, had a similar experience: "At that time [during elementary school], I wasn't with my parents, so I was staying with my elder sister, I told her, but she just laughed over it. She said: That's how they do, they flog students in school when they misbehave. So, she advised me not to do anything that leads to them flogging me again, not to go against the school rules and regulations". CPS lead to primary and compounded trauma as well as secondary trauma.

12. School Culture and Peer Effects

The only consistent thing about corporal punishment in Mississippi was how often it was administrated to students and how it negatively impacted the students who received the corporal punishment and their peers who did not. One student recounts that a peer was punished for stealing something: "He was flogged severely. They flogged him mercilessly. He had wounds, he sustained some wounds on his body... I was scared". Another student, 21-year-old Jamal, recounts a traumatic experience for him when his friend was beaten for something he did not do: "He had a marks on his back, and he cried. I actually helped him to the school clinic. He actually needed treatment. And then his dad came and picked him up. And that was the last I saw of him... I felt angry because he [the teacher] was actually punishing the wrong person, and it was not really that necessary to actually beat him". Other students were punished for making noise/talking, missing or performing poorly on assignments, tardiness, not being where they were supposed to be at a certain time, etc. Another student, Rally, a 21-year-old Black American man, believes that "corporal punishment is like the norm, or like a culture being beaten by the Mississippi personnel". Corporal punishment was part of the school culture and often led to secondary trauma experienced by peers and friends. There is a significant impact of secondary trauma on a child's cognitive ability, their emotional health, their behavior, their physical health, and their personal relationships [27]. Students did not know when to expect CPS for themselves or their peers, which resulted in more trauma.

13. Lack of Consistency

There was a general lack of consistency in how corporal punishment was administered, with incidences ranging from being slapped in the face, made to crawl across pavement, or hold painful positions for long periods of time. Perpetrators were usually teachers and principals, but sometimes even other students, mainly high school seniors, which is a violation of a school law that states that only teachers, assistant teachers, principals, and assistant principals can administer corporal punishment in Mississippi. This inconsistency aligns with the findings of Smith and Hains [46], who emphasize that school discipline policies vary in accordance with the philosophies and beliefs of educators guiding discipline processes. Perpetrators hit students with their hands, paddles, or canes on the buttocks and thighs. Some students were also slapped in the face, pinched, or made to hold painful positions for long periods of time. For example, Mindy, a Black American woman, recounts:

"We were asked to kneel down and carry up a heavy load in our hands, and after sometimes when the teacher when we were getting exhausted, she would then flog us on the back" with a cane. Some students were even asked to crawl back and forth across the floor, which hurt.

14. Racial Biases

There were certain distinctions between White American and Black American participants, with Black American participants often receiving CPS while their White American peers were exempt. For example, Tony, a Black American man who was punished after getting into a heated argument with a fellow student who was a White American, said. "The teacher flogged me, and also asked me to kneel down for a very long time, but the White students was not punished". He believed the incident was racist and that the teacher, who was Black, was operating out of fear: "I felt she was working on the instructions of a White teacher. I felt maybe she was scared of what will happen if she flogged the White student". When talking about how he was paddled seven or eight times for a fight he had with a White American boy, Jim remembers that "The white boy was not punished. . .I can't even, you know, face on the facts that I was beaten. And yeah, I stayed away from the school for like about three days or so before I continued". Black American students often felt that they were being targeted and treated as less than human because they were Black American by both White American and Black American school personnel and students. Overall, former Black American students felt that White American students who committed the same infraction were not punished.

15. Strained Relationships and Push-Out

Following the corporal punishment, students felt dislike or hatred for their teachers, principals, and students. Additionally, they were more likely to skip school or drop out following the incident. Bella, a 25-year-old woman, recounts the strained relationship she experienced with her teacher after she was caned repeatedly all over her body: "It can also lead to emotional distress like fear and anxiety. I couldn't approach her. So that was how it affected my academic performance, because I was always scared of her". Another former student, a 24-year-old Black American man, similarly feels that the incident "really affects my relationship [with the teachers and principal] because most times, if I have any problem, I wish I would have talked to them, but I wasn't able to talk to them because I was actually scared". Other students hated their teacher or principal for inflicting pain on them. Two students recounted that they hated their teachers: "I almost hated the teacher" and "it made me hate that teacher at that moment. I hated her so much for inflicting that bruise on me and I wished that it wasn't that way". Other former students stayed away from school following the incident, while other former students wanted to change schools or drop out.

16. Recommendations for Change

Students had useful insights into recommendations for change, such as more government oversight and scholarly research on CPS as well as more humane treatment and individual therapy and counseling instead of CPS. For example, Jamal, a Black American man, argues that school personnel should recognize the full humanity of their students: "if we are being treated as human, treated as part of the community, yeah, I feel we would actually get along better". Stanley, a 21-year-old Black American man, argues that "it should actually be something the government should look into, because most schools actually misuse corporal punishment for their own benefit, you know. Yeah, like a teacher because he has authority over the student, he would want to punish the kids for his own pleasure". He felt like that was the case for him and his friends. Moreover, Tony believes that "the government should try to oversee what is happening in schools. Try to, you know, try to minimize the rates of corporal punishment in school so that this will not affect the students". This suggestion aligns with the findings of Irby and Clough [43], who highlighted that it is essential that teachers practice consistency in order to ensure that their students are treated fairly and equally. Moreover, Jason believes that more research is needed to ensure that corporal punishment is the best option and whether something else will work better. Lastly, Rally, a Black American man, said that he felt trained professionals (e.g., psychologists and counselors) were needed to address the underlying root causes of student misbehavior. Overall, former students had unique insights into recommendations for change, having experienced corporal punishment and witnessed it among peers.

17. Discussion

We found the following overarching themes: (1) students experienced primary trauma at school following CPS and compounded trauma when their parents found out about their misbehavior; (2) students often did not tell their parents about their punishment for fear of an additional punishment, and instead shouldered the burden alone; (3) there was a lack of consistency in how corporal punishment was administered; (4) corporal punishment was part of the school culture and negatively affected peers, leading to secondary trauma; (5) many Black American participants felt that there were racial biases at play wherein their White American peers were exempt from punishment, but they were not for committing the same infractions; and (6) former students had multiple recommendations for change. The most common were more academic research, government oversight, and individual counseling for the misbehaving student over corporal punishment, specifically, more research on corporal punishment and disparities and more government oversight of the execution of corporal punishment.

These findings align with and extend prior findings. For example, Cruz et al. [9] found that students who experienced physical trauma felt less faith in their perpetrators and in authority figures more generally. Likewise, our participants felt less trust in school officials, parents, and guardians due to corporal punishment. Additionally, the American Psychiatric Association studied the psychological consequences of traumatic exposure and found that youth who experienced trauma had post-traumatic stress [12]. Likewise, our participants felt fear, anxiety, and depression following their instance(s) of trauma. Lastly, Benight and Bandura [29] found that following a traumatic incident, youth had an inability to recover. Likewise, former students often recounted how the event(s) scarred them for life—how they will never forget their experiences with corporal punishment. It is imperative that children be provided with a safe, nonthreatening environment in which safety and the establishment of trust are prioritized in order to heal trauma such as secondary trauma. They also felt that the instances affected their current behavior as adults.

Though our findings align well with the previous literature, we also make valuable contributions to it. First, students experienced compounded trauma on campus by both parents and teachers, and at home by parents and guardians. While prior research finds that students who experience corporal punishment at home are more likely to experience it at school, prior research has yet to find how students are beaten on campus and off-campus by their parents or guardians following and related to incidents of corporal punishment. In that context, students felt fear that if they told their parents, they would be beaten twice—once at school and once at home. As such, students often kept their instances of corporal punishment at school a secret.

More research is needed on the administration and effects of CPS: for example, "corporal punishment in public schools persists in over a third of U.S. states, yet very little is known about how it is administered or what potential unintended effects it may have on students" [34], p. 8. We found that there was a general lack of consistency in how punishment was administered and who was allowed to administer it. While research has previously documented physical assault, there is limited information on students' experiences with painful positions (sitting on the wall) or tasks (crawling on gravel). These instances of corporal punishment reflect a keen form of school torture that should be further explored in the literature. Moreover, while research has well documented the level of trauma felt by victims who receive corporal punishment at school, there is an acute gap in research on the peer effects of trauma. Overall, secondary trauma among children is limited, but it is important to fully theorize the phenomenon of childhood trauma. We found that students experienced trauma when they saw their friends or classmates being beaten regardless of whether they themselves were in immediate danger.

Moreover, while research has quantified racial disparities particularly between White American and Black American students, there is a lack of research on the racial demographics of the perpetrator. Here, we find that both Black American and White American teachers and principals are guilty of beating Black American children for the same infractions that White American children are not punished for and how that negatively impacted the punished students' participation in school and psychological well-being. Lastly, we share recommendations for change from those who have experienced corporal punishment. While research aligns well with these recommendations, it is critical to give voice and space to those who were traumatized to share recommendations for change.

Although not discussed explicitly, we also found that participants experienced a lack of trust in the government (e.g., a reluctance to speak to school personnel or ask for help) and in their parents and guardians (e.g., a tendency to keep the CPS a secret). While research aligns with this finding, we extend it to include the parents (e.g., not just the school personnel). These findings are important to understanding the full scope of trauma experienced by students in Mississippi, which we believe generalizes to the other 22 states that allow corporal punishment. Our last contribution and arguably the most important is this: corporal punishment is still happening in American schools. We hope that this contemporary analysis of corporal punishment practices in American schools published in a flagship journal will remind the world of the legally state-sanctioned violence happening every day in American schools—a practice that is antithetical to American ideals and, we believe, violates our schoolchildren's fundamental human rights.

In terms of implications, we call for the abolishment of CPS. We ask educational stakeholders to push for the reversal of CPS legality because it is ineffective and traumatic. At the very least, students and families should be allowed due process. CPS takes an emotional and psychological toll on students, which demonstrates the need for comprehensive support systems in schools. There is a lack of information and resources available to teachers to address trauma in their daily practice [59]. Additionally, the measurement of secondary trauma has received relatively little research attention, and most of the assessment devices available are designed for therapists rather than for the general public or for children [26]. To facilitate the development of trauma-informed instructional practices, educators will need to gain a deeper understanding of the implications that complex trauma can have for brain development [60]. A teacher or teaching assistant with appropriate training can achieve results similar to those provided by a trained therapist [61].

Implications of the study call for concerted efforts from educators, policymakers, and parents to prioritize the well-being and dignity of all students. Addressing fear, eliminating gender and racial disparities, providing support for affected children, and promoting parental engagement will create safer and more nurturing learning environments for every child in US schools. Schools should not use corporal punishment as a disciplinary strategy because it has negative psychological effects, is ineffective, poses a risk of physical injury, and negatively impacts students' academic performance. Rather, educators should implement nonviolent disciplinary methods that promote positive behavior, respect children's rights, and ensure a safe and supportive learning environment. Again, so long as corporal punishment is used in schools, students should have an opportunity for due process—something they currently do not have.

18. Conclusions

This study makes an important contribution to our understanding of how former victims of corporal punishment in schools process traumatic events. The findings fill a gap in the literature related to corporal punishment in schools and help us understand the critical role school personnel, parents, and even students play in shaping the academic outcomes, shock, and psychological stress students face when exposed to corporal punishment regularly. This study also demonstrates the value of applying childhood trauma theories to K-12 research, in this case, by focusing on archaic educational structures and practices as problematic rather than placing all blame on misbehaving children. Future research on the topic of corporal punishment in American schools should deepen and extend the use of childhood trauma as a conceptual framework to guide study design, research methods, and analysis. Our capacity to create positive, instead of traumatic, experiences for students is dependent on our ability to think in new ways about old laws like corporal punishment in schools.

Author Contributions: Conceptualization, D.T.; Methodology, J.R.F.; Formal analysis, D.T. and R.K.; Data curation, B.V.; Writing—original draft, D.T.; Writing—review & editing, D.T., R.K., B.V. and J.R.F.; Supervision, J.R.F.; Funding acquisition, D.T. All authors have read and agreed to the published version of the manuscript.

Funding: This research was generously funded by Helping Hand's Social Justice Award.

Institutional Review Board Statement: The study was conducted in accordance with the Institutional Review Board of California Lutheran University, IRB-FY2024-20, 27 September 2024.

Informed Consent Statement: Informed consent was obtained from all subjects involved in the study.

Data Availability Statement: The raw data supporting the conclusions of this article will be made available by the authors on request due to privacy of the participants.

Conflicts of Interest: There are no conflicts of interest.

References

1. Whitaker, A.; Losen, D.J. The Striking Outlier: The Persistent, Painful and Problematic Practice of Corporal Punishment in Schools; K-12 Racial Disparities in School Discipline, Issue U. T. C. R. Project. 2019. Available online: https://escholarship.org/uc/item/9d19p8wt (accessed on 5 April 2025).
2. Cardona, M.A. Key Policy Letters Signed by the Education Secretary or Deputy Secretary. 2023. Available online: https://www.ed.gov/laws-and-policy/education-policy/key-policy-letters-signed-by-the-education-secretary-or-deputy-secretary/march-24-2023--letter-from-secretary-cardona-calling-for-an-end-to-corporal-punishment-in-schools (accessed on 28 March 2025).
3. AACAP Corporal Punishment in Schools. 2014. Available online: https://www.aacap.org/aacap/Policy_Statements/1988/Corporal_Punishment_in_Schools.aspx (accessed on 7 April 2025).
4. Gershoff, E.T.; Font, S.A. Corporal punishment in US public schools: Prevalence, disparities in use, and status in state and federal policy. *Soc. Policy Rep.* **2016**, *30*, 1. [CrossRef] [PubMed]
5. Heekes, S.-L.; Kruger, C.B.; Lester, S.N.; Ward, C.L. A Systematic Review of Corporal Punishment in Schools: Global Prevalence and Correlates. *Trauma Violence Abus.* **2022**, *23*, 52–72. [CrossRef] [PubMed]
6. McLoyd, V.C.; Kaplan, R.; Hardaway, C.R.; Wood, D. Does endorsement of physical discipline matter? Assessing moderating influences on the maternal and child psychological correlates of physical discipline in African American families. *J. Fam. Psychol.* **2007**, *21*, 165. [CrossRef]

7. Gershoff, E.; Sattler, K.M.; Holden, G.W. School corporal punishment and its associations with achievement and adjustment. *J. Appl. Dev. Psychol.* **2019**, *63*, 1–8. [CrossRef] [PubMed]
8. Laskey, A.L. Corporal Punishment and Children's Report Cards—Failing Our Children. *JAMA Pediatr.* **2019**, *173*, 132–133. [CrossRef]
9. Cruz, D.; Lichten, M.; Berg, K.; George, P. Developmental trauma: Conceptual framework, associated risks and comorbidities, and evaluation and treatment. *Front. Psychiatry* **2022**, *13*, 800687. [CrossRef]
10. Fairbank, J.A.; Fairbank, D.W. Epidemiology of child traumatic stress. *Curr. Psychiatry Rep.* **2009**, *11*, 289–295. [CrossRef]
11. Sideli, L.; Mule, A.; La Barbera, D.; Murray, R.M. Do child abuse and maltreatment increase risk of schizophrenia? *Psychiatry Investig.* **2012**, *9*, 87. [CrossRef]
12. Kawa, S.; Giordano, J. *A Brief Historicity of the Diagnostic and Statistical Manual of Mental Disorders: Issues and Implications for the Future of Psychiatric Canon and Practice*; Springer: Berlin/Heidelberg, Germany, 2012; Volume 7, pp. 1–9.
13. de Bellis, M.D.; Zisk, A. The biological effects of childhood trauma. *Child Adolesc. Psychiatr. Clin.* **2014**, *23*, 185–222. [CrossRef]
14. Bethell, C.; Jones, J.; Gombojav, N.; Linkenbach, J.; Sege, R. Positive childhood experiences and adult mental and relational health in a statewide sample: Associations across adverse childhood experiences levels. *JAMA Pediatr.* **2019**, *173*, e193007. [CrossRef]
15. Craig, S.E. The trauma-sensitive teacher. *Educ. Leadersh.* **2016**, *74*, 28–32.
16. Craig, S.E. *Trauma-Sensitive Schools for the Adolescent Years: Promoting Resiliency and Healing, Grades 6–12*; Teachers College Press: New York, NY, USA, 2017.
17. Rossen, E.; Cowan, K. The role of schools in supporting traumatized students. *Princ. Res. Rev.* **2013**, *8*, 1–8.
18. Smith, L. *Adverse Childhood Experiences (ACEs): Interventions in Education*; IRSS: Scotland, UK, 2018. Available online: https://www.iriss.org.uk/resources/esss-outlines/aces (accessed on 5 April 2025).
19. Pellegrini, S.; Moore, P.; Murphy, M. Secondary trauma and related concepts in psychologists: A systematic review. *J. Aggress. Maltreatment Trauma* **2022**, *31*, 370–391. [CrossRef]
20. Figley, C.R. Compassion fatigue as secondary traumatic stress disorder-An overview. In *Compassion Fatigue*; Routledge: New York, NY, USA, 1995.
21. National Child Traumatic Stress Network, S.T.S.C. *Secondary Traumatic Stress: A Fact Sheet for Child-Serving Professionals*; The Learning Center: Los Angeles, CA, USA, 2011.
22. Marshall, R.; Galea, S. Special issue: Update on posttraumatic stress disorder. *J. Clin. Psychiatry* **2004**, *65*, 37–43.
23. Propper, R.E.; Stickgold, R.; Keeley, R.; Christman, S.D. Is television traumatic?: Dreams, stress, and media exposure in the aftermath of September 11, 2001. *Psychol. Sci.* **2007**, *18*, 334–340. [CrossRef]
24. Newell, J.M.; MacNeil, G.A. Professional burnout, vicarious trauma, secondary traumatic stress, and compassion fatigue. *Best Pract. Ment. Health* **2010**, *6*, 57–68. [CrossRef]
25. Bride, B.E.; Kintzle, S. Secondary traumatic stress, job satisfaction, and occupational commitment in substance abuse counselors. *Traumatology* **2011**, *17*, 22–28. [CrossRef]
26. Motta, R.W. Secondary trauma in children and school personnel. *J. Appl. Sch. Psychol.* **2012**, *28*, 256–269. [CrossRef]
27. ACF. Secondary Traumatic Stress. 2024. Available online: https://www.acf.hhs.gov/trauma-toolkit/secondary-traumatic-stress (accessed on 5 April 2025).
28. Deb, S.; Kumar, A.; Holden, G.W.; Simpson Rowe, L. School corporal punishment, family tension, and students' internalizing problems: Evidence from India. *Sch. Psychol. Int.* **2017**, *38*, 60–77. [CrossRef]
29. Benight, C.C.; Bandura, A. Social cognitive theory of posttraumatic recovery: The role of perceived self-efficacy. *Behav. Trust. Res. Ther.* **2004**, *42*, 1129–1148. [CrossRef]
30. Devries, K.M.; Child, J.C.; Allen, E.; Walakira, E.; Parkes, J.; Naker, D. School violence, mental health, and educational performance in Uganda. *Pediatrics* **2014**, *133*, e129–e137. [CrossRef] [PubMed]
31. Han, S. Corporal punishment and student outcomes in rural schools. *Educ. Res. Policy Pract.* **2014**, *13*, 221–231. [CrossRef]
32. Talwar, V.; Carlson, S.M.; Lee, K. Effects of a punitive environment on children's executive functioning: A natural experiment. *Soc. Dev.* **2011**, *20*, 805–824. [CrossRef]
33. 3UNICEF. Protecting Children from Violence in School. 2021. Available online: https://www.unicef.org/protection/violence-against-children-in-school (accessed on 5 April 2025).
34. Ward, G.; Petersen, N.; Kupchik, A.; Pratt, J. Historic Lynching and Corporal Punishment in Contemporary Southern Schools. *Soc. Probl.* **2021**, *68*, 41–62. [CrossRef]
35. Patton, S.; Rollo, T.; Curry, T.J. "The first mark of pain": Toward a child-centered methodological reorientation of social theory, race and corporal punishment in American life. *Sociol. Compass* **2021**, *15*, e12943. [CrossRef]
36. LeCuyer, E.A.; Christensen, J.J.; Kearney, M.H.; Kitzman, H.J. African American mothers' self-described discipline strategies with young children. *Issues Compr. Pediatr. Nurs.* **2011**, *34*, 144–162. [CrossRef]
37. Taylor, C.A.; Hamvas, L.; Paris, R. Perceived instrumentality and normativeness of corporal punishment use among black mothers. *Fam. Relat.* **2011**, *60*, 60–72. [CrossRef]

38. Lorber, M.F.; O'Leary, S.G.; Smith Slep, A.M. An initial evaluation of the role of emotion and impulsivity in explaining racial/ethnic differences in the use of corporal punishment. *Dev. Psychol.* **2011**, *47*, 1744. [CrossRef]
39. Su, D.; Toure, D.; Do, K.; Ramos, A.K. Assessing racial and ethnic differences in attitudes towards the use of physical discipline in parenting: A mixed-methods approach. *J. Soc. Serv. Res.* **2019**, *45*, 455–465. [CrossRef]
40. Klevens, J.; Mercer Kollar, L.; Rizzo, G.; O'Shea, G.; Nguyen, J.; Roby, S. Commonalities and differences in social norms related to corporal punishment among Black, Latino and White parents. *Child Adolesc. Soc. Work. J.* **2019**, *36*, 19–28. [CrossRef]
41. Duong, H.T.; Monahan, J.L.; Mercer Kollar, L.M.; Klevens, J. Examining sources of social norms supporting child corporal punishment among low-income Black, Latino, and White Parents. *Health Commun.* **2022**, *37*, 1413–1422. [CrossRef] [PubMed]
42. Welsh, R.O. Navigating tensions in school discipline: Examining school leaders, teachers, and the conversion of referrals into suspensions. *Am. J. Educ.* **2023**, *129*, 237–264. [CrossRef]
43. Irby, D.; Clough, C. Consistency rules: A critical exploration of a universal principle of school discipline. *Pedagog. Cult. Soc.* **2015**, *23*, 153–173. [CrossRef]
44. Williams, J.A., III. Middle School Teachers' Perceptions of School Administrators' Enforcement of School Rules for African American Students. *J. Classr. Interact.* **2022**, *56*, 4–16.
45. Griffith, D.; Tyner, A. *Discipline Reform Through the Eyes of Teachers*; Thomas, B., Ed.; Fordham Institute: Washington, DC, USA, 2019.
46. Smith, B.N.; Hains, B.J. Examining administrators' disciplinary philosophies: A conceptual model. *Educ. Adm. Q.* **2012**, *48*, 548–576. [CrossRef]
47. Kennedy, B.L.; Murphy, A.S.; Jordan, A. Title I middle school administrators' beliefs and choices about using corporal punishment and exclusionary discipline. *Am. J. Educ.* **2017**, *123*, 243–280. [CrossRef]
48. Shabazian, A.N. Voices That Matter: Chief Administrative Officers' Role in the Student Discipline Gap. *Urban Educ.* **2020**, *55*, 66–94. [CrossRef]
49. MDE. Discipline. 2023. Available online: https://msrc.mdek12.org/discipline?EntityID=0000-000&SchoolYear=2022 (accessed on 5 April 2025).
50. CRDC. Corporal Punishment in Public Schools. 2023. Available online: https://civilrightsdata.ed.gov/assets/downloads/Corporal_Punishment_Part4.pdf (accessed on 5 April 2025).
51. James, J. Corporal Punishment Was Used in Schools 4300 Times Last Year. Here's What Districts Are Doing to Change That. 2023. Available online: https://mississippitoday.org/2023/02/07/corporal-punishment-mississippi-schools/ (accessed on 5 April 2025).
52. MDE. Student Enrollment Data. *Mississippi Department of Education*. 2024. Available online: https://newreports.mdek12.org/DataExplorer (accessed on 5 April 2025).
53. Gülirmak Güler, K.; Uzun, S.; Emirza, E.G. Secondary Traumatic Stress and Coping Experiences in Psychiatric Nurses Caring for Trauma Victims: A Phenomenological Study. *J. Psychiatr. Ment. Health Nurs.* **2025**, *32*, 402–413. [CrossRef]
54. Strauss, A.L.; Corbin, J.M. *Basics of Qualitative Research: Grounded Theory Procedures and Techniques*; Sage Publications: Newbury Park, CA, USA, 1990.
55. Silverman, D.; Marvasti, A. *Doing Qualitative Research: A Comprehensive Guide*; Sage: New York, NY, USA, 2008.
56. Miles, M.B.; Huberman, A.M.; Saldaña, J. *Qualitative Data Analysis: A Methods Sourcebook and the Coding Manual for Qualitative Researchers*; SAGE Publication Inc.: New York, NY, USA, 2015.
57. Saldana, J. *Writing Qualitatively: The Selected Works of Johnny Saldaña*; Routledge: Oxfordshire, UK, 2018.
58. Krefting, L. Rigor in qualitative research: The assessment of trustworthiness. *Am. J. Occup. Ther.* **1991**, *45*, 214–222. [CrossRef]
59. Crosby, S.D.; Day, A.; Baroni, B.A.; Somers, C. Examining trauma-informed teaching and the trauma symptomatology of court-involved girls. *Urban Rev.* **2019**, *51*, 582–598. [CrossRef]
60. Wolpow, R.; Johnson, M.; Hertel, R.; Kincaid, S. *Learning and Teaching: Compassion, Resiliency, and Academic Success*; Office of the Superintendent of Public Instruction: Olympia, WA, USA, 2011.
61. Luthar, S.S.; Mendes, S.H. Trauma-informed schools: Supporting educators as they support the children. *Int. J. Sch. Educ. Psychol.* **2020**, *8*, 147–157. [CrossRef]

children

MDPI

Article

Teacher Personality Predicts Emotional Well-Being and Academic Achievement in Students with Specific Learning Disorders

Wanqin Yu, Olivia F. Ward, Brianna Paquette, Sylvie Mrug and Caroline G. Richter *

Department of Psychology, The University of Alabama at Birmingham, 1720 2nd Ave S, Birmingham, AL 35294, USA; yuw@uab.edu (W.Y.); oward@uab.edu (O.F.W.); bristein@uab.edu (B.P.); sylva@uab.edu (S.M.)
* Correspondence: carolinerichter@uab.edu; Tel.: +1-205-934-9897

Abstract: Background/Objectives: Students with specific learning disorders (SLDs) are at increased risk for emotional and academic difficulties. While teacher characteristics can influence student outcomes, few studies have examined the role of teacher personality in supporting students with SLDs. This study investigated whether teacher personality traits predicted student emotional well-being and academic achievement in a school-based intervention context. **Methods**: Participants were 64 students with SLDs (Mage = 13.28) nested within 21 teachers. Students completed measures of emotional well-being at baseline and post-intervention, and grade point average (GPA) was obtained from school records at the end of the school year. Teachers completed the Big Five Inventory mid-intervention. Two-level multilevel models were conducted in Mplus using maximum likelihood estimation with robust standard errors (MLR). The models controlled for student and teacher demographics, baseline emotional well-being, and the intervention group. Missing data were addressed using full information maximum likelihood (FIML). **Results**: Teacher female sex, higher neuroticism, and lower teaching experience were associated with higher student emotional well-being post-intervention. Follow-up analyses confirmed that teacher sex, neuroticism, and conscientiousness each explained substantial between-teacher variance. In the GPA model, student sex and teacher openness were significant predictors, with female students and students taught by more open teachers earning higher GPAs. **Conclusions**: Teacher personality traits, specifically neuroticism, conscientiousness, and openness, were associated with emotional and academic outcomes among students with SLDs. The findings highlight the importance of considering teacher characteristics in designing school-based interventions to support the development of learners with SLDs or other neurodevelopmental disorders.

Keywords: teacher personality; big five traits; emotional well-being; academic achievement; specific learning disorders; multilevel modeling

1. Introduction

Because students spend a significant portion of their lives in school, teachers are key figures in promoting both their emotional well-being and academic achievement [1,2]. Given the pivotal role teachers play in children's lives, understanding teacher-related factors, such as personality, may inform how education systems tailor support to foster positive student outcomes. This is particularly critical for students who are at heightened risk for school-related challenges, such as those with specific learning disorders (SLDs) [3,4]. The present study examined how teacher personality traits relate to emotional well-being and academic achievement in students with SLDs.

 https://doi.org/10.3390/children12060764

SLDs are a group of neurodevelopmental disorders characterized by difficulties in academic domains such as reading, comprehension, spelling, written expression, and/or mathematics [5]. SLDs are among the most prevalent disorders in school-aged children, with rates estimated between 5% and 15% [6,7]. These disorders can negatively impact not only students' academic performance but also their social and emotional development [3,8,9]. Because many students with SLDs face ongoing academic struggles and repeated failure in school, they are more likely to experience frustration, lowered self-esteem, and negative perceptions of their abilities. These experiences contribute to elevated levels of internalizing problems, such as anxiety, depression, and general psychological distress, that are widely reported in this population. In particular, SLDs have been identified as a risk factor for internalizing problems that contribute to poorer emotional well-being [4,9–12]. These challenges often persist into adulthood and are associated with lower rates of college completion, underemployment, and increased interaction with the criminal justice system [13]. Nonetheless, many students with SLDs go on to achieve success and often attribute their progress to positive relationships with teachers, peers, and mentors [14,15]. This aligns with a cumulative risk and resilience perspective, which emphasizes that the presence of protective factors, such as supportive relationships, can buffer the negative effects of learning difficulties [16].

Insights from attachment theory support the importance of teacher–student relationships in shaping emotional outcomes. Attachment theory suggests that behaviors aimed at establishing closeness and contact with adult figures (e.g., parents) are maintained to aid in meeting the child's needs [17]. Teacher–student relationships mimic parent–child relationships in that they both involve care, teaching, and discipline [18]. As such, teachers can become a secure base as children navigate the world [19]. Previous studies have found that greater perceived teacher support positively predicts students' abilities to navigate academic challenges [20], greater student academic efficacy [21], and greater student academic achievement [22]. Given the integral role teachers play in students' lives, it is critical to understand how teacher characteristics, such as personality traits, may influence outcomes for students with SLDs.

1.1. Teacher Personality in an Educational Context

While much of the literature has focused on the instructional or relational roles teachers play, emerging research highlights the importance of teacher personality in shaping students' school experiences. Personality theory, particularly the Five-Factor Model, offers a valuable framework for understanding how individual differences among teachers may influence educational processes [23]. In particular, traits such as conscientiousness, emotional stability, and extraversion are identified as especially relevant for effective teaching, with conscientiousness supporting structured and goal-oriented classroom management, emotional stability helping teachers manage negative emotions, and extraversion contributing to classroom engagement and positive teacher–student interactions [23].

Meta-analytic evidence underscores the relevance of teacher personality in relation to teacher effectiveness, a construct closely tied to classroom organization, instructional quality, and professional competence [24]. Among the Big Five traits, extraversion demonstrates the strongest overall association with teacher effectiveness, followed by conscientiousness, emotional stability, and openness. These traits are consistently linked to positive teaching behaviors across multiple rating sources. Agreeableness, in contrast, is not significantly associated with teacher effectiveness; it is also not consistently linked to key instructional or classroom outcomes across studies [24]. In addition, researchers have found that teachers with a "well-adjusted" personality profile, characterized by high conscientiousness, extraversion, agreeableness, and openness, and low neuroticism, report greater self-efficacy, engagement with students, and job satisfaction [25]. These qualities may help foster emotionally supportive and structured classrooms that are particularly beneficial for students with SLDs. Indeed, research has shown that teacher self-efficacy plays a central role in shaping instructional quality, classroom climate, and student academic adjustment [26].

1.2. Teacher Personality and Student Emotional Well-Being

Many individuals with SLDs experience elevated levels of anxiety, depression, poor mental health, and lower self-esteem in addition to their academic challenges [12]. These internalizing difficulties can further hinder academic success [27,28], creating a negative cycle that compounds the challenges already faced by students with SLDs. However, not all students with SLDs report poor emotional well-being; many demonstrate positive adjustment despite risk factors associated with their SLD [15,29]. Teacher support, in particular, has been identified as a key protective factor in this process [30,31]. Among typically developing students, positive student–teacher relationships are associated with greater student emotional well-being [32]. When compared to support from caregivers and peers, teacher support has been shown to demonstrate the strongest association with students' emotional well-being [33]. Therefore, understanding teacher-related factors is critical for fostering emotional well-being in students with and without SLDs.

Research suggests that positive student–teacher relationships are characterized by high levels of closeness and warmth and low levels of conflict [34,35]. Therefore, teachers who are able to foster closeness and minimize conflict may be better positioned to support students with SLDs. Additionally, students who perceive greater teacher support report higher levels of emotional well-being, both in general school populations [33] and among students with SLDs [30]. As such, teacher personality traits, such as agreeableness, extraversion, conscientiousness, and openness, that facilitate supportive, low-conflict relationships may be particularly important for promoting emotional well-being in students with SLDs.

1.3. Teacher Personality and Student Academic Achievement

In addition to well-being, teacher support may also contribute to improved academic outcomes. For example, emotional support from homeroom teachers has been shown to positively predict class-level academic achievement, in part by fostering a more emotionally positive classroom climate [36,37]. Similarly, teacher emotional support has been linked to improved student math performance, with effects mediated by students' academic self-efficacy and behavioral engagement [38]. Extensive meta-analytic evidence supports the link between teacher–student relationships and academic achievement, including GPA. Positive affective relationships have been shown to promote school engagement and learning outcomes [39], while emotionally supportive classroom climates have been associated with higher academic performance and reduced socioemotional distress [37]. These findings suggest that teacher traits promoting supportive, emotionally responsive interactions may be beneficial not only for students' well-being but also their academic success.

Among students without academic difficulties, positive student–teacher relationships are associated with higher academic achievement [40]. Students with SLDs tend to demonstrate lower academic performance than their typically developing peers, as their learning difficulties often affect information processing and subject-specific skills [41]. However, research suggests that with appropriate instruction, accommodations, and contextual supports, students with SLDs can achieve academic outcomes comparable to their peers [6,16,42]. These findings underscore the importance of identifying factors that influence academic achievement in this population. One such factor may be teachers' personality traits.

Research has yielded mixed findings regarding the impact of teachers' personality traits on student outcomes. Some studies suggest that traits such as extraversion, conscientiousness, agreeableness, and openness to experience are associated with greater student academic achievement in general education settings [43–47]. In contrast, other research has shown that teacher personality traits are more predictive of subjective measures of teaching effectiveness than of students' objective academic achievement [24,48]. These findings suggest that while certain teacher traits may help students feel more supported, this does not always translate into measurable academic gains. Notably, most of this research has been conducted with general student populations, leaving open questions about whether these patterns hold for students with SLDs. Because students with SLDs often benefit from individualized and sustained teacher support, it is important to examine how teacher personality traits may influence their academic achievement.

1.4. Current Study

The present study aimed to examine the associations between teacher personality traits and student outcomes, specifically, emotional well-being and academic achievement, among adolescents with SLDs. Demographic variables, including the age and sex of both students and teachers, and teachers' years of teaching experience, were included as covariates due to their previously documented associations with student outcomes [49,50]. Based on previous studies [23–25,44,46,47], it was hypothesized that teacher traits of openness, conscientiousness, extraversion, and agreeableness would positively predict student academic achievement and emotional well-being over time, controlling for baseline characteristics. In contrast, teacher neuroticism was expected to negatively predict both student outcomes.

2. Methods

2.1. Procedure

Data for the current study were collected as part of a larger longitudinal project evaluating the biopsychosocial outcomes of mindfulness-based instruction on adolescents with SLDs. Participants were randomly assigned to one of two social and emotional learning (SEL) curricula: a mindfulness-based SEL curriculum (MindUP) [51], or "Normal Isn't Real" (NIR), which aimed to promote neurodiversity awareness [52]. Both programs were administered by the teachers for 17 weeks. This study was publicly preregistered on ClinicalTrials.gov, https://clinicaltrials.gov/study/NCT05787483 (accessed on 1 June 2025), including the research design and planned analyses, prior to data collection and analysis. The study protocol was reviewed and approved by the university's Institutional Review Board. Parents or legal guardians of all participants provided written informed consent, and participants provided written assent. Children completed the measures at their school, which were administered by trained doctoral students or research assistants and scored according to standardized procedures. For this study, surveys completed at specific timepoints were used: students completed surveys at baseline and at post-intervention (week 18), while teachers completed surveys at the intervention midpoint (week 9).

2.2. Participants

The initial sample included 68 students nested within 22 teachers. One teacher was excluded due to missing data on all Big Five personality traits, resulting in the removal of their three corresponding students. Additionally, one student was excluded prior to analysis after being identified as a statistical outlier, with a standardized residual of −2.70 and a disproportionate influence on residual normality. The final analytic sample consisted of 64 students nested within 21 teachers.

Participants included in this study were 64 students enrolled in Grades 5 through 12 at a private school in Alabama serving children and adolescents with learning disorders. Students ranged in age from 10 to 19 years ($M = 13.28$, $SD = 2.24$), with equal distribution by sex (50% female, 50% male) and a near-even split between intervention groups (46.9% MindUP, 53.1% NIR). Students in the MindUP group did not differ significantly from those in the NIR group in terms of age, $t(62) = 0.38$, $p = 0.703$; sex, $t(62) = 0.49$, $p = 0.623$; or baseline emotional well-being, $t(61) = 0.47$, $p = 0.643$.

A total of 21 teachers were included in this study, each responsible for an average of 4.39 students ($SD = 0.89$). Teachers ranged in age from 26 to 62 years ($M = 39.05$, $SD = 11.86$), with one participant missing age data. Most teachers were female (66.7%), and all identified as White and non-Hispanic. All teachers held at least a bachelor's degree, and 42.9% reported more than 10 years of teaching experience. Teachers in the MindUP and NIR groups did not differ significantly on sex, $t(19) = 1.56$, $p = 0.135$; years of teaching experience, $t(19) = -0.73$, $p = 0.473$; or any of the Big Five personality traits (all $ps > 0.05$).

2.3. Measures

2.3.1. Big Five Inventory-10 (BFI-10)

Teachers' personality traits were assessed using the BFI-10 [53], a brief 10-item self-report inventory designed to measure the Big Five personality domains: openness, conscientiousness, extraversion, agreeableness, and neuroticism. Each domain is assessed with two items. Teachers rated items on a 5-point Likert scale ranging from 1 (disagree strongly) to 5 (agree strongly), and trait scores were computed by averaging the two items corresponding to each domain. The BFI-10 has demonstrated strong part–whole correlations with the BFI-44 scales ($rs = 0.74$–0.89), acceptable test–retest reliability over 6–8 weeks ($rs = 0.65$–0.87), and good convergent and external validity [53]. Although internal consistency estimates were not reported in the original validation study, consistent with psychometric literature cautioning against the use of Cronbach's alpha for two-item scales [54], recent large-sample research has provided strong support for the BFI-10′s reliability. In a nationally representative Brazilian sample ($n = 3565$), the BFI-10 showed good reliability for all five traits, with omega coefficients ranging from 0.72 to 0.88 [55]. However, in the present sample ($n = 21$), only the extraversion subscale demonstrated acceptable internal consistency ($\alpha = 0.62$). The remaining subscales showed poor internal consistency: openness ($\alpha = 0.52$), neuroticism ($\alpha = 0.43$), agreeableness ($\alpha = 0.36$), and conscientiousness ($\alpha = 0.11$), likely reflecting both the scale's brevity and the small sample size.

2.3.2. Brief Multidimensional Students' Life Satisfaction Scale (BMSLSS-PTPB)

Students' emotional well-being was assessed using the Brief Multidimensional Students' Life Satisfaction Scale–Peabody Treatment Progress Battery version (BMSLSS–PTPB) [56]. This 6-item self-report measure was administered at baseline and post-intervention. Items were rated on a 5-point Likert scale ranging from 0 (very dissatisfied) to 5 (very satisfied). One item assesses overall life satisfaction, while the remaining five items assess satisfaction across specific life domains: family life, friendships, school experience, self-perception, and living environment. Scores were averaged to create a total emotional well-being score, with higher scores indicating greater life satisfaction. Internal consistency in the current sample was good at both timepoints, with Cronbach's alpha increasing from baseline ($\alpha = 0.80$) to post-intervention ($\alpha = 0.88$). This aligns with, and slightly exceeds, the previously reported reliability in clinical samples ($\alpha = 0.77$) [57] and falls within the range observed in normative school-based samples ($\alpha = 0.76$–0.85) [58].

2.3.3. Grade Point Average (GPA)

GPA was utilized to measure students' academic achievement. Students' GPA was reported by the school on a scale ranging from 0.0 to 4.0; grades of A (3.1–4.0) were reported as 4.0, grades of B (2.1–3.0) as 3.0, grades of C (1.1–2.0) as 2.0, grades of D (0.1–1.0) as 1.0, and grades of F as 0.0. Students' end-of-year GPA was calculated as the arithmetic mean of first-semester letter grades and second-semester letter grades. The courses considered in the calculation were math, English, history, science, and health. Students' school-reported GPA was obtained at the end of the school year, which corresponds to a few months post-intervention. Of the twenty-one teachers, five taught math, five taught English, three taught history, three taught science, and five were reading intervention teachers.

2.3.4. Demographics Survey

Student demographic information was collected through parent-reported data. Teacher demographic information was collected through self-reported surveys, including race, sex, years of teaching experience, and highest level of education. Teachers selected the label that best described their highest level of education from the following list: high school diploma or General Equivalency Diploma (GED), associate's degree, bachelor's degree, some graduate coursework (but no degree), master's degree, education specialist or professional diploma (post-master's), or doctorate.

2.4. Statistical Analyses

Missing data were examined, and cases with any vs. no missing data were compared on all variables using independent samples t-tests for continuous variables and chi-square tests of independence for categorical variables. Descriptive statistics were examined. Pearson's bivariate correlations were conducted among all primary study variables, evaluating three sets of associations among (1) student-level variables, (2) teacher-level variables, and (3) cross-level correlations between student and teacher characteristics.

Assumptions of multilevel modeling (MLM) were evaluated in SPSS (Version 30) prior to model estimation in Mplus. Restricted maximum likelihood (REML) was used during assumptions testing, as it provides unbiased estimates of variance components. Intraclass correlation coefficients (ICCs) were calculated using random intercept models to assess the proportion of variance attributable to the teacher level. The assumption of homoscedasticity was examined via residual plots and the Breusch–Pagan test. Normality of residuals was tested with Kolmogorov–Smirnov and Shapiro–Wilk tests. The linearity between continuous predictors and outcomes was evaluated with bivariate scatterplots. Finally, the absence of multicollinearity was verified with the variance inflation factor (VIF) and tolerance.

Main models were estimated in Mplus Version 8.1 using full information maximum likelihood (FIML) with the robust maximum likelihood (MLR) estimator to appropriately handle missing data and assumption violations. Two multilevel models with two levels were estimated to predict students' emotional well-being and GPA, respectively. In both models, students (Level 1) were nested within teachers (Level 2), and random intercepts were specified to account for this clustering. In the first model predicting students' post-intervention emotional well-being, student-level (within) predictors included age, sex at birth, intervention group, and baseline emotional well-being. Teacher-level (between) predictors included sex, years of teaching experience, and Big Five personality traits (extraversion, agreeableness, conscientiousness, neuroticism, and openness). In the second model predicting students' end-of-school-year GPA, student-level predictors were age, sex at birth, and intervention group, while teacher-level predictors were identical to those in the emotional well-being model. All continuous predictors were centered prior to analysis to facilitate interpretation of the results: student-level variables were group-mean-centered, and teacher-level variables were grand-mean-centered. Categorical predictors were dummy coded.

3. Results

3.1. Preliminary Analyses

Among the 64 students included in the analytic sample, 10.9% ($n = 7$) had missing data on emotional well-being variables used in the multilevel models. Specifically, six students were missing post-intervention emotional well-being scores, and one was missing baseline emotional well-being. Independent samples t-tests were conducted to examine whether this missingness was associated with any study variables. There was no significant difference in post-intervention emotional well-being between those with and without missing data, $t(56) = 0.32$, $p = 0.751$. A corrected t-test was used for end-of-school-year GPA due to unequal variances, which also revealed no significant difference, $t(6.50) = 1.46$, $p = 0.190$. Additionally, missingness was unrelated to all student-level covariates, including age, sex, intervention group, and baseline emotional well-being (all $ps > 0.05$), supporting the assumption that data were missing at random (MAR).

At the teacher level, there was a significant difference in years of teaching experience, $t(55.35) = -5.22$, $p < 0.001$, such that students with missing data had teachers with more experience ($M = 9.57$, $SD = 0.54$) than those with complete data ($M = 7.21$, $SD = 3.06$). No significant differences were found for teacher sex, $t(8.65) = -1.44$, $p = 0.185$; extraversion, $t(62) = 1.86$, $p = 0.068$; agreeableness, $t(62) = 0.19$, $p = 0.850$; conscientiousness, $t(62) = -1.36$, $p = 0.178$; neuroticism, $t(62) = 0.97$, $p = 0.335$; or openness, $t(62) = 1.15$, $p = 0.254$.

Descriptives (see Table 1) showed that students reported moderately high levels of post-intervention emotional well-being ($M = 4.08$, $SD = 0.77$) on a scale ranging from 0 to 5. Their academic performance, assessed via school-reported GPA, averaged 3.70 ($SD = 0.35$). Teachers had an average of 7.81 years of teaching experience ($SD = 2.89$). On average, teachers scored slightly above the midpoint (i.e., neither agree nor disagree) on the Big Five personality traits of agreeableness ($M = 3.24$, $SD = 0.87$), conscientiousness ($M = 3.93$, $SD = 0.75$), neuroticism ($M = 3.38$, $SD = 0.91$), and openness ($M = 3.83$, $SD = 0.93$), but slightly below the midpoint on extraversion ($M = 2.52$, $SD = 1.03$), based on a scale ranging from 1 to 5.

Pearson's bivariate correlations (see Table 1) revealed that at the student level, older students reported significantly lower emotional well-being at both timepoints, $r = -0.37$, $p = 0.003$ (baseline), and $r = -0.38$, $p = 0.003$ (post-intervention). Baseline emotional well-being was strongly and positively associated with post-intervention emotional well-being, $r = 0.78$, $p < 0.001$.

Correlations among teacher-level variables were computed using a dataset aggregated at the teacher level to preserve independence. More years of teaching experience were significantly associated with lower extraversion, $r = -0.47$, $p = 0.032$. Female teachers reported significantly lower levels of openness, $r = -0.47$, $p = 0.033$. Openness was also negatively associated with conscientiousness, $r = -0.45$, $p = 0.040$.

Several significant correlations emerged between student-level and teacher-level variables. Older students were more likely to have male teachers, $r = -0.49$, $p < 0.001$, and teachers who scored lower on agreeableness, $r = -0.44$, $p < 0.001$. Students in the MindUP group were more likely to have male teachers, $r = -0.38$, $p = 0.002$, and teachers who scored higher on openness, $r = 0.32$, $p = 0.011$. Additionally, students with female teachers reported higher levels of emotional well-being at both timepoints, $r = 0.26$, $p = 0.037$ (baseline), and $r = 0.40$, $p = 0.002$ (post-intervention).

Table 1. Descriptive statistics and correlations for study variables.

Variable	*n*	*M*	*SD*	Range	1	2	3	4	5	6	7	8	9	10	11	12	13
Student																	
1. Age	64	13.28	2.24	10–19	-												
2. Sex	64	0.50	0.50	0–1	−0.03	-											
3. Group	64	0.47	0.50	0–1	−0.05	−0.06	-										
4. Baseline EWB	63	4.11	0.72	2–5	−0.37 **	−0.06	−0.06	-									
5. Post EWB	58	4.08	0.77	2.17–5	−0.38 **	−0.12	−0.08	0.78 **	-								
6. Student GPA	64	3.70	0.35	2.8–4.0	−0.21	0.16	−0.06	−0.07	−0.15	-							
Teacher																	
7. Sex	21	0.67	0.48	0–1	−0.49 **	0.07	−0.38 **	0.26 *	0.40 **	0.08	-						
8. Teaching experience	21	7.81	2.89	1–10	−0.19	0.09	0.15	0.04	0.09	0.02	0.35	-					
9. Extraversion	21	2.52	1.03	1–5	0.14	−0.13	0.03	−0.12	−0.16	0.03	−0.13	−0.47 *	-				
10. Agreeableness	21	3.24	0.87	1.5–4.5	−0.44 **	−0.23	−0.09	0.16	0.20	−0.05	0.26	−0.16	0.29	-			
11. Conscientiousness	21	3.93	0.75	2.5–5	−0.04	−0.16	−0.05	0.05	0.19	−0.14	0.00	0.16	−0.14	0.31	-		
12. Neuroticism	21	3.38	0.91	2–5	−0.24	0.04	−0.07	0.24	0.24	0.04	0.02	0.25	0.02	−0.20	−0.01	-	
13. Openness	21	3.83	0.93	2–5	0.02	−0.10	0.32 *	−0.11	−0.25	0.22	−0.47 *	−0.24	0.28	−0.41	−0.45 *	0.14	-

Note. EWB = emotional well-being; GPA = grade point average; post = post-intervention. Sex was coded as 0 = male, 1 = female. Group was coded as 0 = Normal Isn't Real, 1 = MindUP.
* $p < 0.05$. ** $p < 0.01$.

Assumption testing indicated that for emotional well-being, the ICC was 0.181, and for GPA, the ICC was 0.054, indicating that 18.1% and 5.4% of the variance, respectively, were due to differences between teachers. Both values fell within the range of 0.05 to 0.25, commonly observed in educational research, supporting the use of MLM to account for the nested structure of students within teachers [59].

Residual plots suggested homoscedasticity for emotional well-being but heteroscedasticity for GPA. This violation was confirmed by a significant Breusch–Pagan test for GPA, $F(1, 62) = 29.80$, $p < 0.001$. Attempts to correct the heteroscedasticity through data transformations were unsuccessful. As a result, both models were estimated using the MLR estimator in Mplus to account for this violation. The normality of residuals was supported for emotional well-being, as indicated by non-significant results from both the Kolmogorov–Smirnov test, $p = 0.200$, and the Shapiro–Wilk test, $p = 0.645$. For GPA, residual normality was less clear, with the Kolmogorov–Smirnov test indicating a significant deviation from normality, $p = 0.013$, while the Shapiro–Wilk test was not significant, $p = 0.060$. Minor non-normality in GPA residuals was addressed using robust maximum likelihood estimation. Visual inspection confirmed linear relationships between continuous predictors and outcomes. Multicollinearity diagnostics indicated no concerns, with all VIF values below 2.40 and tolerance values above 0.40.

3.2. Main Analyses

All 64 students had complete data for the GPA full model, while only 57 students had complete data for the emotional well-being full model. Both models were estimated in Mplus using the MLR estimator with FIML to handle missing data. The emotional well-being model has an average cluster size of 2.71 and an ICC of 0.380, while the academic achievement model has an average cluster size of 3.05 and an ICC of 0.114.

3.2.1. Emotional Well-Being Model

A two-level multilevel model was estimated to examine predictors of students' post-intervention emotional well-being, accounting for the nesting of students (Level 1) within teachers (Level 2). Complete model results, including unstandardized estimates, standard errors, and significance levels, are presented in Table 2, along with standardized coefficients to facilitate interpretation of effect sizes (see Figure 1). At the student level, higher baseline emotional well-being significantly predicted greater post-intervention emotional well-being ($b = 0.70$, $SE = 0.10$, $p < 0.001$). Students assigned to the MindUP group also reported significantly higher emotional well-being compared to those in the NIR group ($b = 0.33$, $SE = 0.16$, $p = 0.034$). Student age and sex were not significant predictors ($b = 0.03$, $SE = 0.08$, $p = 0.708$; $b = -0.02$, $SE = 0.12$, $p = 0.860$, respectively).

At the teacher level, students taught by female teachers reported significantly higher emotional well-being ($b = 0.89$, $SE = 0.19$, $p < 0.001$). Higher teacher neuroticism was positively associated with student emotional well-being ($b = 0.25$, $SE = 0.08$, $p = 0.003$), whereas more years of teaching experience was negatively associated with student emotional well-being ($b = -0.09$, $SE = 0.03$, $p = 0.001$). Teacher conscientiousness was not a significant predictor ($b = 0.28$, $SE = 0.14$, $p = 0.055$). Teacher extraversion, agreeableness, and openness were all not significant ($ps > 0.10$). While these non-significant results may reflect true null effects, it is also possible that the small number of teacher-level observations limited our ability to detect associations of modest size. After accounting for covariates and predictors, the residual variance at the student level was 0.22 ($SE = 0.06$, $p < 0.001$), and the residual between-teacher variance was negligible and non-significant (0.002, $SE = 0.06$, $p = 0.978$). The model explained 47.4% of the variance in emotional well-being at the student level ($p < 0.001$) and 99.3% at the teacher level ($p < 0.001$).

Table 2. Multilevel model predicting post-intervention emotional well-being.

Predictor	*b*	*SE*	95% CI for *b*	*β*	*p*
Level 1 (Student Level)					
Age	0.03	0.08	[−0.12, 0.18]	0.04	0.708
Sex	−0.02	0.12	[−0.25, 0.21]	−0.02	0.860
Intervention Group	0.33	0.16	[0.03, 0.64]	0.26	0.034
Baseline EWB	0.70	0.10	[0.50, 0.90]	0.65	<0.001
Level 2 (Teacher Level)					
Sex	0.89	0.19	[0.53, 1.25]	0.83	<0.001
Teaching Experience	−0.09	0.03	[−0.15, −0.04]	−0.52	0.001
Extraversion	−0.15	0.09	[−0.33, 0.04]	−0.29	0.114
Agreeableness	0.03	0.05	[−0.06, 0.13]	0.06	0.478
Conscientiousness	0.28	0.14	[−0.01, 0.56]	0.40	0.055
Neuroticism	0.25	0.08	[0.09, 0.42]	0.44	0.003
Openness	−0.04	0.10	[−0.24, 0.16]	−0.07	0.701

Note. EWB = emotional well-being; *b* = unstandardized regression coefficient; *SE* = standard error; CI = confidence interval; *β* = standardized coefficient; *p* = significance value. Student-level predictors were group-mean centered; teacher-level predictors were grand-mean centered. Sex was coded as 0 = male, 1 = female. Intervention group was coded as 0 = Normal Isn't Real, 1 = MindUP. *n* = 57 students with complete data.

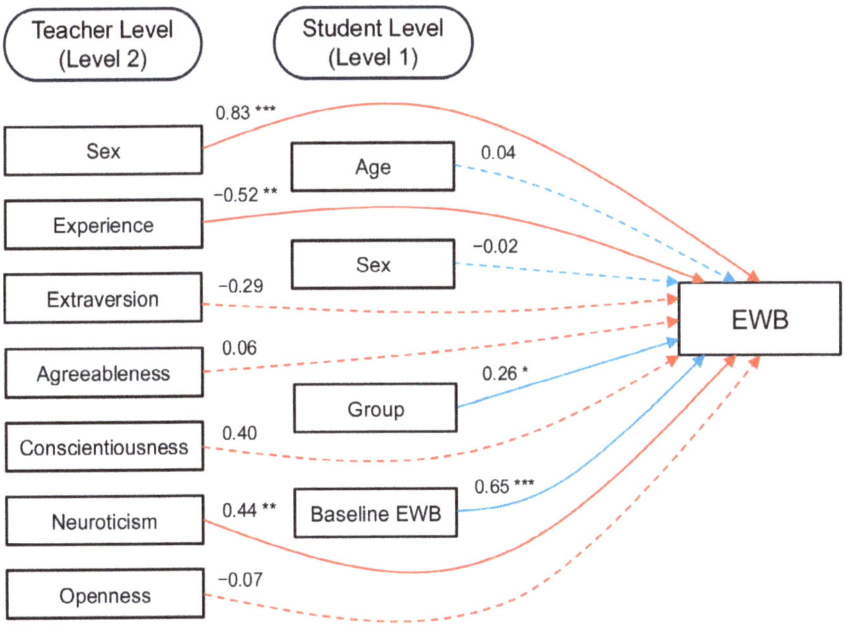

Figure 1. Graphical representation of MLM predicting post-intervention EWB. *Note.* MLM = multilevel model; EWB = emotional well-being; Experience = years of teaching experience. Sex was coded as 0 = male, 1 = female. Group was coded as 0 = Normal Isn't Real, 1 = MindUP. *n* = 57 students with complete data. All coefficients are standardized. * $p < 0.05$. ** $p < 0.01$. *** $p < 0.001$.

Given the unusually high R-square at the between level, several follow-up models were tested to examine the plausibility of this value. First, individual teacher-level predictors were entered separately into four additional models. When teacher sex, neuroticism, and conscientiousness were tested as individual predictors while controlling for covariates, each emerged as significant. Teacher sex alone significantly predicted emotional well-being ($b = 0.75$, $SE = 0.28$, $p = 0.006$) and explained 53.8% of the between-level variance ($p = 0.005$).

Teacher neuroticism was a significant positive predictor ($b = 0.19$, $SE = 0.08$, $p = 0.012$), accounting for 70.4% of the between-level variance ($p = 0.001$). Teacher conscientiousness also significantly predicted emotional well-being ($b = 0.32$, $SE = 0.15$, $p = 0.029$), explaining 79.8% of the between-level variance ($p < 0.001$). In contrast, teaching experience was not a significant predictor ($b = 0.03$, $SE = 0.03$, $p = 0.376$) and explained only 2.7% of the between-level variance ($p = 0.666$). These findings suggest that teacher sex, neuroticism, and conscientiousness may be driving a large portion of the between-level variance, and that the high R-square observed in the full model likely reflects a combination of overlapping contributions from multiple teacher-level characteristics.

3.2.2. Academic Achievement Model

A second two-level multilevel model examined predictors of students' academic achievement (end-of-school-year GPA). Complete model results, including unstandardized estimates, standard errors, and significance levels, are presented in Table 3, along with standardized coefficients to facilitate interpretation of effect sizes (see Figure 2). At the student level, sex was a significant predictor, with school records showing that girls achieved a higher GPA than boys ($b = 0.14$, $SE = 0.07$, $p = 0.038$). Student age and intervention group were not significantly associated with GPA ($b = -0.02$, $SE = 0.05$, $p = 0.772$; $b = -0.10$, $SE = 0.09$, $p = 0.256$, respectively). At the teacher level, greater teacher openness significantly predicted higher GPA ($b = 0.17$, $SE = 0.07$, $p = 0.022$). No other teacher-level predictors reached significance, including teacher sex ($b = 0.09$, $SE = 0.11$, $p = 0.393$), teaching experience ($b = 0.01$, $SE = 0.02$, $p = 0.560$), and the remaining personality traits (all $ps > 0.10$).

Table 3. Multilevel model predicting end-of-school-year GPA.

Predictor	b	SE	95% CI for b	β	p
Level 1 (Student-Level)					
Age	−0.02	0.05	[−0.11, 0.08]	−0.04	0.772
Sex	0.14	0.07	[0.01, 0.28]	0.21	0.038
Intervention Group	−0.10	0.09	[−0.26, 0.07]	−0.14	0.256
Level 2 (Teacher-Level)					
Sex	0.09	0.11	[−0.12, 0.30]	0.37	0.393
Teaching Experience	0.01	0.02	[−0.02, 0.04]	0.24	0.560
Extraversion	−0.01	0.06	[−0.12, 0.11]	−0.05	0.923
Agreeableness	0.05	0.08	[−0.10, 0.20]	0.37	0.498
Conscientiousness	0.02	0.07	[−0.11, 0.15]	0.14	0.731
Neuroticism	−0.02	0.04	[−0.10, 0.07]	−0.11	0.736
Openness	0.17	0.07	[0.03, 0.31]	1.29	0.022

Note. GPA = grade point average; b = unstandardized regression coefficient; SE = standard error; CI = confidence interval; β = standardized coefficient; p = significance value. Student-level predictors were group-mean centered; teacher-level predictors were grand-mean centered. Sex was coded as 0 = male, 1 = female. Intervention group was coded as 0 = Normal Isn't Real, 1 = MindUP. $n = 64$ students with complete data.

After accounting for covariates and predictors, the residual variance in GPA remained significant at the student level ($b = 0.10$, $SE = 0.02$, $p < 0.001$), while the between-teacher residual variance was negligible and non-significant ($b = 0.00$, $SE = 0.01$, $p = 0.967$). The model explained 7.3% of the variance in GPA at the student level ($p = 0.196$) and 96.9% at the teacher level ($p = 0.190$); however, neither R-square value reached statistical significance. To examine the robustness of the significant effect for openness, a follow-up model tested openness as the only teacher-level personality predictor while controlling for teacher sex and teaching experience. In this model, teacher openness remained a significant predictor of student GPA ($b = 0.13$, $SE = 0.06$, $p = 0.033$), suggesting this effect is not dependent on other personality traits in the model. However, the between-level R-square was not significant (0.961, $p = 0.353$), indicating that substantial unexplained variance remained.

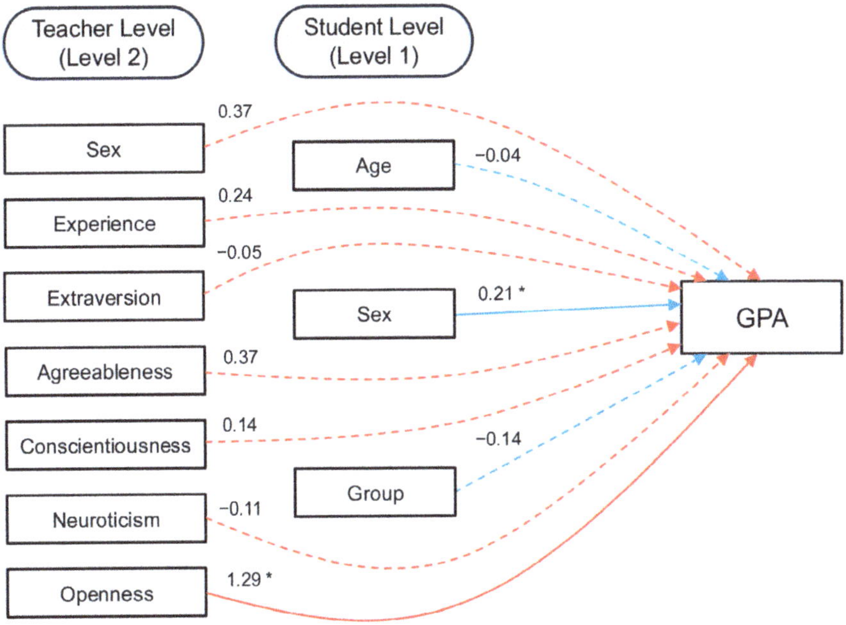

Figure 2. Graphical representation of MLM predicting end-of-school-year GPA. *Note.* MLM = multilevel model; GPA = grade point average; Experience = years of teaching experience. Sex was coded as 0 = male, 1 = female. Group was coded as 0 = Normal Isn't Real, 1 = MindUP. n = 64 students with complete data. All coefficients are standardized. * $p < 0.05$.

4. Discussion

4.1. Summary of Findings

The present study investigated how teacher personality traits influence emotional well-being and academic achievement among students with SLDs, a population often underrepresented in research on teacher–student dynamics [15,16,29]. While previous studies have examined the relationship between teacher personality and student outcomes in general populations [23,24,44,46–48], this study extends the literature by focusing on students with SLDs and using a multilevel framework to capture teacher-level effects.

Findings partially supported the initial hypotheses and offered nuanced insights into the influence of teacher personality traits on student outcomes [23]. Contrary to expectations, higher teacher neuroticism significantly predicted greater student emotional well-being following the intervention [23–25,44,46]. Although this finding diverges from prior literature linking teacher depressive symptoms to poorer student achievement [60], it may reflect the benefits of emotional sensitivity. Neuroticism reflects a tendency toward emotional sensitivity, anxiety, and self-consciousness [61]. While often associated with negative outcomes, certain facets of neuroticism, such as heightened emotional awareness, may enhance a teacher's ability to recognize and respond to students' emotional needs. Teachers higher in neuroticism may be more emotionally attuned and better able to create classroom environments that are validating and responsive to students' affective experiences. This interpretation aligns with research suggesting that teachers who develop greater emotional awareness and regulation through mindfulness training can foster psychologically safe and supportive classroom environments [62]. Notably, of the 21 teachers, 9 scored at or below the midpoint and 12 scored above it, indicating that neuroticism levels in this sample were generally moderate rather than extreme. It is possible that moderate levels of neuroticism are adaptive, whereas higher levels may produce different effects. Future research should explore potential nonlinear (e.g., U-shaped) associations between teacher neuroticism and student well-being.

It is also important to consider the non-significant findings in light of this study's statistical power. Although traits such as agreeableness and extraversion have been linked to student outcomes in prior studies [23,24,44,46,47], these traits did not reach significance in our models. This may reflect a true lack of association in this context, or it may be due to the modest number of clusters, which reduces power to detect smaller effects. By reporting confidence intervals alongside estimates, we aim to transparently communicate the level of uncertainty around these findings and encourage cautious interpretation.

Teacher conscientiousness did not significantly predict student emotional well-being in the full model but did emerge as a significant predictor when examined in isolation. This finding supports prior research suggesting that conscientious teachers, who tend to be organized, responsible, and attentive, are more likely to demonstrate effective classroom management, greater support for students, and adaptability to diverse learning needs [23–25,48]. These qualities may function as protective factors for students with SLDs, promoting their socioemotional resilience [29–31]. In particular, teacher conscientiousness may contribute to the creation of structured yet flexible learning environments that are especially beneficial for students requiring additional support [23,24].

As hypothesized, greater teacher openness significantly predicted higher student GPA post-intervention [23–25,44,46,47]. This finding aligns with prior work indicating that more open teachers, who are often imaginative, flexible, and intellectually curious, are more likely to implement adaptive and inclusive instructional strategies [23,24,61,63]. Such characteristics may be especially beneficial for students with SLDs, who are known to benefit from creative, individualized, and differentiated instructional approaches [42]. In contrast, teacher agreeableness and extraversion were not significantly associated with student outcomes in this study. This aligns with prior research indicating that while these personality traits may enhance students' perceptions of teacher support and foster greater self-efficacy, they do not directly predict objective measures such as academic achievement [24,48]. These findings suggest that although interpersonal warmth and sociability are important for relational aspects of teaching [23], they may not be sufficient to influence academic or emotional outcomes in students with SLDs.

Beyond personality traits, several student and teacher characteristics also contributed to post-intervention outcomes. Students with higher baseline emotional well-being showed higher post-intervention emotional well-being, as expected. Participation in the MindUP intervention was also associated with increased emotional well-being. This finding is in line with previous research demonstrating the positive effects of MindUP and other SEL programs on students' emotional well-being [64,65], highlighting the program's potential value for supporting students with diverse learning needs. Female teachers were associated with higher student emotional well-being, consistent with literature suggesting that female teachers often display higher levels of emotional support [66]. Notably, fewer years of teaching experience predicted greater student emotional well-being, potentially due to reduced burnout or increased enthusiasm among early-career teachers. Teacher burnout, which tends to increase with years of service, has been linked to decreased emotional support and may negatively impact both teacher and student well-being [1,67].

Finally, female students demonstrated a higher end-of-school-year GPA than male students, consistent with national trends showing higher academic performance among girls [49,68]. These findings underscore the importance of considering both teacher and student characteristics when evaluating how teacher personality influences developmental outcomes in students with SLDs. Building on the attachment theory, our results suggest that teacher personality traits, particularly openness, neuroticism, and conscientiousness, may shape the emotional and academic outcomes of students with SLDs by influencing how secure, supported, and understood students feel in the classroom [17–22].

4.2. Implications

The findings of this study offer meaningful implications for educational practice, particularly for supporting the success of students with SLDs. First, the observed associations between teacher personality traits and student outcomes highlight the importance of considering personality dimensions in teacher recruitment, training, and ongoing professional development [23]. Teacher openness reflects qualities such as adaptability, creativity, and openness to experience, all of which are traits that may enhance a teacher's ability to differentiate instruction and respond to diverse learners' needs [23,24,61,63]. Integrating strategies that cultivate these qualities in professional learning settings may improve student academic outcomes, especially in inclusive classrooms.

The unexpected positive association between teacher neuroticism and student emotional well-being suggests that emotionally sensitive teachers might create more validating and emotionally attuned environments, particularly beneficial for students with SLDs who may be at greater risk for emotional challenges. Teacher preparation programs may benefit from helping educators channel emotional sensitivity into supportive classroom practices [23–25] while also ensuring appropriate emotional regulation strategies are in place to protect teacher well-being [62].

Additionally, the association between teacher conscientiousness and greater student emotional well-being in exploratory analyses suggests that structured, responsible, and dependable teacher behaviors may foster emotional safety and predictability in the classroom, all of which are key components of well-being for students requiring additional support [1,23–25,69]. This highlights the potential value of embedding classroom management, organization, and relationship-building skills within teacher development programs.

Organizations have long used personality assessments to guide personnel decisions [70]. However, the findings from the present study suggest that teacher personality traits may not consistently predict student outcomes, particularly for students with SLDs. While certain traits, such as openness and conscientiousness, showed positive associations with student outcomes, others, like agreeableness and extraversion, did not. The unexpected positive link between teacher neuroticism and student emotional well-being further underscores the complexity of teacher–student interactions and cautions against overly simplistic interpretations of personality effects in the classroom.

Rather than relying solely on personality profiles, teacher selection and training processes might benefit more from emphasizing adaptive interpersonal and instructional behaviors [23,62]. For example, traits commonly associated with female teachers, such as empathy and emotional responsiveness [66], were indirectly supported by findings showing that students of female teachers reported higher emotional well-being. These qualities could be more effectively cultivated through targeted professional development than predicted through trait-based assessments alone.

Beyond personality, the findings that female teachers and less experienced teachers were associated with higher student emotional well-being raise important considerations for mentoring and workplace support. It may be that newer teachers, despite having less classroom experience, exhibit higher enthusiasm or lower levels of burnout, which benefits student mental health [71–73]. Schools might consider supporting mid- and late-career teachers with emotional wellness initiatives or job re-engagement strategies to mitigate burnout and sustain effective emotional support over time.

Finally, the positive effect of participation in the MindUP program reinforces the value of implementing structured mindfulness-based SEL interventions in middle and high school settings [64,65]. Given the unique academic and emotional needs of students with SLDs, embedding SEL into standard curricula, especially when delivered by emotionally attuned and adaptable teachers, may optimize both academic and psychosocial outcomes. Taken together, these findings point to the need for a more comprehensive approach to teacher development—one that integrates relational competencies, classroom adaptability, and evidence-based intervention delivery to better support students with neurodevelopmental disorders.

4.3. Limitations and Future Directions

Several limitations should be considered when interpreting the findings of this study. First, the relatively small sample size, particularly at the teacher level, may have limited statistical power to detect smaller effects and increased the potential for over- or underestimating associations. To address this limitation, we employed a two-level multilevel modeling design, limited the number of predictors to theoretically grounded variables to reduce the risk of overfitting, reported effect sizes (standardized beta coefficients) alongside 95% confidence intervals, and used FIML with the MLR estimator to handle missing data. Although multilevel modeling accounted for the nested data structure, the modest number of clusters (i.e., teachers) may constrain the generalizability and stability of the estimates. Future research should aim to replicate these findings using larger samples across multiple schools or districts to enhance both statistical power and external validity.

One key limitation in the present study was the absence of baseline GPA data. As a result, the multilevel model predicting end-of-school-year academic achievement could not control for students' prior academic performance. This prevents making any causal inferences about the impact of teacher characteristics on student academic achievement. Future studies should incorporate pre-intervention academic data to better assess change over time.

Additionally, the teachers included in this study taught very different academic subjects at the school, such as math and reading. Considering that SLDs can be specific to a single academic domain, it is possible that the influence of teacher personality may differ depending on subject area and the particular domain of student difficulty. Future research may consider how content-area instruction (e.g., reading vs. math) interacts with teacher traits to shape academic or emotional outcomes in students with SLDs.

Another limitation involves how students were assigned to teachers. Students had different teachers for core subjects such as math, English, and science. Although all teachers delivered the same SEL curriculum (MindUP or NIR), the teacher who completed the personality assessment was not directly tied to the specific subject grades used to calculate each student's GPA. As a result, multiple teachers contributed to each student's GPA, but this study focused only on SEL teachers. This creates some uncertainty when interpreting the finding that teacher personality predicted student achievement, since the measured teacher may have influenced only a portion of the student's GPA. Future research should aim to more directly link teacher characteristics to the specific subjects and outcomes they influence.

This study also relied on a brief self-report personality inventory (BFI-10) [53], which includes only two items per trait and showed limited internal consistency for several subscales in our small sample. The BFI-10 was selected due to its widespread use and practical advantages in survey research, particularly in contexts with limited assessment time [53,55,74,75]. Indeed, the BFI-10 has demonstrated acceptable psychometric properties in large, population-based studies across different countries [55,75,76]. However, consistent with prior cautions in the literature, very brief scales may show attenuated reliability, especially in small samples, and may not fully capture the breadth of each personality domain [77]. Thus, the limited reliability observed in this study may be due in part to the short scale length and small teacher sample size, potentially introducing measurement error. Future research would benefit from using longer, more psychometrically robust personality assessments when feasible to enhance measurement precision and construct validity.

Lastly, the lack of direct assessment of teaching practices and teacher–student relationship quality limits understanding of the mechanisms linking teacher personality to student outcomes. Including such variables in future studies would help clarify these pathways. Despite the above limitations, this study offers valuable insights into how teacher characteristics relate to emotional well-being and academic achievement among students with SLDs. Continued investigation in this area can inform teacher preparation programs, classroom interventions, and inclusive education practices aimed at promoting well-being and success among students with neurodevelopmental disorders.

5. Conclusions

This study contributes to the growing body of research on teacher influences in inclusive education by examining how teacher personality traits relate to academic and emotional outcomes among students with SLDs. Using a multilevel framework, the findings revealed that teacher neuroticism and conscientiousness were associated with greater student emotional well-being, while teacher openness was associated with higher student GPAs. The findings highlight the importance of considering teacher characteristics in designing school-based interventions to support the development of learners with SLDs or other neurodevelopmental disorders. In addition to teacher traits, student and teacher demographic variables such as sex, teaching experience, and participation in a mindfulness-based SEL intervention also emerged as important contributors to student outcomes. These results underscore the multifaceted nature of classroom dynamics and the need to consider both interpersonal and contextual factors in supporting the success of students with SLDs. Although limitations related to measurement reliability and sample size warrant caution, the findings offer meaningful implications for teacher training, intervention implementation, and inclusive education policy. These findings contribute to the broader literature on children's well-being and mental health in educational contexts, emphasizing the importance of teacher characteristics in designing school-based strategies that support the holistic development of students with neurodevelopmental disorders.

Author Contributions: Conceptualization, W.Y. and C.G.R.; Methodology, W.Y., S.M., and C.G.R.; Software, W.Y.; Validation, O.F.W.; Formal Analysis, W.Y.; Investigation, W.Y. and B.P.; Resources, B.P. and C.G.R.; Data Curation, W.Y.; Writing—Original Draft Preparation, W.Y. and O.F.W.; Writing—Review and Editing, B.P., S.M., and C.G.R.; Visualization, W.Y.; Supervision, C.G.R.; Project Administration, B.P. and C.G.R.; Funding Acquisition, C.G.R. All authors have read and agreed to the published version of the manuscript.

Funding: This work was supported by the University of Alabama at Birmingham (UAB) Center for Engagement in Disability Health and Rehabilitation Sciences (CEDHARS; awarded to Caroline G. Richter).

Institutional Review Board Statement: This study was conducted according to the guidelines of the Declaration of Helsinki and approved by the Institutional Review Board of the University of Alabama at Birmingham (IRB#300010662, approved on 15 August 2023).

Informed Consent Statement: Informed consent was obtained from all subjects involved in this study.

Data Availability Statement: The data presented in this study are available on request from the corresponding author due to privacy reasons.

Acknowledgments: We thank all the students and teachers who took part in this study, along with the school administrators and caregivers who supported their participation. We are also grateful to the research assistants who helped with data collection, and to the school for allowing us to conduct this research on site.

Conflicts of Interest: The authors declare no conflicts of interest.

References

1. Jennings, P.A.; Greenberg, M.T. The prosocial classroom: Teacher social and emotional competence in relation to student and classroom outcomes. *Rev. Educ. Res.* **2009**, *79*, 491–525. [CrossRef]
2. Zheng, F. Fostering students' well-being: The mediating role of teacher interpersonal behavior and student-teacher relationships. *Front. Psychol.* **2022**, *12*, 796728. [CrossRef] [PubMed]
3. Bonuomo, M.; Marini, M.; Vegni, N.; Melogno, S.; Torregiani, G.; Livi, S.; Di Filippo, G. Analysis of psychological and social functioning in undergraduate students with a specific learning disorder (SLD). *Brain Sci.* **2023**, *13*, 1020. [CrossRef] [PubMed]
4. Matteucci, M.C.; Scalone, L.; Tomasetto, C.; Cavrini, G.; Selleri, P. Health-related quality of life and psychological wellbeing of children with specific learning disorders and their mothers. *Res. Dev. Disabil.* **2019**, *87*, 43–53. [CrossRef]
5. American Psychiatric Association. *Diagnostic and Statistical Manual of Mental Disorders*, 5th ed.; Text Rev.; American Psychiatric Publishing: Washington, DC, USA, 2022.
6. Grigorenko, E.L.; Compton, D.L.; Fuchs, L.S.; Wagner, R.K.; Willcutt, E.G.; Fletcher, J.M. Understanding, educating, and supporting children with specific learning disabilities: 50 years of science and practice. *Am. Psychol.* **2020**, *75*, 37–51. [CrossRef]
7. Piko, B.F.; Dudok, R. Strengths and difficulties among adolescent with and without specific learning disorders (SLD). *Children* **2023**, *10*, 1741. [CrossRef]
8. Mugnaini, D.; Lassi, S.; La Malfa, G.; Albertini, G. Internalizing correlates of dyslexia. *World J. Pediatr.* **2009**, *5*, 255–264. [CrossRef]
9. Visser, L.; Kalmar, J.; Linkersdörfer, J.; Görgen, R.; Rothe, J.; Hasselhorn, M.; Schulte-Körne, G. Comorbidities between specific learning disorders and psychopathology in elementary school children in Germany. *Front. Psychiatry* **2020**, *11*, 292. [CrossRef]
10. Carroll, J.M.; Maughan, B.; Goodman, R.; Meltzer, H. Literacy difficulties and psychiatric disorders: Evidence for comorbidity. *J. Child Psychol. Psychiatry* **2005**, *46*, 524–532. [CrossRef]
11. Francis, D.A.; Caruana, N.; Hudson, J.L.; McArthur, G.M. The association between poor reading and internalising problems: A systematic review and meta-analysis. *Clin. Psychol. Rev.* **2019**, *67*, 45–60. [CrossRef]
12. Hendren, R.L.; Haft, S.L.; Black, J.M.; White, N.C.; Hoeft, F. Recognizing psychiatric comorbidity with reading disorders. *Front. Psychiatry* **2018**, *9*, 101. [CrossRef] [PubMed]
13. Cortiella, C.; Horowitz, S.H. *The State of Learning Disabilities: Facts, Trends and Emerging Issues*, 3rd ed.; National Center for Learning Disabilities: New York, NY, USA, 2014.
14. Orr, A.C.; Goodman, N. "People like me don't go to college:" The legacy of learning disability. *J. Ethnogr. Qual. Res.* **2010**, *4*, 213–225.
15. Stein, B.; Hoeft, F.; Richter, C.G. Stress, resilience, and emotional well-being in children and adolescents with specific learning disabilities. *Curr. Opin. Behav. Sci.* **2024**, *58*, 101410. [CrossRef]
16. Catts, H.W.; Petscher, Y. A cumulative risk and resilience model of dyslexia. *J. Learn. Disabil.* **2021**, *55*, 171–184. [CrossRef]
17. Bowlby, J. The nature of the child's tie to his mother. *Int. J. Psychoanal.* **1958**, *39*, 350–373.
18. Verschueren, K.; Koomen, H.M.Y. Teacher–child relationships from an attachment perspective. *Attach. Hum. Dev.* **2012**, *14*, 205–211. [CrossRef]
19. García-Rodríguez, I.; Carracedo, C.H.; Suárez, Á.L.; González-Castro, P.; Álvarez-García, D. Teacher–student attachment relationships and academic and emotional outcomes in children: A systematic review. *Educ. Res. Rev.* **2023**, *38*, 100488. [CrossRef]
20. Li, X.; Duan, S.; Liu, H. Unveiling the predictive effect of students' perceived EFL teacher support on academic achievement: The mediating role of academic buoyancy. *Sustainability* **2023**, *15*, 10205. [CrossRef]
21. He, L.; Feng, L.; Ding, J. The relationship between perceived teacher emotional support, online academic burnout, academic self-efficacy, and online English academic engagement of Chinese EFL learners. *Sustainability* **2024**, *16*, 5542. [CrossRef]
22. Huang, L.; Wang, D. Teacher support, academic self-efficacy, student engagement, and academic achievement in emergency online learning. *Behav. Sci.* **2023**, *13*, 704. [CrossRef]
23. Göncz, L. Teacher personality: A review of psychological research and guidelines for a more comprehensive theory in educational psychology. *Open Rev. Educ. Res.* **2017**, *4*, 75–95. [CrossRef]
24. Kim, L.E.; Jörg, V.; Klassen, R.M. A meta-analysis of the effects of teacher personality on teacher effectiveness and burnout. *Educ. Psychol. Rev.* **2019**, *31*, 163–195. [CrossRef] [PubMed]

25. Perera, H.N.; McIlveen, P. Profiles of teacher personality and relationships with teacher self-efficacy, work engagement, and job satisfaction. *Pers. Individ. Dif.* **2018**, *120*, 171–178. [CrossRef]
26. Zee, M.; Koomen, H.M.Y. Teacher self-efficacy and its effects on classroom processes, student academic adjustment, and teacher well-being: A synthesis of 40 years of research. *Rev. Educ. Res.* **2016**, *86*, 981–1015. [CrossRef]
27. Brännlund, A.; Strandh, M.; Nilsson, K. Mental-health and educational achievement: The link between poor mental-health and upper secondary school completion and grades. *J. Ment. Health* **2017**, *26*, 318–325. [CrossRef]
28. McLeod, J.D.; Kaiser, K. Childhood emotional and behavioral problems and educational attainment. *Am. Sociol. Rev.* **2004**, *69*, 636–658. [CrossRef]
29. Haft, S.L.; Myers, C.A.; Hoeft, F. Socio-emotional and cognitive resilience in children with reading disabilities. *Curr. Opin. Behav. Sci.* **2016**, *10*, 133–141. [CrossRef]
30. Al-Yagon, M. Perceived close relationships with parents, teachers, and peers: Predictors of social, emotional, and behavioral features in adolescents with LD or comorbid LD and ADHD. *J. Learn. Disabil.* **2016**, *49*, 597–615. [CrossRef]
31. Kiuru, N.; Poikkeus, A.-M.; Lerkkanen, M.-K.; Pakarinen, E.; Siekkinen, M.; Ahonen, T.; Nurmi, J.-E. Teacher-perceived supportive classroom climate protects against detrimental impact of reading disability risk on peer rejection. *Learn. Instr.* **2012**, *22*, 331–339. [CrossRef]
32. Baker, J.A.; Grant, S.; Morlock, L. The teacher-student relationship as a developmental context for children with internalizing or externalizing behavior problems. *Sch. Psychol. Q.* **2008**, *23*, 3–15. [CrossRef]
33. Danielsen, A.G.; Samdal, O.; Hetland, J.; Wold, B. School-related social support and students' perceived life satisfaction. *J. Educ. Res.* **2010**, *102*, 303–320. [CrossRef]
34. Furrer, C.J.; Skinner, E.A.; Pitzer, J.R. The influence of teacher and peer relationships on students' classroom engagement and everyday motivational resilience. *Teach. Coll. Rec.* **2014**, *116*, 101. [CrossRef]
35. Hamre, B.K.; Pianta, R.C. Early teacher-child relationships and the trajectory of children's school outcomes through eighth grade. *Child Dev.* **2003**, *72*, 625–638. [CrossRef]
36. Kashy-Rosenbaum, G.; Kaplan, O.; Israel-Cohen, Y. Predicting academic achievement by class-level emotions and perceived homeroom teachers' emotional support. *Psychol. Sch.* **2018**, *55*, 770–782. [CrossRef]
37. Wang, M.-T.; Degol, J.L.; Amemiya, J.; Parr, A.; Guo, J. Classroom climate and children's academic and psychological well-being: A systematic review and meta-analysis. *Dev. Rev.* **2020**, *57*, 100912. [CrossRef]
38. Yang, Y.; Li, G.; Su, Z.; Yuan, Y. Teacher's emotional support and math performance: The chain mediating effect of academic self-efficacy and math behavioral engagement. *Front. Psychol.* **2021**, *12*, 651608. [CrossRef]
39. Roorda, D.L.; Koomen, H.M.Y.; Spilt, J.L.; Oort, F.J. The influence of affective teacher–student relationships on students' school engagement and achievement: A meta-analytic approach. *Rev. Educ. Res.* **2011**, *81*, 493–529. [CrossRef]
40. McCormick, M.P.; O'Connor, E.E.; Cappella, E.; McClowry, S.G. Teacher–child relationships and academic achievement: A multilevel propensity score model approach. *J. Sch. Psychol.* **2013**, *51*, 611–624. [CrossRef]
41. Mattison, R.E.; Woods, A.D.; Morgan, P.L.; Farkas, G.; Hillemeier, M.M. Longitudinal trajectories of reading and mathematics achievement for students with learning disabilities. *J. Learn. Disabil.* **2022**, *56*, 132–144. [CrossRef]
42. Sideridis, G.D. International approaches to learning disabilities: More alike or more different? *Learn. Disabil. Res. Pract.* **2007**, *22*, 210–215. [CrossRef]
43. Eilam, B.; Vidergor, H.E. Gifted Israeli students' perceptions of teachers' desired characteristics: A case of cultural orientation. *Roeper Rev.* **2011**, *33*, 86–96. [CrossRef]
44. Eryilmaz, A. Perceived personality traits and types of teachers and their relationship to the subjective well-being and academic achievements of adolescents. *Educ. Sci. Theory Pract.* **2014**, *14*, 2049–2062. [CrossRef]
45. Goldstein, G.S.; Benassi, V.A. Students' and instructors' beliefs about excellent lecturers and discussion leaders. *Res. High. Educ.* **2006**, *47*, 685–707. [CrossRef]
46. Kell, H.J. Do teachers' personality traits predict their performance? A comprehensive review of the empirical literature from 1990 to 2018. *ETS Res. Rep. Ser.* **2019**, *2019*, 1–27. [CrossRef]
47. Nkomo, N.N.; Ochiche, U.P.; Akpan, E.M. The influence of teachers' agreeableness and openness to experience on secondary school students' English language academic achievement in Ogoja Education Zone of Cross River State, Nigeria. *J. Educ. Pract.* **2022**, *6*, 5. [CrossRef]
48. Kim, L.E.; Dar-Nimrod, I.; MacCann, C. Teacher personality and teacher effectiveness in secondary school: Personality predicts teacher support and student self-efficacy but not academic achievement. *J. Educ. Psychol.* **2018**, *110*, 309–323. [CrossRef]
49. Hwang, N.; Fitzpatrick, B. Student–teacher gender matching and academic achievement. *AERA Open* **2021**, *7*, 23328584211040058. [CrossRef]
50. Kini, T.; Podolsky, A. Does teaching experience increase teacher effectiveness? A review of the research. *Learn. Policy Inst.* **2016**. [CrossRef]

51. Maloney, J.E.; Lawlor, M.S.; Schonert-Reichl, K.A.; Whitehead, J. A mindfulness-based social and emotional learning curriculum for school-aged children: The MindUP program. In *Handbook of Mindfulness in Education: Integrating Theory and Research into Practice*; Springer Nature: New York, NY, USA, 2016; pp. 313–334. [CrossRef]
52. Banerjee, M.; Lalor, A.R. *Toolkit for Normal Isn't Real: Succeeding with Learning Disabilities & ADHD*; 4-D Productions, Inc.: Los Angeles, CA, USA, 2021.
53. Rammstedt, B.; John, O.P. Measuring personality in one minute or less: A 10-item short version of the Big Five Inventory in English and German. *J. Res. Pers.* **2007**, *41*, 203–212. [CrossRef]
54. Eisinga, R.; Te Grotenhuis, M.; Pelzer, B. The reliability of a two-item scale: Pearson, Cronbach, or Spearman-Brown? *Int. J. Public Health* **2012**, *58*, 637–642. [CrossRef]
55. Costa Mastrascusa, R.; de Oliveira Fenili Antunes, M.L.; de Albuquerque, N.S.; Virissimo, S.L.; Foletto Moura, M.; Vieira Marques Motta, B.; de Lara Machado, W.; Moret-Tatay, C.; Quarti Irigaray, T. Evaluating the complete (44-item), short (20-item) and ultra-short (10-item) versions of the Big Five Inventory (BFI) in the Brazilian population. *Sci. Rep.* **2023**, *13*, 7372. [CrossRef]
56. Bickman, L.; Athay, M.M.; Riemer, M.; Lambert, E.W.; Kelley, S.D.; Breda, C.; Tempesti, T.; Dew-Reeves, S.E.; Brannan, A.M.; Vides de Andrade, A.R. (Eds.) *Manual of the Peabody Treatment Progress Battery*, 2nd ed.; Vanderbilt University: Nashville, TN, USA, 2010; Available online: http://vueinnovations.com/overview-ptpb (accessed on 8 June 2025).
57. Athay, M.M.; Kelley, S.D.; Dew-Reeves, S.E. Brief multidimensional students' life satisfaction scale—PTPB version (BMSLSS-PTPB): Psychometric properties and relationship with mental health symptom severity over time. *Adm. Policy Ment. Health Ment. Health Serv. Res.* **2012**, *39*, 30–40. [CrossRef]
58. Huebner, E.S.; Seligson, J.L.; Valois, R.F.; Suldo, S.M. A review of the Brief Multidimensional Students' Life Satisfaction Scale. *Soc. Indic. Res.* **2006**, *79*, 477–484. [CrossRef]
59. Hedges, L.V.; Hedberg, E.C. Intraclass correlation values for planning group-randomized trials in education. *Educ. Eval. Policy Anal.* **2007**, *29*, 60–87. [CrossRef]
60. McLean, L.; Connor, C.M. Depressive symptoms in third-grade teachers: Relations to classroom quality and student achievement. *Child Dev.* **2015**, *86*, 945–954. [CrossRef]
61. John, O.P.; Srivastava, S. The Big Five trait taxonomy: History, measurement, and theoretical perspectives. In *Handbook of Personality: Theory and Research*, 2nd ed.; Pervin, L.A., John, O.P., Eds.; Guilford Press: New York, NY, USA, 1999; pp. 102–138.
62. Roeser, R.W.; Skinner, E.; Beers, J.; Jennings, P.A. Mindfulness training and teachers' professional development: An emerging area of research and practice. *Child Dev. Perspect.* **2012**, *6*, 167–173. [CrossRef]
63. Decker, D.M.; Rimm-Kaufman, S.E. Personality characteristics and teacher beliefs among pre-service teachers. *Teach. Educ. Q.* **2008**, *35*, 45–64.
64. Schonert-Reichl, K.A.; Oberle, E.; Lawlor, M.S.; Abbott, D.; Thomson, K.; Oberlander, T.F.; Diamond, A. Enhancing cognitive and social–emotional development through a simple-to-administer mindfulness-based school program for elementary school children: A randomized controlled trial. *Dev. Psychol.* **2015**, *51*, 52–66. [CrossRef]
65. Taylor, R.D.; Oberle, E.; Durlak, J.A.; Weissberg, R.P. Promoting positive youth development through school-based social and emotional learning interventions: A meta-analysis of follow-up effects. *Child Dev.* **2017**, *88*, 1156–1171. [CrossRef]
66. Graziano, F.; Mastrokoukou, S.; Monchietto, A.; Marchisio, C.; Calandri, E. The moderating role of emotional self-efficacy and gender in teacher empathy and inclusive education. *Sci. Rep.* **2024**, *14*, 22587. [CrossRef]
67. Chang, M.L. An appraisal perspective of teacher burnout: Examining the emotional work of teachers. *Educ. Psychol. Rev.* **2009**, *21*, 193–218. [CrossRef]
68. Duckworth, A.L.; Seligman, M.E.P. Self-discipline gives girls the edge: Gender in self-discipline, grades, and achievement test scores. *J. Educ. Psychol.* **2006**, *98*, 198–208. [CrossRef]
69. Iznardo, M.; Ryan, J.; Rogers, M.; McKibbin, S.; Piers, L.; Hogan, T. Examining resiliency in children with learning disabilities and co-occurring ADHD symptoms: The protective role of a close teacher-student relationship. *Learn. Disabil. Contemp. J.* **2023**, *21*, 1–16.
70. Salgado, J.F.; De Fruyt, F. Personality in personnel selection. In *The Blackwell Handbook of Personnel Selection*; Evers, A., Anderson, N., Voskuijl, O., Eds.; John Wiley & Sons: Chichester, UK, 2017; pp. 174–198. [CrossRef]
71. Harding, S.; Morris, R.; Gunnell, D.; Ford, T.; Hollingworth, W.; Tilling, K.; Evans, R.; Bell, S.; Grey, J.; Brockman, R.; et al. Is teachers' mental health and wellbeing associated with students' mental health and wellbeing? *J. Affect. Disord.* **2019**, *242*, 180–187. [CrossRef]
72. Madigan, D.J.; Kim, L.E. Towards an understanding of teacher attrition: A meta-analysis of burnout, job satisfaction, and teachers' intentions to quit. *Teach. Teach. Educ.* **2021**, *105*, 103425. [CrossRef]
73. Oberle, E.; Schonert-Reichl, K.A. Stress contagion in the classroom? The link between classroom teacher burnout and morning cortisol in elementary school students. *Soc. Sci. Med.* **2016**, *159*, 30–37. [CrossRef]
74. Gaisendrees, L.; John, O.P.; Rammstedt, B. Measuring the Big Five with single items using the BFI-S: A replication and extension. *Adv. Open Educ.* **2022**, *3*, 1–12.

75. Rammstedt, B.; Kemper, C.J.; Klein, M.C.; Beierlein, C.; Kovaleva, A. Eine kurze Skala zur Messung der fünf Dimensionen der Persönlichkeit: BFI-10 [A short scale for assessing the Big Five dimensions of personality: BFI-10]. *Methods Data Anal.* **2013**, *7*, 233–249. [CrossRef]
76. Courtois, R.; Petot, J.-M.; Plaisant, O.; Allibe, B.; Lignier, B.; Réveillère, C. Validation française du Big Five Inventory à 10 items (BFI-10) [French validation of the Big Five Inventory–10 (BFI-10)]. *L'Encéphale* **2020**, *46*, 455–462. [CrossRef]
77. Chapman, B.P.; Elliot, A.J. Brief report: How short is too short? An ultra-brief measure of the big-five personality domains implicates "agreeableness" as a risk for all-cause mortality. *J. Health Psychol.* **2017**, *24*, 1568–1573. [CrossRef]

children

MDPI

Article

Parents' and Teachers' Perspectives on Children's Socio-Emotional Well-Being During Transition from Home to Kindergarten

Sanja Tatalović Vorkapić [1,*] and Tamara Komadina [2]

[1] Faculty of Teacher Education, University of Rijeka, 51000 Rijeka, Croatia
[2] Kindergarten Fijolica, 51250 Novi Vinodolski, Croatia; tamara.komadina@dv-fijolica.hr
* Correspondence: sanjatv@uniri.hr

Abstract

Background: As the social-emotional well-being of children as a whole and specifically during the transition to kindergarten is of paramount importance, it is important to continuously research this topic using a multi-informant approach. Moreover, a further contribution of this study lies in addressing the substantial gap in the existing literature within this important field. Objectives: Starting from the Ecological-Dynamic Transition Model and the Positive Development and Resilience in Kindergarten (PERIK) Model, the main aim of this research was to analyze parents' and teachers' perceptions of children's social-emotional well-being during the transition and adjustment, and the quality of transition and adjustment. Methods: The study was conducted on a sample of parents (N = 154; 147 mothers) and teachers from 4 kindergartens (N = 12, all female) as raters of children's (N = 202; 82 girls) social-emotional well-being, using PERIK scale and four questions on the quality of transition. Results: All PERIK-dimensions were rated as elevated based on parents' ratings and moderate based on teachers' ratings. Ratings of difficulties during transition decreased, and satisfaction with transition and adjustment and cooperation between parents and caregivers during transition increased (teachers' ratings were lower than parents' ratings). The average duration of adjustment in kindergarten was three weeks. Correlation analyses showed the expected significant correlations between the PERIK dimensions and the quality of transitions and adjustment of children. Inter-rater agreement analyses showed the effect sizes were predominantly large and poor to medium agreement between parent and teacher ratings was determined. Conclusions: Although the study found that there are significant differences in perceptions of the relationship between PERIK-dimensions and satisfaction with children's transition between teachers and parents, which was expected due to the assessment of children in different contexts, it is important to consider them both in future research.

Keywords: children; parents; satisfaction with transition; social-emotional well-being; kindergarten teachers

1. Introduction

For children at early and preschool age, the transition from the family home to daycare or kindergarten represents the first significant step into the world [1]. In order to ensure that this transition is as smooth and supportive as possible, for the child as well as for their family, and to facilitate the continuation of expected developmental and learning trajectories, thorough preparation for this upcoming phase is essential [2]. During early childhood, children feel safest in the arms of their parents. However, as they begin to spend most of their day in early childhood care and education institutions, this role of providing emotional security is gradually assumed by kindergarten teachers, and, over time, by peers within the kindergarten [3]. Most kindergartens organize parent orientation meetings before a child's first day of attendance, during which detailed information is provided regarding institutional routines, expectations, and essential guidelines for the transition [4–6]. According to the Croatian early childhood education system, children are eligible to enter nursery programs upon reaching one year of age (in some institutions from as early as six months of age). Throughout the preschool period, children may enroll in programs at any point as decided by their parents. The first mandatory participation in the formal education system in Croatia occurs in the year preceding entry into primary school (typically at age six), when children are enrolled in the compulsory preschool program [7]. The child's first day at daycare initiates the formation of relationships between teachers, parents, and children, based on mutual trust, collaboration, and support, which are the elements essential for a successful adaptation process [8].

This transition marks the beginning of the adaptation within the institution, which is often more challenging for younger children due to their increased developmental needs and other influencing factors [9,10]. While the education system is expected to ensure pedagogical continuity to support development and learning in early and preschool-aged children, thereby facilitating transitions and adaptation, this is not always achieved in practice [11]. As a result, a wide array of challenges may arise, affecting not only children but also their caregivers, family members, teachers, and professional associates. Accordingly, the adaptation process is defined as *an individual's capacity to adjust to their environment or novel circumstances* [12] (p. 272). Importantly, the contemporary paradigm shifts the focus from *adaptation to* the institution to *adaptation within* the institution [13], highlighting the central role and responsibility of early childhood education institutions in facilitating high-quality transitions and child adjustment.

Educational transitions and adjustments are embedded in an already dynamic sequence of developmental changes that naturally occur throughout early childhood [14]. This period is thus marked by numerous anticipated changes, with a particular emphasis on ensuring the socio-emotional well-being of children. The National Curriculum for Early and Preschool Education in Croatia [15] identifies one of the main objectives of early childhood care and education as the support of children's socio-emotional well-being, particularly during critical periods such as transitions. In this process, the roles of significant adults, especially teachers and parents, are paramount for ensuring the quality of transitions and subsequent adjustment [16]. Their perceptions of transition quality can serve as a foundation for the development of effective guidelines and support mechanisms. Therefore, it is essential that both teachers' and parents' evaluations are integrated into research on this topic. In light of these considerations, the present study focuses on evaluating the quality of transitions and adjustment processes for children entering kindergartens, with particular attention to their socio-emotional well-being. Furthermore, it aims to explore the relationship between transition and adjustment quality and six dimensions of children's socio-emotional well-being, using a multi-informant approach which encompasses ratings from two perspectives: teachers' and parents'.

1.1. An Ecological Perspective on Children's Transitions from Home to Kindergarten and Their Adjustment in Kindergarten

A transition is a dynamic process of change that begins the moment children (and their families) move from one set of circumstances to another [17] (p. 3) and continues until the child becomes a well-adjusted member of their new environment [18]. Upon entering kindergarten, children are exposed to unfamiliar situations. As they begin constructing a new identity within this new context, they attempt to make sense of the new rules and routines while integrating their prior knowledge and experiences with the current setting [19]. The outcomes of such early experiences are both short- and long-term, as the strategies children develop to adapt in a new environment are often employed in future contexts. The effectiveness of these strategies is of paramount importance. Numerous studies have shown that positive experiences during these crucial educational transitions are predictive of future success in social, emotional, and academic domains [20–22].

As described in earlier studies [6,23,24], the theoretical foundation for understanding childhood transitions is based on Bronfenbrenner's ecological systems theory, which views development as occurring within a series of nested systems: micro-, meso-, exo-, and macro-systems [25]. Additionally, the temporal aspect, shaped by the specific historical, cultural, and social context in which children grow up, can strongly influence the developmental paths of different cohorts. By viewing transitions as ecological events, current literature has developed a comprehensive ecological model for understanding key factors related to early childhood transitions. Rimm-Kaufman and Pianta [26] were among the first to see the transition to kindergarten as a period marked by significant developmental vulnerability, during which children experience numerous major changes that create new expectations, such as the ability to follow structured routines and work more independently. It is therefore not surprising that their research found that about 16% of children were reported by teachers to have experienced serious adjustment difficulties during the transition to kindergarten, with another third facing moderate challenges [27,28].

From an ecological perspective, the child's move to kindergarten is best understood as the result of interactions between intra- (e.g., characteristics of the child, parents, family, classroom, and broader community) and inter-personal factors (e.g., child–teacher relationships, family–kindergarten connections, parent–teacher collaboration), both synchronically and diachronically [27]. While all these factors are important for a full understanding of the quality of transitions, the ecological model highlights that the main focus is on establishing relationships between the family environment and the kindergarten setting, with the child's optimal development as the key goal [27]. The basis of this ecological transition model is deeply rooted in the work of Bronfenbrenner and Morris [29], who elaborated on the two-way influences between children and the contexts they inhabit.

This framework provides a strong basis for examining relevant research questions, especially those related to children's perceived socio-emotional well-being during transitions and adjustment, as well as strategies to improve it [6,9,23,30–32]. Importantly, such research must consider the different perceptions of key stakeholders. Analyzing the transition from home to kindergarten helps researchers and practitioners think about how these contexts change over time and what these changes mean. Central to the transition is creating meaningful contact and overlap between the family and kindergarten systems, most notably, developing parent-teacher relationships and collaborative practices. These newly formed relationships are vital for children's successful adjustment in kindergarten [33]. In this way, the ecological transition model acts as a valuable analytical tool, capable of capturing the complexity of diverse situations and perspectives that characterize children's transitional experiences.

1.2. Children's Socio-Emotional Well-Being During Transition and Adjustment: A Multi-Informant Approach

The concept of child well-being refers to the state of optimal psychological functioning and experience, and is widely recognized as a central indicator of the quality of an educational process [34]. Child well-being is a multidimensional construct encompassing physical, motor, cognitive, emotional, and social dimensions that focus not only on the child's present but also on their future life outcomes [35]. Drawing from the theoretical model of socio-emotional well-being and resilience developed by Mayr and Ulich [36], this construct is understood as a multidimensional phenomenon with a significant influence on child development, framed within a positive developmental perspective. It is grounded in three theoretical foundations: children's mental health, resilience, and school readiness. Within the domain of mental health, the model integrates three core concepts: life skills, adult conceptions of well-being (hedonic and eudaimonic; [37]), and Becker's work on mental health [38,39]. Life skills [40,41] refer to competencies enabling children to interact effectively with others and manage challenges. According to hedonic and eudaimonic frameworks, high-quality mental health requires satisfaction of both subjective internal drives and objective environmental needs, often a complex balance to achieve. The third concept views mental health through physical well-being, high energy levels, and expansiveness, traits later reflected in model dimensions such as assertiveness and initiative. In terms of resilience, the model highlights children's ability to cope effectively with life challenges and emerge without manifest or latent cognitive, emotional, or behavioral impairment, showing continued positive developmental progress despite adversity [42,43]. In educational contexts, school readiness is another key concept, defined by environmental demands and essential child competencies: regulatory abilities, impulse control, emotional regulation, and self-directed exploratory behavior [44].

Based on these conceptual foundations and empirical validation, Mayr and Ulich [45] developed six factors of socio-emotional well-being and resilience. Self-control and thoughtfulness refer to children's ability to manage their behavior, show empathy, and care for others. Social competence and relationship skills encompass the ability to form and maintain positive social relationships, engage in play, initiate communication, and involve peers in shared activities. Task/Activity orientation captures the child's capacity to take responsibility for planning and execution of developmentally appropriate tasks or activities. While originally termed "task orientation," a Croatian validation study [46] suggested the term "activity orientation" is more appropriate in early childhood settings, where structured tasks are replaced by free and guided activities. Assertiveness describes children's capacity to express their emotions, needs, intentions, and desires in a confident and appropriate verbal manner. Emotional stability and stress management combine the ability to maintain emotional balance in challenging situations with the ability to regulate emotional reactivity and find effective coping strategies for calming down. Curiosity and pleasure in exploration, as the name suggests, refer to children's enthusiasm for learning, openness to new situations, and positive emotional engagement with the world around them. Building upon this theoretical model, Mayr and Ulich [45] developed a standardized measurement instrument, which was later adapted and validated for use in Croatia [46] and employed in the present research.

The multi-informant approach to scientific assessment is widely utilized in developmental research, especially in studies of child mental health and well-being [34]. To obtain a comprehensive understanding of a child's functioning, it is common to use assessments from multiple informants, ideally including both parents, teachers, and, where possible, the children themselves [47,48]. Multi-informant reports are a hallmark of high-quality developmental research because they offer multiple perspectives across different contexts, such as home and kindergarten, thus providing a more holistic view of the child [49]. While parents are often the primary informants due to their intimate knowledge of the child, their assessments are typically limited to the home environment and may carry a high degree of subjectivity. In contrast, kindergarten teachers serve as secondary informants who offer critical insights into the child's behavior in educational settings, often characterized by structured social interactions and peer dynamics. There are three key advantages of using teachers as informants: (a) familiarity with each child, developed through substantial time spent together in daily routines; (b) objectivity, fostered by professional training in child observation; and (c) access to comparative data, based on classroom peer groups, allowing for relative assessments of behavior.

Thus, whenever feasible, collecting data from multiple relevant sources is essential, especially when the findings inform early interventions or educational programming. Overreliance on a single informant can lead to poor decision-making in school contexts [50]. While both parents and teachers contribute valuable insights, each carries distinct biases and limitations in expertise. Teachers may lack in-depth knowledge of children's mental health and well-being, despite having access to peer-based behavioral benchmarks [51]. Screening processes that rely solely on one type of informant, either parent or teacher, often result in misidentification of children with mental health difficulties [52,53]. A key question arises: What should be done once data are collected from multiple informants? De Los Reyes et al. [54,55] argue that discrepancies between informants should not be automatically treated as measurement error to be minimized. In fields such as education [48], such differences often reflect valid, context-specific insights and may be uniquely meaningful [56,57]. Attempting to suppress these differences can be counterproductive.

To design and implement effective educational programs that support children's socio-emotional well-being during transitions and adjustment in kindergarten, it is essential to integrate multi-informant data, a methodological principle that underpins the present study.

2. Research Aim, Tasks, and Hypotheses

The main aim of this study was to examine the levels of transition and adjustment quality in kindergarten and children's socio-emotional well-being using a multi-informant approach, their relationship, and the level of inter-rater agreement. This comprehensive research covers these tasks:

(1) To assess the levels of transition and adjustment quality in kindergarten (measured by four questions about difficulties, satisfaction, collaboration, and adjustment duration) and children's socio-emotional well-being (measured by six dimensions) through multiple informants, and to compare mean scores between parents' and teachers' ratings;
(2) To evaluate inter-rater agreement in transition quality and children's socio-emotional well-being using correlation and reliability analyses;
(3) To investigate the relationship between transition quality and children's socio-emotional well-being, including examining differences in two sets of correlations based on parents' and teachers' ratings.

Based on established theoretical models and prior research findings, the following hypotheses are postulated:

(1) It is expected to determine moderate to high levels of transition quality and socio-emotional well-being in children during their move from home to kindergarten and their adjustment process, with notable differences between parents' and teachers' ratings;
(2) Small to moderate inter-rater agreement in assessing transition quality and socio-emotional well-being during this period is expected to be found;
(3) Medium to high positive correlations between these variables, indicating a significant relationship between higher transition quality and better socio-emotional well-being in children, with noticeable differences depending on whether ratings are from parents or teachers' ratings are expected to be determined.

3. Materials and Methods

3.1. Participants

The study included a total of 202 children from 12 kindergarten groups located across four towns in Croatia: Novi Vinodolski, Bribir, Tribalj, and Crikvenica. Among the participating children, 82 were girls and 110 were boys, with a mean age of M = 4.17 years (SD = 1.67; range = 1–7 years). Of the total sample, three children were identified as having special needs, primarily related to autism spectrum disorders, and one child had been born prematurely. Twelve kindergarten teachers and 154 parents participated in the study. Each teacher assessed the children in her respective group, while each parent evaluated their child. The teachers had a mean age of M = 39.75 years (SD = 10.76; range, 24–59 years) and an average professional experience of M = 16.75 years (SD = 10.39; range, 3–38 years). Of the 154 parents who participated, seven were fathers. The parents' average age was M = 34.90 years (SD = 5.11; range = 24–50 years). Regarding marital status, 121 parents were married, 29 were in cohabiting partnerships, one was single, one was widowed, and two were divorced. Participants' demographics could be observed in Table 1.

Table 1. Participants' (teachers, parents, children) demographics.

	Kindergarten Teachers	Parents	Children
N	12	154	202
Gender (frequencies)			
Female	12	147	82
Male	0	7	110
Age			
Mean	39.75	34.90	4.17
SD	10.76	5.11	1.67
Range	24–59	24–50	1–7
Teachers' professional experience			
Mean	16.75		
SD	10.39		
Range	3–38		
Parents' marital status (frequencies)			
Married		121	
Cohabiting partnerships		29	
Single		1	
Widowed		1	
Divorced		2	

3.2. Measures

To assess the quality of children's transition and adjustment to kindergarten, four items were used: (1) the level of difficulties children experienced during the transition and adjustment period, (2) the level of satisfaction with the transition and adjustment process, (3) the perceived quality of cooperation between parents and teacher during the transition and adjustment, and (4) the duration of the adjustment period. The first three items were rated for each child by both teachers and parents using a 5-point Likert-type scale, while the fourth item was open-ended, requiring respondents to indicate the number of weeks the adjustment process lasted for each child. The rating scales used were as follows: (a) Level of difficulties during transition and adjustment—from 1 (*completely absent*) to 5 (*completely present*); (b) Level of satisfaction with transition and adjustment—from 1 (*unsatisfactory*) to 5 (*satisfactory*); and (c) Quality of parent-teacher cooperation—from 1 (*very low*) to 5 (*very high*). The fourth item, regarding adjustment duration, was open-ended, with both teachers and parents instructed to specify the number of weeks.

To measure children's socio-emotional well-being and resilience, the study used the Positive Development and Resilience in Kindergarten (PERIK) scale [45], specifically its

Croatian adaptation and validation [46]. Originally, the PERIK scale existed in both German and English versions and included six subscales, each consisting of six items, for a total of 36 items. During translation and cultural adaptation to Croatian, two items were added to each subscale, except for the "Establishing Contact and Social Skills" subscale, which remained unchanged, and the "Assertiveness" subscale, which had three additional items, bringing the total number of items to 45. Kindergarten teachers and parents rated each item using a 5-point Likert-type scale: (1 = NO—*Strongly disagree*, 2 = no—*Partially disagree*, 3 = maybe—*Neither agree nor disagree*, 4 = yes—*Partially agree*, 5 = YES—*Strongly agree*). The original validation study [45] reported high and satisfactory reliability for each subscale: Making Contact/Social Skills (α = 0.88), Self-Regulation and Thoughtfulness (α = 0.86), Self-Assertiveness (α = 0.81), Emotional Stability (α = 0.82), Pleasure in Exploration (α = 0.86) and Task/Activity Orientation (α = 0.85). These findings were confirmed in the Croatian validation study [46]: Making Contact/Social Skills (α = 0.92), Self-Regulation and Thoughtfulness (α = 0.92), Self-Assertiveness (α = 0.87), Emotional Stability (α = 0.85), Pleasure in Exploration (α = 0.92). Reliability analysis conducted in the present study supported these previous findings. The results are presented in Table 2.

Table 2. Descriptive parameters (M = Mean, SD = Standard Deviation, Range, and Cronbach alpha α) for 4 transition quality variables and 6 dimensions of socio-emotional well-being of children rated by parents and kindergarten teachers.

		Parents				Kindergarten Teachers			
		M	SD	RANGE	α	M	SD	RANGE	α
Satisfaction with the quality of transition from home to kindergarten	Difficulties during transition and adjustment	2.38	1.16	1–5		2.43	1.15	1–5	
	Satisfaction with transition and adjustment	4.60	0.65	1–5		4.11	0.93	1–5	
	Quality of parent-teacher cooperation	4.48	0.80	1–5		4.19	0.76	2–5	
	Adjustment duration (in weeks)	3.24	4.04	0–24		2.56	5.54	0.2–24	
Socio-emotional well-being and resilience	Social skills	4.05	0.77	1.33–5.00	0.866	3.55	1.06	1.00–5.00	0.946
	Self-regulation	3.90	0.68	1.13–5.00	0.867	3.70	0.98	1.00–5.00	0.947
	Self-assertiveness	3.98	0.77	1.14–5.00	0.861	3.45	0.96	1.14–5.00	0.912
	Emotional stability	3.74	0.64	2.00–5.00	0.805	3.37	0.71	1.00–5.00	0.847
	Activity orientation	3.77	0.66	1.75–4.88	0.781	3.42	0.78	1.25–5.00	0.863
	Pleasure in exploration	4.44	0.60	1.00–5.00	0.884	3.79	0.83	1.00–5.00	0.923

3.3. Procedure

This study represents an integral component of a larger research project supported by the University of Rijeka, Croatia. Concurrently, this part of the research formed a part of the master's thesis of one of the co-authors. Before data collection, the Faculty of Teacher Education at the University of Rijeka issued an official request for collaboration with kindergartens, with which previous cooperation had been established within the framework of the broader research project, specifically within the Primorje-Gorski Kotar County. Following informed consent from the principals of the contacted kindergartens, kindergarten teachers agreed to participate in the study. Notices about the research were posted on bulletin boards intended for parents, ensuring they were informed about key aspects of the study. As parents had already provided general consent at the beginning of the pedagogical year for the collection of developmental data on their children (which aligns with the objectives of this study), they were only asked to notify the teachers if they did not wish to participate in this specific research, given that both teachers and parents were expected to complete assessments. After obtaining consent and providing detailed assessment instructions, each educational group received a set of rating scales. Teachers conducted their assessments using a paper-and-pencil method throughout 7 to 10 days. Once completed, the researchers collected the filled-out scales. Teachers generated unique identification codes for each child and assigned these codes accordingly. They then communicated the relevant code to each child's parent. In this way, only teachers had access to the actual identities of the children, ensuring that researchers remained blinded to the participants' identities, thus preserving anonymity and confidentiality. Based on the suggestion of kindergarten staff, parents were provided with a digital version of the scales via a link to a Google Forms application. They completed the questionnaires online. The collected data were processed using JASP 0.17.2.1. and SPSS 29, employing statistical techniques such as descriptive analysis, correlation analysis, intraclass reliability analysis, and paired-sample difference testing, along with effect size estimations.

4. Results

4.1. Parents' and Kindergarten Teachers' Ratings of the Transition and Adjustment Quality and Children's Socio-Emotional Well-Being

Table 2 presents the results of the descriptive analysis, including means, standard deviations, ranges, and Cronbach's alpha reliability coefficients for four transition quality variables: difficulties during transition and adjustment; satisfaction with the transition and adjustment process; quality of parent–teacher cooperation during the transition; and duration of adjustment (in weeks); as well as six dimensions of children's socio-emotional well-being: social skills, self-regulation, self-assertiveness, emotional stability, activity orientation, and pleasure in exploration, as evaluated by both parents and kindergarten teachers.

Parents generally reported few difficulties during the adjustment period (M = 2.38), a perception shared by kindergarten teachers (M = 2.43), who likewise assessed the adjustment process as largely smooth with a low level of difficulties. Based on the collected data, parents rated the transition process as highly satisfactory (M = 4.60), whereas teachers assessed it as moderately to highly satisfactory (M = 4.11). A key component contributing to a successful adjustment process is the quality of parent–teacher cooperation. In this regard, parents reported a high level of collaboration with teachers (M = 4.48). Similarly, teachers also perceived an elevated level of cooperation with parents, highlighting the mutual importance of this relationship (M = 4.19). Both parents (M = 3.24) and teachers (M = 2.56) estimated the duration of the adjustment process to vary considerably, ranging from a single day to as long as six months, with an estimated average of 3 weeks of adjustment duration.

Regarding the children's socio-emotional well-being during the transition and adjustment period, the highest-rated dimension, according to both parents (M = 4.44) and teachers (M = 3.79), was pleasure in exploration, while emotional stability received the lowest ratings (parents: M = 3.74; teachers: M = 3.37). When analyzing the parental assessments separately, elevated levels were observed across all six socio-emotional dimensions, indicating a generally positive perception of children's adjustment. Teacher evaluations revealed the same relative pattern among the dimensions; however, overall ratings were lower than those provided by parents. Specifically, parents reported elevated levels in all dimensions, while teachers reported elevated levels only in pleasure in exploration and self-regulation (other dimensions were rated by teachers as moderate).

4.2. Inter-Rater Agreement on the Transition and Adjustment Quality and Children's Socio-Emotional Well-Being

The second stage of the analysis focused on examining differences between parent and teacher mean scores for each of the four transition quality variables and the six dimensions of children's socio-emotional well-being. A series of one-way repeated measures analyses of variance (ANOVAs) were conducted for this purpose. In addition, effect sizes were calculated for each variable using partial eta squared (η^2_p), and these are presented in Table 3 alongside the corresponding ANOVA statistics (F and *p* values). To interpret the magnitude of effect sizes, the classification proposed by Cohen [58] was applied: $\eta^2_p = 0.01$ indicates a small effect, $\eta^2_p = 0.06$ a medium effect, and $\eta^2_p = 0.14$ a large effect. The analysis revealed statistically significant differences in two of the four transition quality variables: satisfaction with the transition and adjustment process, and the quality of cooperation between parents and teachers.

Table 3. Mean differences (F, *p*), effect sizes (η^2_p), Pearson (r) and Spearman (rho) inter-rater correlations, and inter-rater agreement (ICC, lower and upper bound) for 4 transitions quality variables and 6 dimensions of socio-emotional well-being.

		ANOVA			Parents and Teachers	Inter-Rater Agreement 95% Confidence Interval		
		F	*p*	η^2_p	r (rho)	ICC	Lower Bound	Upper Bound
Satisfaction with the quality of transition from home to kindergarten	Difficulties during transition and adjustment	1.48	0.23	0.01	**0.21 * (0.22 *)**	0.21	0.09	0.33
	Satisfaction with transition and adjustment	22.51	**0.001**	0.17	**0.24 ** (0.20 *)**	0.25	0.12	0.36
	Quality of parent-teacher cooperation	9.29	**0.002**	0.08	**0.25 ** (0.27 **)**	0.25	0.13	0.36
	Adjustment duration (in weeks)	3.08	0.08	0.03	**0.54 *** (0.27 **)**	0.44	0.33	0.54
Socio-emotional well-being and resilience	Social skills	42.29	**0.000**	0.27	**0.52 *** (0.48 ***)**	0.52	0.42	0.60
	Self-regulation	9.61	**0.002**	0.08	**0.46 *** (0.45 ***)**	0.45	0.34	0.54
	Self-assertiveness	34.78	**0.000**	0.24	**0.31 ** (0.30 **)**	0.34	0.22	0.44
	Emotional stability	27.04	**0.000**	0.19	**0.19 *** (0.15)	0.20	0.07	0.32
	Activity orientation	23.69	**0.000**	0.18	**0.34 ** (0.28 **)**	0.36	0.25	0.47
	Pleasure in exploration	53.89	**0.000**	0.32	0.13 (−0.04)	0.13	0.01	0.25

* $p < 0.05$, ** $p < 0.01$, *** $p < 0.001$. Note: Bolded values are significant

Specifically, parents reported significantly higher levels of satisfaction with the transition process and perceived a higher quality of cooperation with teachers than teachers did. Moreover, for all six dimensions of socio-emotional well-being, parents consistently rated their children's adjustment significantly more positively than teachers. The effect sizes for these differences were predominantly large, indicating a robust discrepancy in perception between the two groups. In contrast, the effect sizes for differences in the variables difficulties during transition and adjustment, and adjustment duration were small. The effect size for the quality of parent–teacher cooperation was medium to large, while the effect size for satisfaction with transition and adjustment was large. To assess the degree of agreement between parent and teacher evaluations, two types of analyses were performed: (a) Pearson's and Spearman's correlation coefficients, to examine the strength and direction of the relationships between raters' scores on both the transition quality variables and socio-emotional well-being dimensions, and (b) intraclass correlation coefficients (ICCs), to measure the absolute level of agreement between raters. The results of these analyses are presented in Table 3.

For the four transition quality variables, all correlations between parent and teacher ratings were statistically significant, indicating a shared perception to some degree. However, for the socio-emotional well-being dimensions, the results were more nuanced. Significant correlations were found for social skills, self-regulation, self-assertiveness, and activity orientation, while the correlation for emotional stability was marginally significant. No significant correlation was observed for pleasure in exploration. ICCs were calculated using a two-way random-effects model based on absolute agreement. The interpretation of ICC values followed Cicchetti's [59] guidelines: values below 0.40 indicate poor agreement, 0.40 to 0.59 fair agreement, 0.60 to 0.74 good agreement, and values above 0.75 excellent agreement. Based on these criteria, poor agreement between parent and teacher ratings was observed for the following variables: difficulties during transition and adjustment, satisfaction with transition and adjustment, quality of parent–teacher cooperation, self-assertiveness, emotional stability, activity orientation, and pleasure in exploration. Fair agreement was established for adjustment duration, social skills, and self-regulation.

4.3. *Parents' and Kindergarten Teachers' Perspective on the Correlation Between the Transition and Adjustment Quality and Children's Socio-Emotional Well-Being*

Finally, to explore the relationship between quality transition variables and dimensions of socio-emotional well-being among children during transition and adjustment in kindergarten, two separate correlation analyses were run, based on parents' and teachers' ratings, and Spearman's correlation coefficients (due to significant deviations regarding Skewness and Kurtosis) with significance probability flags as can be seen in Table 4.

Table 4. Spearman's correlation coefficients and flagged probability for 4 transition quality variables, socio-demographic variables, and 6 dimensions of socio-emotional well-being of children based on parents' (N = 145; upper row) and kindergarten teachers' ratings (N = 202; lower row) with z-scores and probability levels for significance of difference testing (cells with significant z-scores are marked in grey colour).

	Difficulties During Transition and Adjustment		**Satisfaction with Transition and Adjustment**		**Quality of Parent-Teacher Cooperation**		**Adjustment Duration (In Weeks)**		**Children's Gender**		**Children's Age**		**Parents' or Teachers' Age**	
Social skills	−0.06 **−0.23 *****	1.61 (0.11)	0.14 **0.22 ****	−0.77 (0.44)	0.09 **0.29 *****	**−1.93** **(0.05)**	**−0.27 ***** **−0.19 ****	−0.78 (0.43)	0.05 0.09	0.37 (0.71)	**0.28 ***** **0.45 *****	−1.82 (0.07)	−0.03 0.05	−0.74 (0.46)
Self-regulation	−0.06 **−0.20 ****	1.32 (0.19)	0.09 **0.18 ***	−0.85 (0.40)	0.11 **0.30 *****	−1.84 (0.06)	−0.07 −0.11	0.37 (0.71)	**0.16 *** **0.21 ****	−0.48 (0.63)	**0.32 ***** **0.48 *****	−1.77 (0.08)	0.03 0.12	−0.84 (0.40)
Self-assertiveness	0.06 **−0.17 ***	**2.14** **(0.03)**	0.08 0.15	−0.66 (0.51)	−0.02 **0.22 ****	**−2.26** **(0.02)**	**−0.16 *** **−0.17 ***	0.10 (0.92)	**0.16 *** 0.07	0.84 (0.40)	**0.30 ***** **0.51 *****	**−2.34** **(0.02)**	−0.05 **0.16 ***	**−1.96** **(0.05)**
Emotional stability	−0.11 **−0.28 *****	1.64 (0.10)	0.12 **0.32 *****	**−1.95** **(0.05)**	0.08 **0.32 *****	**−2.33** **(0.02)**	−0.13 **−0.18 ***	0.47 (0.64)	0.12 **0.14 ***	−0.19 (0.85)	0.05 **0.26 *****	**−2.00** **(0.05)**	−0.02 0.01	−0.28 (0.78)
Activity orientation	−0.08 −0.14	0.56 (0.57)	0.15 **0.17 ***	−0.19 (0.85)	0.16 **0.28 *****	−1.17 (0.24)	**−0.18 *** −0.05	−1.22 (0.22)	0.05 **0.25 *****	−1.90 (0.06)	0.15 **0.36 *****	**−2.08** **(0.04)**	−0.00 0.10	−0.93 (0.35)
Pleasure in exploration	−0.09 **−0.14 ***	0.47 (0.64)	**0.19 *** **0.27 *****	−0.78 (0.43)	0.08 **0.26 *****	−1.72 (0.09)	−0.09 **−0.14 ***	0.47 (0.64)	0.04 0.12	−0.74 (0.46)	−0.09 **0.29 *****	**−3.60** **(0.001)**	−0.09 0.03	−1.11 (0.27)
Children's gender	0.01 0.06	−0.46 (0.64)	0.00 −0.03	−0.28 (0.78)	**0.20 *** 0.08	1.14 (0.26)	0.05 0.03	0.19 (0.85)						
Children's age	−0.11 **−0.24 *****	1.24 (0.21)	−0.14 −0.11	−0.28 (0.78)	**−0.24 **** 0.05	**−2.73** **(0.01)**	**−0.25 **** **−0.28 *****	0.30 (0.76)						
Parents' or teachers' age	−0.06 −0.06	0.00 (1.00)	0.01 **−0.23 ****	**2.26** **(0.02)**	−0.04 0.03	−0.65 (0.52)	−0.05 −0.10	0.47 (0.64)						

* $p < 0.05$, ** $p < 0.01$, *** $p < 0.001$. Note: Bolded values are significant

The parents' ratings (upper rows in the cells) showed no significant relations between the first three transitions' quality variables and dimensions of socio-emotional well-being, except in the case of pleasure in exploration. They evaluated that with the greater pleasure in exploration in children, a higher level of satisfaction with the transition and adjustment will be present, similar to what kindergarten teachers evaluated. In contrast to that, based on kindergarten teachers' ratings, several significant correlations were determined: greater difficulties during transition and adjustment were related with lower social skills, self-regulation, self-assertiveness, emotional stability and pleasure in exploration; greater satisfaction with transition and adjustment was related with higher level of social skills, self-regulation, emotional stability, activity orientation and pleasure in exploration; and greater collaboration with parents was related with all six dimensions of socio-emotional well-being of children during transition and adjustment. Regarding the variable of adjustment duration in kindergarten, longer adjustment was related to lower social skills, self-assertiveness, and activity orientation based on parents' ratings. Based on teachers' ratings, it was determined that longer adjustment was related to lower social skills, self-assertiveness, emotional stability, and pleasure in exploration.

To analyze the significance of the difference between two correlations, an online calculator created by Daniel Soper [60] was applied. By this, it was possible to explore whether two correlation coefficients are significantly different from each other, those from parents' and teachers' ratings, given the two correlation coefficients and their associated sample sizes. Calculations resulted in z-scores and their probability level. A probability value of less than 0.05 indicates that the two correlation coefficients are significantly different from each other. Therefore, analyzing the determined findings showed in Table 4, it could be seen that there are five significant differences between correlation coefficients regarding the connection between transition quality and socio-emotional well-being: parents and teachers. Significantly greater correlation coefficients are determined in teachers than in parents' ratings in these relationships: difficulties during transition-self-assertiveness; satisfaction with transition and adjustment-emotional stability; quality of parent-teacher collaboration-social skills; quality of parent-teacher collaboration-self-assertiveness; quality of parent-teacher collaboration-emotional stability.

Found significant correlations between quality transition and socio-demographic variables showed that parents perceive greater collaboration with kindergarten teachers if they are parents of girls and younger children, and longer adjustment in younger children. Based on teachers' ratings, the significant correlations are determined related to greater difficulties during transition and adjustment, and longer adjustment in kindergarten among younger children; and the greater satisfaction with the transition and adjustment if they were younger, regarding their age. Within this set of correlations, parents' and teachers' ratings significantly differed in two relationships: parents rated the relationship between younger children and higher quality of collaboration with teachers as significant, while teachers didn't; and teachers rated the relationship between their greater age and less satisfaction with transition and adjustment of children as significant, while parents didn't.

Finally, analyzing the determined correlation between socio-emotional well-being and socio-demographic variables, it was determined that girls and older children have greater self-regulation and self-assertiveness, while older children also show greater social skills, based on parents' ratings. Based on the teachers' ratings, more correlations were found to be significant: girls were rated as more self-regulated, emotionally stable, and activity oriented, while older children showed higher all sic dimensions of socio-emotional well-being during transition and adjustment. In addition, based on teachers' ratings, it was found that the self-assertiveness of children was dependent on teachers' age: older teachers rated children as more self-assertive. Mostly, parents' and teachers' ratings significantly differed in correlations between children's age and four dimensions of socio-emotional well-being: self-assertiveness, emotional stability, activity orientation, and pleasure in exploration, within which, correlations were significantly higher based on teachers' ratings. In addition, teachers rated the relationship between their greater age and children's greater self-assertiveness as significant, while parents didn't.

5. Discussion

5.1. Children's Socio-Emotional Well-Being During Transition and Adjustment, and the Transition and Adjustment Quality: Parents' and Kindergarten Teachers' Perspectives

In general, the observed levels of transition quality from home to preschool and children's adjustment within preschool settings revealed results consistent with prior expectations and previously established findings. Specifically, these included lower levels of difficulties experienced by children during the transition and adjustment processes, a high level of collaboration between parents and teachers, and very high ratings of satisfaction during the transition and adjustment. These results are comparable to those from the national five-year longitudinal study [9], which was conducted on a sample of 795 children aged 1 to 5 years. In that study, both teachers (N = 77) and parents (N = 247) assessed the quality of transition and adjustment using identical quality transition variables. When comparing teachers' assessments, the present study indicated slightly higher levels of difficulties experienced by children (M = 2.81), suggesting a moderate level of challenge. Meanwhile, satisfaction with the transition (M = 4.22) and collaboration between parents and teachers (M = 3.92) were both rated as elevated. In terms of parental evaluations, the national study reported a higher level of perceived difficulty (M = 2.93), but equally high levels of satisfaction with the transition and adjustment process (M = 4.60) and with parent-teacher collaboration (M = 4.43). It may thus be concluded that the findings are highly similar and largely expected, given that the majority of children experience a low level of difficulty during transitions and adjustment. Consequently, this contributes to increased satisfaction with the transition itself as well as with the collaboration between parents and teachers [16,27,28]. In addition, similar findings have been reported in studies beyond the domestic context, based on the perspectives of kindergarten teachers, parents, and children. Various international empirical studies have demonstrated that the majority of children experience positive and successful transitions when adequate support for their socio-emotional well-being is provided, characterized by satisfactory adjustment to kindergartens and effective cooperation with parents [61–64].

The implications of these findings point to the need for future research focusing on the detailed collection of qualitative data regarding the types and frequencies of difficulties encountered by children during transitions and adjustment. Moreover, it is necessary to examine how these difficulties vary according to institutional characteristics and other potentially significant variables. Such insights could inform the development of targeted support programs for children and parents during the transition process, ultimately reducing difficulties and enhancing satisfaction with both the transition and parent-teacher collaboration.

It is essential to consider both parental and teacher assessments, as statistical analyses revealed that teachers rated satisfaction with the transition and collaboration significantly lower than parents did. Given the large effect sizes observed, these differences should not be overlooked. Future studies employing qualitative methodologies may help to uncover the underlying reasons for these divergent perceptions. Interestingly, assessments did not significantly differ in terms of the estimated duration of children's adjustment in kindergarten, which was reported as approximately three weeks. This finding aligns with previous research conducted in Croatia, in which 34 teachers estimated the average adjustment period as one month (i.e., four weeks) [6]. Stojić and colleagues [65] suggest that the adjustment period can range from 10–15 days up to two months, emphasizing the highly individual nature of adjustment, which is influenced by numerous factors, including the child's age, developmental stage, emotional and health status, and temperament.

Moderate to high levels of social-emotional well-being dimensions, as rated by teachers, largely confirm findings from previous validation studies [45,46] as well as from the national study [9]. However, parental assessments indicated even higher levels across all dimensions compared to teacher assessments, which is again consistent with findings from the national study based on parental data. Statistical analyses, including significance testing and effect size analysis, revealed substantial differences between parental and teacher evaluations of all dimensions of children's social-emotional well-being, with large effect sizes. This suggests a fundamental divergence in how these two groups perceive children's social-emotional well-being during transitions. Overall, parents consistently rated their children's well-being during transition and adaptation significantly higher than teachers did. This result aligns with prior expectations given the greater subjectivity typically present in parental assessments [47].

5.2. The Transition and Adjustment Quality and Children's Socio-Emotional Well-Being During Transition: What Is the Level of Inter-Rater Agreement?

Conducting two types of analyses, Pearson's and Spearman's correlation coefficients, and intraclass correlation coefficients (ICCs) to assess inter-rater agreement revealed notable discrepancies between parents and kindergarten teachers in their evaluations of transition and adjustment quality, as well as children's socio-emotional well-being during this period. With regard to the strength and direction of relationships between raters' scores on the key variables, significant positive correlations were found for all four transition quality variables and the dimensions of socio-emotional well-being, with the exception of pleasure in exploration. These findings are consistent with ICC results, which indicated mostly poor to fair agreement between raters concerning both transition quality and socio-emotional well-being. Although low inter-rater agreement could potentially be attributed to low reliability, this explanation does not hold in this case. While slightly lower for parents, both groups' ratings demonstrated high and satisfactory levels of internal consistency. Therefore, the observed discrepancies likely stem from children's situation-specific behaviors and the differing evaluative standards used by informants [47,55,57].

Interestingly, the variables adjustment duration, social skills, and self-regulation showed fair levels of inter-rater agreement. This raises an important question: Are these particular behaviors easier to observe and therefore more consistently rated, or do these variables reflect dimensions that are more reliably and validly measured, or possibly both? Notably, reliability levels for social skills and self-regulation were highest in teacher ratings. However, regardless of reliability, children's behavior appears to be highly context-dependent, varying significantly between the home and kindergarten environments. This underscores the importance of employing a multi-informant approach in studies of children's socio-emotional well-being during transition and adjustment periods to capture a more comprehensive and nuanced understanding. Although there are currently no published studies focusing specifically on inter-rater agreement in the assessment of children's socio-emotional well-being during transition to kindergarten, related studies in the field of child mental health report similar discrepancies between parent and teacher ratings [47,48,56,57]. In light of these findings, future research should incorporate the child's perspective alongside those of parents and teachers [66]. Moreover, it is essential to include an equal representation of mothers and fathers to allow for more detailed analysis of multi-informant data. Each informant provides unique and valuable insight that, when considered together, can lead to a richer and more accurate understanding of children's developmental experiences.

5.3. Parents' and Kindergarten Teachers' Perspectives on the Correlation Between the Transition and Adjustment Quality and Children's Socio-Emotional Well-Being

Finally, given that previous research phases identified significant differences in mean scores for transition quality and children's socio-emotional well-being during the transition and adjustment period, accompanied by large effect sizes, statistically significant yet low correlations, and poor inter-rater agreement based on calculated intraclass correlation coefficients (ICCs), the findings regarding significant differences in correlation coefficients reflecting the relationship between transition quality and socio-emotional well-being are to be expected. Overall, based on teacher ratings, more consistent and statistically significant correlations were observed between transition quality and all six dimensions of socio-emotional well-being, compared to parent ratings. These findings indicate that higher levels of socio-emotional well-being are significantly associated with higher-quality transitions from home to kindergarten and more successful child adjustment within the kindergarten setting. These relationships are consistent with previous research [9,32,67].

The study found that children assessed as having higher levels of social skills, self-regulation, pleasure in exploration, assertiveness, emotional stability, and activity orientation experienced significantly fewer difficulties during the transition process, as well as greater satisfaction with the transition and higher quality of collaboration between parents and teachers. Consistent with previous research, this study confirms that children in early and preschool education exhibit higher levels of social-emotional well-being and resilience across all dimensions when the transition process is perceived as highly satisfactory, collaboration with parents is of higher quality, and the number of experienced difficulties is lower. This finding represents one of the key outcomes of this complex study, which is primarily focused on children's well-being during transitions and adaptation in preschool and primary school settings.

Given the significance of the identified correlations, it is critically important to ensure a high quality of transitions and adjustment, as these have a direct effect on children's social-emotional well-being. Although these correlations were less pronounced in parental assessments, significant differences were observed in the relationships between difficulties and assertiveness, satisfaction with the transition and emotional stability, as well as between the quality of parent-teacher collaboration and three dimensions of social-emotional well-being: social skills, assertiveness, and emotional stability. The significance of these associations, as perceived by teachers, may be explained by the unique context in which teachers interact directly with children during the transition and adjustment periods, an experience that is only partially accessible to parents, for instance, during joint parent–child visits to the kindergarten setting. It is important to acknowledge that even in such shared contexts, parents do not have full insight into their child's behavior in the new environment, since children typically behave differently in kindergarten settings depending on whether a parent is present or not. Consequently, differing perceptions between parents and teachers regarding children's social-emotional well-being during transition and adjustment are to be expected. Additionally, Lopez and Benner [68] and Fukkink et al. [69] emphasize that the support provided by teachers during transitions is significantly associated with children's social-emotional well-being in kindergarten. Effective collaboration and mutual respect between teachers and parents facilitate easier adjustment for the child, foster a sense of security and trust, and promote a higher level of social-emotional well-being. This is further supported by the findings on the variable measuring the quality of teacher-parent collaboration and its relationship to children's social-emotional well-being, where the association was significantly stronger from the teachers' perspective.

Furthermore, notable differences were found between parent and teacher perceptions in terms of the quality of transition, social-emotional well-being, and socio-demographic variables. Original validation studies demonstrated the expected significant associations between children's general social-emotional well-being and their gender and age [45,46], as well as the association between these same variables and well-being during transition and adjustment [9,32,67], based on teacher assessments, differing from parental perspectives. Regarding age-related correlations, it is developmentally expected that younger children would experience more difficulties and lower satisfaction during the transition and adjustment period, along with lower levels of social-emotional well-being. This is due to the developmental trajectory of social-emotional competencies, which are directly related to children's ability to cope with and adjust in new situations [45]. Teachers, due to their professional knowledge of developmental milestones and their ability to observe and compare behaviors across different age groups, are more sensitive to age-related correlations. Most parents lack access to these two key points of reference, which fundamentally affects their baseline for evaluating such constructs. Interestingly, although gender was found to affect collaboration quality, where cooperation was perceived as more effective with girls (according to parents), and higher dimensions of social-emotional well-being were observed in girls, these findings remain an open question. While gender-related correlational differences were identified in this study, there were no statistically significant differences between parent and teacher assessments in this regard. Previous research on transitional periods indicates that gender strongly influences all aspects of childhood development, although the degree and specific nature of its influence on transitions vary across families, communities, and cultures [14,70]. Moreover, studies on gender differences in children's academic and behavioral outcomes, as indicators of effective adjustment, consistently show that girls outperform boys [2,71]. Therefore, future research should continue to explore the effects of gender and age on children's social-emotional well-being during transitions and adjustment periods.

6. Conclusions

The primary aim of this study was to examine the quality of transition and children's socio-emotional well-being, their interrelationship, as well as the inter-rater agreement between parents and teachers. In summary, the findings confirmed previous research indicating moderate to elevated levels of children's socio-emotional well-being during the transition and adjustment period, as well as overall high quality of these transitions in kindergarten settings. As expected, although there are notable similarities in parents' and teachers' perceptions of these important aspects of transition and adaptation, which can serve as a basis for creating guidelines to facilitate the process, the study revealed a small to fair level of inter-rater agreement regarding parents' and teachers' ratings of transition quality and children's socio-emotional well-being during this period. The explanation offered by Fält et al. [47] is applied in this study as well: parents and teachers possess distinct characteristics that significantly determine their assessments. Moreover, their evaluations are also shaped by context-specific situational factors. Therefore, when designing educational guidelines for practice, such as those aimed at facilitating smooth transitions and ensuring high levels of children's socio-emotional well-being, it is crucial to employ a multi-informant approach in studies assessing children's behavior.

Despite the study's significant contribution, it is important to address its limitations, particularly when designing future research. As the sample was not randomly selected and included a relatively small number of parents (predominantly mothers), replication with a larger, randomly selected sample of children, parents, and teachers is warranted. As previously suggested, future studies should aim to include both parents in the assessment process, thereby enabling an examination of inter-rater agreement between mothers and fathers. Furthermore, as certain variables were not controlled, such as early childhood educators' level of education and prior experience with similar assessments, they should be considered in future studies. Additionally, given that transition quality in this study was measured using only four items, future research should employ comprehensive transition quality assessment scales that capture multiple dimensions of this construct, allowing for a more nuanced understanding of the transition process. To develop practical guidelines, it would also be beneficial to apply qualitative methodologies to explore the causes and types of difficulties children experience during transitions. In addition, it would be useful to explore possible predictors of children's socio-emotional well-being during transition and adjustment, and to see whether there are any differences in perceived predictors by parents and teachers. Such an approach could increase both child and parent satisfaction and enhance children's socio-emotional well-being. Taken together, the findings of this study have significant implications for the professional practice of kindergarten teachers. The results provide both parents and teachers with a deeper understanding of children's socio-emotional well-being during transitions and highlight the value of employing a multi-informant approach. Importantly, this study represents a rare contribution within the Croatian context and, for the first time, offers a detailed analysis of both parents' and teachers' perceptions of the transition process.

Author Contributions: Conceptualization, methodology, statistical analyses and writing, S.T.V.; data collecting and writing, T.K. All authors have read and agreed to the published version of the manuscript.

Funding: This research was funded by the University of Rijeka, grant number PU-180, uniri-iz-25-115: "ADJUST_WELL: Adjustment in kindergarten: Enhancement of educational practice as a facilitator of early transitions and children's well-being".

Institutional Review Board Statement: This research study was approved by the Croatian Ministry of Science and Education (number: 602-01/19-01/00501, 533-05-19-0005, date: 19 September 2019) and the Ethical Committee of the Faculty of Humanities and Social Sciences, University of Rijeka (number: 640-01/19-01/113, 2170-24-02-19-2, date: 28 August 2019).

Informed Consent Statement: Informed consent was obtained from all subjects involved in the study.

Data Availability Statement: The data underlying this article cannot be shared publicly because of the privacy and confidentiality of the study participants, which are protected. The data of this study are available upon reasonable request from the corresponding author.

Acknowledgments: We would like to express our gratitude to all kindergarten teachers who participated in this study.

Conflicts of Interest: The authors declare no potential conflicts of interest related to the research, authorship, or publication of this article. Additionally, the authors report no relevant financial or nonfinancial interests.

References

1. Early, D.M.; Pianta, R.C.; Taylor, L.C.; Cox, M.J. Transition Practices: Findings from a National Survey of Kindergarten Teachers. *Early Child. Educ. J.* **2001**, *28*, 199–206. [CrossRef]
2. Tatalović Vorkapić, S.; LoCasale-Crouch, J. *Supporting Children's Well-Being During Early Childhood Transition to School*; IGI Global: Hershey, PA, USA, 2021.
3. Mihić, I. *Vrtić Kao Sigurna Baza: Adaptacija Dece Nakon Jaslenog Uzrasta (Kindergarten as a Secure Base: Adaptation of Children After Toddlers' Age)*; University of Novi Sad, Faculty of Philosophy, Department of Psychology (Center for Applied Psychology): Novi Sad, Serbia, 2016.
4. Mašković, T.; Droždan, D.; Sokač, M.; Josić, M. *Od Jaslica do Škole, Vodič za Lakši Proces Prilagodbe na Jaslice, Vrtić I Školu (from Nursery to School, a Guide to Making the Process of Adjusting to Nursery, Kindergarten and School Easier)*; RTL kockica: Zagreb, Croatia, 2018.
5. Einarsdóttir, J.; Perry, B.; Dockett, S. Transition to school practices: Comparisons from Iceland and Australia. *Early Years Int. Res. J.* **2008**, *28*, 47–60. [CrossRef]
6. Tatalović Vorkapić, S. *Psihologija Privrženosti I Prilagodba U Dječjemu Vrtiću, Psihologija Dobrobiti Djece Vol. 1 (the Attachment Psychology and Adjustment in Kindergarten, the Psychology of Children's Well-Being, Vol. 1)*; University of Rijeka, Faculty of Teacher Education: Rijeka, Croatia, 2020.

7. Eurydice 2024. Available online: https://eurydice.eacea.ec.europa.eu/eurypedia/croatia/organisation-education-system-and-its-structure (accessed on 25 July 2025).
8. Došen-Dobud, A. *S Djecom U Jaslicama (with Children in Nursery)*; Alinea: Zagreb, Croatia, 2004.
9. Tatalović Vorkapić, S. *Dobrobit Djece Tijekom Prijelaznih Perioda: Empirijska Provjera Ekološko-Dinamičkog Modela; Psihologija Dobrobiti Djece Vol. 3 (The Well-Being of Children in Transitional Periods: Empirical Validation of the Ecological-Dynamic Model, The Psychology of Children's Well-Being Vol. 3)*; University of Rijeka, Faculty of Teacher Education: Rijeka, Croatia, 2024.
10. Then, D.; Pohlmann-Rother, S. Adaptivity in the inclusive transition to school. *Front. Educ.* **2024**, *8*, 1304918. [CrossRef]
11. Downes, P. Transition as a displacement from more fundamental system concerns: Distinguishing four different meanings of transition in education. *Educ. Philos. Theory* **2019**, *51*, 1465–1476. [CrossRef]
12. Anić, V.; Brozović Rončević, D.; Goldstein, I.; Goldstein, S.; Jojić, G.; Matasović, R.; Pranjković, I. *Hrvatski Encikklopedijski Rječnik: Pes-Pro (Croatian Encyclopedic Dictionary: Pes-Pro)*; EPH d.o.o.: Zagreb, Croatia; Novi Liber d.o.o.: Zagreb, Croatia, 2004.
13. Lam, M.S.; Pollard, A. A conceptual framework for understanding children as agents in the transition from home to kindergarten. *Early Years Int. J. Res. Dev.* **2006**, *26*, 123–141. [CrossRef]
14. Vogler, P.; Crivello, G.; Woodhead, M. *Early Childhood Transitions Research: A Review of Concepts, Theory and Practice*; Bernard van Leer Foundation: The Hague, The Netherlands, 2008.
15. *Nacionalni Kurikulum Za Rani I Predškolski Odgoj I Obrazovanje—National Curriculum for Early and Preschool Care and Education*; Narodne Novine, 5/2015; Ministarstvo Znanosti i Obazovanja: Zagreb, Croatia, 2015. Available online: https://mzo.gov.hr/UserDocsImages/dokumenti/Obrazovanje/Predskolski/Nacionalni%20kurikulum%20za%20rani%20i%20predskolski%20odgoj%20i%20obrazovanje%20NN%2005-2015.pdf (accessed on 26 July 2025).
16. Mashburn, A.J.; LoCasale-Crouch, J.; Pears, K.C. *Kindergarten Transition and Readiness: Promoting Cognitive, Social-Emotional, and Self-Regulatory Development*; Springer International Publishing AG, Part of Springer Nature: Cham, Switzerland, 2018.
17. Fabian, H.; Dunlop, A.-W. *Outcomes of Good Practice in Transition Processes for Children Entering Primary School*; Working Papers in Early Childhood Development; Bernard van Leer Foundation: The Hague, The Netherlands, 2007; No. 42.
18. Mihić, I. Vrtić kao sigurna baza: Primer modela tranzicije u vrtić temeljenog na teoriji afektivne vezanosti. (Kindergarten as a safe base: The example of transition to kindergarten model based on the attachment theory). In *The Attachment Psychology and Adjustment in Kindergarten, The Psychology of Children's Well-Being*; Tatalović Vorkapić, S., Ed.; University of Rijeka, Faculty of Teacher Education: Rijeka, Croatia, 2020; Volume 1, pp. 183–219.
19. Ackesjö, H. Transitions—Times of reconstructions. *Int. J. Transit. Child.* **2013**, *6*, 16–27.
20. Dockett, S.; Perry, B. Starting school: Effective transitions. *Early Child. Res. Pract.* **2001**, *3*, n2. Available online: https://files.eric.ed.gov/fulltext/ED458041.pdf (accessed on 25 August 2025).
21. Peters, R.S. *The Concept of Education (International Library of the Philosophy of Education)*; Routledge: London, UK, 2010; Volume 17. [CrossRef]
22. Sayers, M.; West, S.; Lorains, J.; Laidlaw, B.; Moore, T.; Robinson, R. Starting school: A pivotal life transition for children and their families. *Fam. Matters* **2012**, *90*, 45–56.
23. Tatalović Vorkapić, S. Children's well-being during transition periods in Croatia: The proposal of empirical validation of Ecological-dynamic model. In *INTED2019 Proceedings, 13th International Technology, Education and Development Conference, Valencia, Spain, 11–13 March 2019*; Gómez Chova, L., López Martínez, A., Candel Torres, I., Eds.; IATED: Valencia, Spain, 2019; pp. 265–276.
24. O'Toole, L.; Hayes, N.; Mhathúna, M.M. A Bio-ecological Perspective on Educational Transition. *Procedia-Soc. Behav. Sci.* **2014**, *140*, 121–127. [CrossRef]
25. Brofenbrenner, U. *The Ecology of Human Development*; Harvard University Press: Cambridge, MA, USA, 1979.
26. Rimm-Kaufman, S.E.; Pianta, R.C. An Ecological Perspective on the Transition to Kindergarten: A Theoretical Framework to Guide Empirical Research. *J. Appl. Dev. Psychol.* **2000**, *21*, 491–511. [CrossRef]
27. Pianta, R.C.; Cox, M.J. *The Transition to Kindergarten*; Paul H. Brookes: Baltimore, MD, USA, 1999.
28. Pianta, R.C.; Cox, M.J.; Taylor, L.; Early, D. Kindergarten teachers' practices related to transition into schools: Results of a national survey. *Elem. Sch. J.* **1999**, *100*, 71–86. [CrossRef]
29. Bronfenbrenner, U.; Morris, P.A. The ecology of developmental processes. In *Handbook of Child Psychology*, 5th ed.; Damon, W., Lerner, R.M., Eds.; Wiley: New York, NY, USA, 1998; Volume 1, pp. 993–1028.
30. Little, M.H.; Cohen-Vogel, L.; Curran, F.C. Facilitating the Transition to Kindergarten: What ECLS-K Dana Tell Us about School Practices Then and Now. *AERA Open* **2016**, *2*, 2332858416655766. [CrossRef]
31. Morawska, A.; Mitchell, A.E.; Etel, E.; Armstrong, R.; McAuliffe, T.; Ma, T.; McBryde, C.; Johnston, L.M. A Systematic Review of Parents' Experiences during their Child's Transition to School. *Early Child. Educ. J.* **2024**, *2014*, 1–12. [CrossRef]
32. Tatalović Vorkapić, S. How to support early educational transitions of children?—An overview of university science project's activities from Croatia. *Rev. Românească Pentru Educ. Multidimens.* **2023**, *15*, 532–556. [CrossRef]
33. Birch, S.H.; Ladd, G.W. The teacher-child relationship and children's early school adjustment. *J. Sch. Psychol.* **1997**, *35*, 61–79. [CrossRef]

34. Ben-Arieh, A.; Casas, F.; Frønes, I.; Korbin, J.E. *Handbook of Child Well-Being: Theories, Methods and Policies in Global Perspective*; Springer: Berlin/Heidelberg, Germany, 2014.
35. Statham, J.; Chase, E. *Childhood Wellbeing: A Brief Overview (Childhood Wellbeing Research Centre)*; Leading Education and Societal Research; Institute of Education, University of London: London, UK; Loughborough University and University of Kent: Canterbury, UK, 2010; Available online: https://www.researchgate.net/publication/242676811_Childhood_Wellbeing_A_Brief_Overview (accessed on 28 July 2025).
36. Mayr, T.; Ulich, M. *Perik: Positive Entwicklung und Resilienz im Kindergartenalltag*; Staatinstitut fur frühpädagogik IFP: Munich, Germany, 2006.
37. Deci, E.L.; Ryan, R.M. The 'what' and 'why' of goal pursuits: Human needs and the self-determination of behaviour. *Psychol. Inq.* **2000**, *11*, 227–268. [CrossRef]
38. Becker, P. *Psychologie der Seelischen Gesundheit. Band 1*; Hogrehe: Göttingen, Germany, 1982.
39. Becker, P. Erste Überprüfung der Theorie der Seelischen Gesundheit. In *Psychologie der Seelischen Gesundheit. Band 2*; Becker, P., Minsel, B., Eds.; Hogrefe: Göttingen, Germany, 1986; pp. 91–119.
40. World Health Organisation. *Life Skills Education in Schools, Parts 1 and 2*; WHO, Division of Mental Health: Geneva, Switzerland, 1994.
41. Asshauer, M.; Hanewinkel, R. Lebenskompetenztraining fu¨r Erst-Zweitkla¨ssler:Ergebnisse einer Interventionsstudie. *Kindh. Entwickl.* **2000**, *9*, 251–263. [CrossRef]
42. Masten, A.S. Resilience Theory and Research on Children and Families: Past, Present, and Promise. *J. Fam. Theory Rev.* **2018**, *10*, 12–31. [CrossRef]
43. Masten, A.S. Resilience from a developmental systems perspective. *World Psychiatry* **2019**, *18*, 101–102. [CrossRef]
44. Blair, C. Integrating cognition and emotion in a neurobiological conceptualization of children's functioning at school entry. *Am. Psychol.* **2002**, *57*, 111–127. [CrossRef]
45. Mayr, T.; Ulich, M. Social-emotional well-being and resilience of children in early childhood settings- PERIK: An empirically based observation scale for practitioners. *Early Years Int. J. Res. Dev.* **2009**, *29*, 45–57. [CrossRef]
46. Tatalović Vorkapić, S.; Lončarić, D. Validacija hrvatske verzije Ljestvice socio-emocionalne dobrobiti i otpornosti predškolske djece (The validation of the Croatian version of the Socio-emotional well-being and resilience scale in preschool children). *Hrvat. Rev. Rehabil. Istraživanja* **2014**, *502*, 102–117. Available online: https://hrcak.srce.hr/file/193745 (accessed on 25 August 2025).
47. Fält, E.; Wallby, T.; Sarkadi, A.; Salari, R.; Fabian, H. Agreement between mothers', fathers', and teachers' ratings of behavioural and emotional problems in 3–5-year-old children. *PLoS ONE* **2018**, *13*, e0206752. [CrossRef]
48. Tobia, V.; Greco, A.; Steca, P.; Marzocchi, G. Children's Wellbeing at School: A Multi-dimensional and Multi-informant Approach. *J. Happiness Stud.* **2019**, *20*, 841–861. [CrossRef]
49. Anderson, J.K.; Ford, T.; Soneson, E.; Coon, J.T.; Humphrey, A.; Rogers, M.; Moore, D.; Jones, P.B.; Clarke, E.; Howarth, E. A systematic review of effectiveness and cost-effectiveness of school-based identification of children and young people at risk of, or currently experiencing mental health difficulties. *Psychol. Med.* **2019**, *49*, 9–19. [CrossRef]
50. Von der Embse, N.; De Los Reyes, A. Advancing equity in access to school mental health through multiple informant decision-making. *J. Sch. Psychol.* **2024**, *104*, 101310. [CrossRef]
51. Stormont, M.; Stebbins, M.S. Preschool teachers' knowledge, opinions, and educational experiences with attention deficit/hyperactivity disorder. *Teach. Educ. Spec. Educ.* **2005**, *28*, 52–61. [CrossRef]
52. Eklund, K.; Dowdy, E. Screening for behavioral and emotional risk versus traditional school identification methods. *Sch. Ment. Health A Multidiscip. Res. Pract. J.* **2014**, *6*, 40–49. [CrossRef]
53. Stefan, C.A.; Miclea, M. Reliability and validity of two brief screening measures of preschoolers' social-emotional competencies. *Sch. Ment. Health* **2017**, *9*, 44–65. [CrossRef]
54. De Los Reyes, A.; Kazdin, A.E. Identifying evidence-based interventions for children and adolescents using the range of possible changes model: A meta-analytic illustration. *Behav. Modif.* **2009**, *33*, 583–617. [CrossRef]
55. De Los Reyes, A.; Thomas, S.A.; Goodman, K.L.; Kundey, S.M.A. Principles underlying the use of multiple informants' reports. *Annu. Rev. Clin. Psychol.* **2013**, *9*, 123–149. [CrossRef]
56. McLeod, B.D.; Porter, N.; Hogue, A.; Becker-Haimes, E.M.; Jensen-Doss, A. What is the Status of Multi-Informant Treatment Fidelity Research? *J. Clin. Child Adolesc. Psychol.* **2022**, *52*, 74–94. [CrossRef]
57. McLean, R.K.; Tully, L.A.; Brinley, S.K.; Carl, T.; Turnell, A.; Northam, J.C.; Dadds, M.R. Multi-Informant Universal Mental Health Screening for Preschool-Aged Children by Parents and Educators: A PRISMA Systematic Review. *Clin. Child Fam. Psychol. Rev.* **2025**, *28*, 1–21. [CrossRef]
58. Cohen, J. *Statistical Power Analysis for the Behavioral Sciences*; Routledge Academic: New York, NY, USA, 1988.
59. Cicchetti, D.V. Guidelines, criteria, and rules of thumb for evaluating normed and standardized assessment instruments in psychology. *Psychol. Assess.* **1994**, *6*, 284–290. [CrossRef]

60. Soper, D.S. *Significance of the Difference Between Two Correlations Calculator*, Version 4.0; Free Statistics Calculators: Fullerton, CA, USA, 2025. Available online: https://www.danielsoper.com/statcalc (accessed on 15 June 2025).
61. Bulkeley, J.; Fabian, H. Wellbeing and belonging during early educational transitions. *Int. J. Transit. Child.* **2006**, *2*, 18–31.
62. Gath, M.E.; Herold, L.; Hunkin, E.; McNair, L.J.; Redder, B.; Rutanen, N.; White, E.J. Infants' emotional and social experiences during and after the transition to early childhood education and care. *J. Early Child. Res.* **2024**, *22*, 88–105. [CrossRef]
63. Murray, L.; Levickis, P.; McFarland, L.; Eadie, P.; Lee-Pang, L.; Quach, J.; Page, J. Supporting Young Children's Social–Emotional Wellbeing in Early Childhood Education and Care: Perspectives from the Sector. *Educ. Sci.* **2025**, *15*, 569. [CrossRef]
64. Zhoc, K.C.H.; Tse, J.K.Y.; King, R.B. The importance of social and emotional learning in facilitating positive transitions from kindergarten to primary school in Hong Kong. *J. Early Child. Res.* **2025**, *2025*, 1476718X251349938. [CrossRef]
65. Stojić, O.; Divljan, S.; Avramov, N. Adaptacija dece jaslenog uzrasta u kontekstu teorije afektivne vezanosti: Iskustva predškolskih ustanova Srema (Nursery school children adaptation in the context of attachment theory: Experiences of preschool institutions in the region of Srem). *Primenj. Psihol.* **2010**, *3*, 357–376. [CrossRef]
66. Demkowicz, O.; Bagnall, C.; Hennessey, A.; Pert, K.; Bray, L.; Ashworth, E.; Mason, C. 'It's scary starting a new school': Children and young people's perspectives on wellbeing support during educational transitions. *Br. J. Educ. Psychol.* **2023**, *93*, 1017–1033. [CrossRef]
67. Tatalović Vorkapić, S. Children's socio-emotional well-being and resilience during transition from family home to kindergarten. In *Contemporary Challenges in Education: Paradoxes & Illuminations; Voices from the Classroom*; Chiou, V., Geunis, L., Holz, O., Ertürk, N.O., Ratkowska-Pasikowska, J., Shelton, F., Eds.; Waxmann Verlag GmbH: Münster, Germany, 2023; Volume 3, pp. 68–79. ISBN 978-3-8309-4697-7.
68. López, B.A.; Benner, A.D. Challenges in the transition to kindergarten and children's well-being through elementary school: Do school transition supports matter? *Early Child. Res. Q.* **2025**, *71*, 193–204. [CrossRef]
69. Fukkink, R.G.; Sluiter, R.M.V.; Fekkes, M. Transition from childcare to school: Surgency, center-based care and caregiver-child relationship predict self-regulation, social competence and well-being. *Learn. Individ. Differ.* **2024**, *110*, 102409. [CrossRef]
70. Rimm-Kaufman, S.E.; Kagan, J. Infant Predictors of Kindergarten Behavior: The Contribution of Inhibited and Uninhibited Temperament Types. *Behav. Disord.* **2005**, *30*, 331–347. [CrossRef]
71. Margetts, K. Transition and Adjustment to School. In *Transitions to School-International Research, Policy and Practice*; International Perspectives on Early Childhood Education and Development; Perry, B., Dockett, S., Petriwskyj, A., Eds.; Springer: Dordrecht, The Netherlands, 2014; Volume 9, pp. 75–87. [CrossRef]

children

MDPI

Article

Schools as Neighborhoods: A Holistic Framework for Student Well-Being, Opportunity, and Social Success

Cordelia R. Elaiho [1,*], Constance Gundacker [2], Thomas H. Chelius [3], Brandon Currie [4] and John R. Meurer [3,*]

[1] School of Medicine, Medical College of Wisconsin, Milwaukee, WI 53226, USA
[2] Department of Pediatrics, Medical College of Wisconsin, Milwaukee, WI 53226, USA
[3] Institute for Health & Humanity, Medical College of Wisconsin, Milwaukee, WI 53226, USA
[4] STRYV365, Milwaukee, WI 53202, USA; bcurrie@stryv365.org
* Correspondence: celaiho@mcw.edu (C.R.E.); jmeurer@mcw.edu (J.R.M.)

Abstract

Background: Schools play a central role in child development and socialization and can function as protective environments that mitigate the effects of adversity. Building on the Social Ecological Model and Community School Transformation, we propose a "Schools-as-Neighborhoods" framework that conceptualizes schools as intentionally designed microenvironments capable of generating social capital, promoting positive childhood experiences, and buffering harmful neighborhood exposures through trauma-informed programming. Methods: We conducted a convergent mixed-methods study across four public and charter schools in Milwaukee, Wisconsin, serving grades five through nine. STRYV365's *peak team* and Brain Agents gamified intervention were implemented between 2022–2024. Quantitative surveys and qualitative data assessed students' lived experiences, exposure to adversity, emotional awareness, coping skills, and school connectedness/climate across multiple waves. Results: Across the four schools (n = 1626 students), baseline academic proficiency was low, and exposure to adversity was high among surveyed participants (n = 321), including bereavement (74%) and family incarceration (56%). Despite these challenges, qualitative findings revealed strengthened emotional regulation, empathy, motivation, and goal setting among students engaged in trauma-informed programming. Teachers reported improved peer interaction and community building during sustained implementation. Conclusion: The Schools-as-Neighborhoods framework highlights the value of trauma-informed, relationship-centered school environments in promoting student well-being. By positioning schools as cohesive ecosystems that foster belonging and cultivate social capital, this approach offers educators and policymakers a pathway for mitigating the effects of hostile lived environments and supporting students' mental health, social development, and engagement in learning.

Keywords: school; adolescents; social capital; neighborhood; socioecological model; social-emotional learning; trauma-informed curricula; school-based health

1. Introduction

Education plays a critical role in shaping children's health, development, and long-term opportunities. Yet persistent disparities in access and outcomes highlight the need to reimagine how schools support students, particularly those facing adversity. Various proposals for bettering neighborhood schools exist. Most involve bettering student and community relations; however, for students in underserved communities and under-resourced schools, the community does not always provide appropriate avenues for self-improvement. Schools provide a unique opportunity to function as a community and neighborhood in their own right, helping to counteract unproductive environments and enhance students' physical and mental well-being.

1.1. Government Involvement in Education

States spend a considerable amount of funding on education, plus an additional amount in United States Federal contributions, with the Department of Education (DoE) having the third-largest discretionary fund [1]. However, this quality and administration of education has caused divisions in scholastic achievement, resources, financial mobility, and health. Urban and lower-resourced schools experience higher rates of truancy, dropout rates, lower-quality education, and lower health outcomes [2].

The DoE and public education at the state and local levels in the United States have long been a topic of contention [3]. The DoE was initially created to collect and condense information about American schools to inform school system effectiveness in teaching and create globally competitive students. Since its origins, the DoE has been responsible for managing federal student loans and ensuring that there is federal support for students in under-resourced areas [1]. Various innovations have occurred to assist these differences, including the Elementary and Secondary Education Act of 1965, the No Child Left Behind law signed in 2002, and the Every Student Succeeds Act signed in 2015 [1,3–5]. However, with each administration, opposing bureaucratic ideals and rhetoric cause inconsistency and slowed progression for students [6–8]. Education is a social driver of health metric, with high school diplomas and higher education allowing for social advancement, adaptability, and increased access, which improve health and economic outcomes [9]. Yet, there has been a continuous achievement gap in under-resourced schools, with shifting national priorities creating challenges for continuity in trauma-informed and social–emotional programming.

1.2. Frameworks for Expanding the Role and Redefining Schools

A sociological definition of a neighborhood incorporates the immediate geographical location of a residence, including physical features and social interactions, cohesion, and shared identity of the neighborhood's individuals [10]. The impact of neighborhoods on the development, lifestyle, and prospects of children and adolescents has been documented in topics including, but not limited to, poverty, crime and violence, socialization, and education [11,12]. The Social Ecological Model (SEM) is a framework that identifies how interpersonal relationships, institutions and organizations, the community, and broader structures and systems impact an individual's attitudes, beliefs, knowledge, behaviors, and overall health [13]. Resourced and socially advancing neighborhoods typically have well-funded institutions with like-minded individuals, which increases social cohesion and social capital. These things being considered, it is paramount to view and orchestrate schools as not just in neighborhoods, but as their own ecosystem/neighborhood within the neighborhood. This allows for a shift in mindset, resources, and outcomes for the school. Schools-as-Neighborhoods is a conceptual framework that defines schools as intentionally designed micro-environments that function as protective neighborhoods for children and adolescents, particularly those facing adversity. The framework emphasizes the school itself as a primary site for generating social capital. The framework distinguishes schools as a standalone community that supports the health, mission, and vision of its students through relationship-centered practices (Figure 1). This contributes to positive childhood experiences (PCEs). By reframing the notion of schools through this framework, schools are positioned as modifiable environments buffering harmful neighborhood exposures while

https://doi.org/10.3390/children13010059

supporting emotional, social, and developmental well-being. Few manuscripts describe the concrete notion of Schools-as-Neighborhoods and social shifters. There are elements of these aspects in social capital and in physical and mental health school resources, such as the Community School Transformation (CST) framework; however, this manuscript seeks to define and reframe schools as standalone neighborhoods that can positively impact students beyond written knowledge [14].

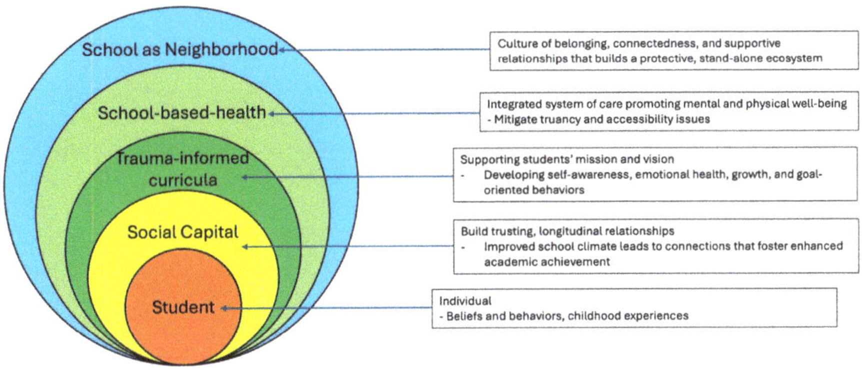

Figure 1. Schools-as-Neighborhoods conceptual framework and key concepts.

Utilizing data from students in Milwaukee, WI, USA, in grades five through nine, and following them into the next school year, we identify vulnerable youth and schools and examine whether trauma-informed interventions—*peak team* and Brain Agents—foster student emotional well-being and school connectedness. Additionally, through this work, we propose a framework of Schools-as-Neighborhoods, building on the community school model [15], in which schools function as cohesive ecosystems supporting social capital, emotional health, and community belonging. With proposed funding cuts to the DoE, it is essential that schools create sustainable and progressive frameworks that support students independent of curriculum, funding, or ideological changes [7,16,17].

2. Materials and Methods

2.1. Literature Review

This study incorporates a scoping review to better understand the individual concepts of a neighborhood and the elements in practice within adolescent education. A literature search utilizing PubMed, the Education Resources Information Center (ERIC), which is managed by the United States Department of Education, SCOPUS, and Google Scholar, assisted in identifying the breadth of literature. Search terms are located in Appendix A, Table A1.

Search results center around urban centers and schools, and the myriad of factors that impact the development of a child/adolescent and the makeup of an advancing neighborhood, including: social capital, health/school-based health, and educational policies. The Community Schools Transformation framework outlines key practices for community schools with a culture of belonging, integrated support, student and family engagement, and expanded learning opportunities.

2.2. Implementation of a Trauma-Informed Curriculum at Four Milwaukee Schools

2.2.1. School Participants and Context

STRYV365 is a non-profit organization based in Milwaukee, Wisconsin, designed to customize non-clinical trauma-informed curricula. STRYV365 utilizes multifaceted approaches to curriculum design, fostering resilience and increasing positive lived experiences for school-aged children. Two SAMHSA-based social–emotional learning curricula, the *peak team* coaching program and the Brain Agents video game, were developed by STRYV365. Both curricula utilize the COPE (Creativity, Optimism, Planning, and Expert Information) and CRAFFT (Care, Relax, Alone, Forget, Family/Friends, and Trouble) frameworks and incorporate physical activities and reflective art-based exercises to promote student self-awareness, decision-making, and relationship building [18–21]. STRYV365 partnered with four schools in Milwaukee: two public and two charter.

2.2.2. Study Design and Conceptual Framework

This study employed a convergent mixed-methods design in which quantitative survey data and qualitative focus group and interview data were collected in parallel across four semesters and integrated at the interpretation stage. Quantitative analyses tested prespecified hypotheses regarding social–emotional learning (SEL) outcomes using a clustered randomized incomplete block factorial design (Appendix B Table A2), with classrooms as the unit of randomization. Qualitative analyses explored students' and teachers' lived experiences of emotional regulation, coping, and school connectedness. Integration occurred through thematic triangulation, whereby quantitative findings for each SEL domain (e.g., emotional regulation, coping strategies) were presented alongside corroborating or explanatory qualitative themes.

Intervention fidelity was supported through standardized curricula, trained coaches, and consistent implementation frameworks across schools. *Peak team* student-coach sessions followed a structured trauma-informed curriculum aligned with the COPE and CRAFFT frameworks. It was delivered over 9–12 sessions within 4–10 weeks, with flexibility to accommodate school schedules and student needs. Brain Agents provides complementary trauma-informed support through the gamification of narrative contexts and minigames. It followed a standardized schedule of 2–3 sessions per week for 4–5 weeks, with usage metrics captured directly from the game platform. Variation in duration and exposure was addressed analytically through the inclusion of cluster indicators.

Sociocultural theory informs the conceptual framework for the study [22,23]. The mixed-methods design operationalizes the Schools-as-Neighborhoods concept by measuring emotional, behavioral, and relational outcomes through surveys and qualitative interviews. We hypothesized that two of STRYV365's school-based programs, the *peak team* coaching program and complementary Brain Agents video game interventions, helped establish and reinforce a safe, supportive, neighborhood/community-building environment that modifies student feelings, attitudes, behavior, and school performance, originally influenced by their lived environment. Research questions included: What did success mean to each of the students, and how did students intend to obtain their goals? How do trauma-informed programs influence students' emotional awareness, coping skills, and school connectedness? How do teachers perceive changes in classroom relationships after implementation?

This work was submitted to and approved by the Medical College of Wisconsin Institutional Review Board (PRO00037500) in Milwaukee, WI, USA.

2.2.3. Recruitment and Participant Consent and Assent

The two interventions were implemented in four Milwaukee, Wisconsin schools for students in grades five through nine between 2022–2024. Students were randomized to one of four groups: Brain Agents, *peak team*, both, or neither intervention. STRYV365 and school staff were CITI-trained in human research protection. Parents and caregivers of students at each school were recruited at back-to-school events, open houses, parent-teacher conferences, and through emails. Informed consent was obtained on digital tablets

https://doi.org/10.3390/children13010059

in English for study participation. Students provided informed assent before completing the baseline REDCap survey and joining focus groups or interviews [24].

2.2.4. Quantitative Analysis

Sample size considerations were informed by a priori power analysis conducted for the primary SEL outcomes. To detect small-to-moderate effects (Cohen's d = 0.3) with 80% power and $\alpha = 0.05$ across four intervention conditions, approximately 175 participants per arm were estimated to be required. Although consent and assent rates resulted in a smaller analytic sample, the repeated measures clustered design increased statistical efficiency. Analyses therefore emphasize effect estimation with appropriate covariate adjustment rather than reliance on dichotomous significance testing alone.

Data collection included a 41-question survey instrument in REDCap derived from validated and reliable items provided by the Life Paths Research Center and aligned with the competencies outlined by the Collaborative for Academic, Social, and Emotional Learning [25,26]. The surveys administered in the fall, winter, and spring of each intervention year assessed key SEL domains such as self-awareness, self-management, relationship skills, responsible decision-making, social awareness, and adversity. The surveys also included recent feelings of depression and anxiety, using items from the Patient Health Questionnaire-2 and Generalized Anxiety Disorder-7 questionnaires [27,28]. Students who reported daily symptoms of anxiety or depression were promptly referred to their school behavioral health counselor and a child psychologist through STRYV365.

Quantitative analysis used mixed-effects regression models with random intercepts for classroom and school to account for clustering and repeated measurements over time. Assessments were conducted at baseline (early fall 2022) and at subsequent waves in late fall, spring, and the following academic year (through spring 2024), corresponding to intervention cycles. Of the 1626 students enrolled across the four schools, 321 consented to complete surveys. Response rates varied by wave, with 225–277 respondents per wave, 70–86% of invited participants. Attrition across waves primarily reflected student absenteeism and school mobility rather than study withdrawal. Rather than imputing missing outcomes, analyses used all available data under a missing-at-random assumption, incorporating baseline scores, cluster indicators, and time effects to reduce bias. This approach is appropriate for longitudinal school-based studies with staggered participation and minimizes distortions that may arise from imputation in the presence of structural absenteeism.

2.2.5. Qualitative Analysis

Qualitative data were collected through semi-structured student focus groups, individual student interviews, and teacher focus groups conducted at the conclusion of intervention semesters. Student focus groups for fifth through seventh grade lasted 45–60 min and were designed to promote peer interaction, while individual interviews with older students, 8th–10th grade, were 30–45 min and allowed for deeper reflection. Teacher focus groups were 60 min in length. Focus group prompts addressed emotional regulation, coping strategies, future aspirations, relationships, school connectedness, and perceptions of program impact (Appendix C). Qualitative data included focus groups with 57 students, individual interviews with 68 students, and focus groups with 29 teachers and school staff.

Qualitative analysis of focus group and interview transcripts used a hybrid deductive-inductive thematic coding approach. An initial deductive codebook was developed based on the same CASEL and emotional intelligence domains as the quantitative analysis. Inductive codes were then added iteratively as novel concepts emerged from the data. Each transcript was independently coded by two coders, with discrepancies resolved through consensus meetings, minimizing bias and enhancing analytic rigor. Thematic saturation

https://doi.org/10.3390/children13010059

was considered achieved when successive focus groups and interviews failed to generate new codes within the predefined SEL/EL domains, and when thematic patterns remained consistent across schools, grade levels, and intervention conditions.

3. Results

3.1. Quantitative Findings

3.1.1. School Statistics and Participant Demographics

A total of 1626 students in grades five through nine collectively attend the four schools. Of those who participated in the interventions of *peak team* and Brain Agents, 61% were Black/African American, 19% White, 11% Hispanic/Latinx, 6% Asian/Hmong, and 3% mixed racial/ethnic background. 69% experience economic disadvantage. In state standardized exam performance, 58% were below basic, 27% basic, and 15% were proficient in English and language arts and math, respectively. 28% were chronically absent, and 88% of students at the schools earn high school diplomas. Baseline statistics of the four schools depict that the majority of students come from economically disadvantaged communities. Economically disadvantaged youth in Milwaukee are defined by direct certification or household income guidelines for free or reduced-price meals under the National School Lunch Program (NSLP) [29]. These schools do not have a school-based health center, integrated alternative, or trauma-informed curriculum. Additionally, the schools have, on average, a 25% chronic absenteeism rate; however, three of the schools have an average 90% graduation rate, while one school has a graduation rate of 47% at baseline (Appendix C Table A3). A subset of participants, $n = 321$, were invited to complete a survey indicating their exposure to adversity. Their demographics are depicted in Appendix C Table A4.

3.1.2. Student Adversity and Resilience

Up to 277 students responded to questions about adverse events. Cyberbullying items were added in fall 2024 and not collected in earlier semesters. At baseline for the first group of participants, in early fall 2022, 74% of students had someone close to them die, 56% had someone close to them go to jail, and almost 30% had someone close to them with substance use issues. About one-third had felt nervous or anxious early every day for a two-week period. About one-fifth had signs of melancholy (Table 1). Notable trends included a decrease in the proportion of participants reporting symptoms of depression or anxiety following implementation of the interventions. Survey responses were analyzed as a cross-sectional series of different students over two years.

Table 1. Survey Results about Adversity by Semester.

Survey Item Responses	**Early Fall 2022**	**Late Fall 2022**	**Late Spring 2023**	**Early Fall 2023**	**Late Fall 2023**	**Late Spring 2024**
Survey participant number	225	277	259	254	223	210
Did you ever have anyone close to you die—yes	74%	73%	72%	73%	74%	69%
Did you every have anyone close to you go to jail—yes	56%	53%	54%	52%	51%	50%
Did you ever have anyone close to you drink or use drugs so often that it caused problems—yes	29%	26%	29%	30%	29%	29%
Over the last 2 weeks, nearly every day and more than half the days have been feeling down, depressed, or hopeless	22%	24%	22%	15%	16%	16%
Over the last 2 weeks, nearly every day and more than half the days have been feeling nervous, anxious, or on edge	30%	24%	23%	20%	18%	20%
Over the last 2 weeks, nearly every day and more than half the days have been bullied, called names, harassed, or abused through texting, social media, or gaming	Not assessed	NA	NA	10%	4%	9%

https://doi.org/10.3390/children13010059

3.2. *Qualitative Findings*

3.2.1. Emotional Awareness and Regulation

Quotes from the qualitative analysis of student focus group and interview data are recorded in Table 2. Participants were asked how the trauma-informed curriculum of *peak team* and Brain Agents helped their emotional awareness, coping mechanisms, future goals, and school connectedness. The trauma-informed learning emphasized student qualities and goals. Students identified intrinsic and extrinsic qualities such as resilience (Quote 4, Table 2), self-regulation (Quote 5, Table 2), and physical activity or spiritual discipline (Quote 6). Notably, participants' future goals spanned education, financial stability, and creating a meaningful life (Quotes 10–12, Table 2). Some students noted that their neighborhood cohesion was lacking outside of school and identified a seeming barrier for social mobility (Quote 15, Table 2). However, students highlighted their anticipation and desire to engage with STRYV365 programming while at school, differing from their outside experience (Quotes 1–2, Table 2).

Table 2. Quotes from the students after interacting with the STRYV365 curriculum.

Overall Comments
Quote 1. "I mean, I like STRYV. It's just something I look forward to in my day."—9th Grade, *peak team* **Quote 2.** "Yes, because I actually want to stay longer. So about STRYV? Yeah. Oh, in my opinion, I think STRYV is a really good thing... And STRYV have a lot of things, a lot of activities to do to get your body moving. If you tired, when you go to gym in the morning, you can do the games that they have printed for you and then you would just be, feel like a brand new person."—FG: *peak team* and Brain Agents/5th grade participant
Qualities most proud of:
a. Intrinsic: **Quote 3.** "creativity" "focusing on other people" "being myself" "helpful" "I'm smart" "good person" **Quote 4.** "nice to people" "being on top of my stuff" "keep pushing forward even when it gets hard" **Quote 5.** "controlling my anger" b. Extrinsic: **Quote 6.** "reading" "sports" "athleticism" "energetic" "I can run fast" "I read the Bible" "my hands" **Quote 7.** "artistic" "how clean I am" "I am strong" c. Unable to name quality (negative self-image): **Quote 8.** "I don't have any."—8th grade **Quote 9.** "No. Is there a hate myself part?"—FG: *peak team* and Brain Agents/5th grade participant
Future goal in 5 years (all class years):
a. Educational Goal **Quote 10.** "college" "learning about cosmetics" "get a degree" "studying as a nurse" "med school" "outside of state" "get a good scholarship" "good grades" "culinary school" "Ivy league" "graduate" "art school" b. Career Goal **Quote 11.** "Orthodontist" "architecture" "doctor" "NBA" "OB" "working at McDonald's" "summer job" "professional NFL player" "manager at a US Bank" "start my own business" c. Stability Goal **Quote 12.** "getting a car" d. Extracurriculars/Hobbies Goal **Quote 13.** "football" "win the NCAA title" "wrestle" "playing basketball" 'I'm going to go D1" "work for the Boys and Girls Club" "baseball" e. Other goal **Quote 14.** "stable lifestyle" "apartment" "out of parent's house" "first car" "get my house" "swimming in money" "Live in Chicago" "driver's license"
Neighborhood Cohesion
Quote 15. "And I was born here, so I'm like, I know that I'm American, but I'm not white, so I don't feel like I'm validated by white people. It's such a thing with... You have American privilege. I have American privilege for which I'm so grateful, but I don't have white privilege."—FG: *peak team*/8th Grade participant

https://doi.org/10.3390/children13010059

3.2.2. School Connectedness and Climate

Teachers were asked to evaluate their understanding of the *peak team* and Brain Agents curricula, noticeable changes in the students, and suggestions for the rollout of the program. Overall, teachers expressed the connection that students make with the coaches of the STRYV365 program. The longitudinal engagement and recognizability of the coaches support the students and the school administrators through stressful times. Consistent coaching and engagement fostered belonging and a positive classroom culture. Teachers noted changes in student behavior when STRYV365 programming was in session. In Quote 18 of Table 3, a teacher expressed how the implementation of the program helped the culture of the school. The students were "high-fiving, greeting coaches, and excited" throughout the school day, but especially after a session. Another teacher reported early-year challenges and observed improvements following implementation of the *peak team* and Brain Agents programming, although she could not scientifically attribute these changes to the intervention (Quote 19, Table 3). One teacher noticed a temporal nature to difficulties with students, noting that "during holidays, breaks, or earlier in the year," when students are away from the school and the intentional curriculum, "you get these more infractions… we've had a brawl at high school" (Quote 21, Table 3).

Table 3. Quotes from teachers discussing their view of student interactions with the STRYV365 curriculum.

Teacher Quotes on School/Programming
Highlighted Theme: *Connection/Community with Schools-Targeted coaching and mentoring*
Quote 16. "Consistency of Engagement. *peak team* at MAS for 4 or 5 years now (compounding years) I can just say they appreciate when y'all are here, when they're working with you, they enjoy it… I know the kids are always exciting when they've got STRYV for a special…, but… to see the consistency throughout the years, the kids are like, "Oh yeah, you're that coach, you're that tall one," and then, the tall one, that's always, I think. Good for them."
Quote 17. "I think this year too, STRYV Specials came in at a perfect time because I had been out for so long for a period and so for me to come back in and when I didn't have that bond with my students anymore, the STRYV, especially in the classroom, helped rebuild [00:26:00] that. It really forces them to work as a team…. What a perfect example of why we should have a year-round for everybody, right?"
Quote 18. "I like those community building things. I feel like that always just helps the culture… because during the day there's a lot of stressful things going on. Sometimes, things get communicated poorly and people get frustrated with other people, but then it's at the end of the day, yeah, we're just all human beings. Playing a goofy game, acting out pictures of someone bowling is really funny, and I think helps, has helped me build better relationships with teachers I think…the staff really engaged well with the students. Students were excited, um, to see staff. They, when they saw them even outside of the classroom, they were given high fives and greeting them. …, they really appreciated the energy that, um, all of the staff from STRYV365 brought into our building"
Quote 19. "I don't know that I would have anything to add, um, to that. It was a rough start to the year…second semester was significantly better than first semester. So STRYV may have played some, some part of that, but I don't, I don't know that I would have data to defend that one way or the other."
Quote 20. "I mean, I think I wish we could have more time than just one special cycle or just one little bit of it. I wish it could be consistent like a regular class. I get it, but that would I think really be powerful too. I think a couple of you guys talked about de-escalation and physical and for me, my vision will be to have them in SEL and then you're getting those multiple intelligences, the physical, just looking at the screen or just talking because some kids just need to talk to somebody in the morning. I think giving them the choices too on how they start their day… Some kids, they come right in and doing some of those activities with STRYV would give them something positive as well as, like you said, do some de-escalation so they don't have as much built up by the time they do get to some of those situations."
Quote 21. "I think that having more exposure with for them as well would allow them to be able to deescalate. There are peak times of the year where we notice, especially in high school and probably across the board, you get these more infractions of these spikes. People start getting messy, the holidays, breaks, and even during the early parts of the year, even probably being during some summer PD, I don't know what y'all would go about that but having you all be a little bit more present when those peak seasons come up because we've had a brawl at high school."

4. Discussion

4.1. STRYV365 Curriculum for Students in At-Risk Schools

This study explored how trauma-informed programs can enhance emotional well-being and connectedness within the conceptual framework of Schools-as-Neighborhoods.

https://doi.org/10.3390/children13010059

Our study of adolescents in four Milwaukee middle and high schools assessed risk profiles and social relationships of vulnerable youth. We utilized a trauma-informed care curriculum to assess their ability to manage their emotions and have better interpersonal outcomes. These skills are a necessary part of education and social mobility.

These four schools ranged in student population size from small to mid-sized, and from true public to charter schools. Another option for parents and students is private choice, which allows parents to use public funds to enroll their students in private schools. These schools generally have smaller class sizes and alternative or expanded curricula [30]. Previous studies suggest that smaller schools and class sizes promote better student outcomes, with the flexibility of charter or private choice schools providing a more supportive or personalized environment [30,31]. Despite these indicated improvements, the schools in this study still had the majority of students well below proficiency in English/Language Arts and Mathematics, and an over 20% chronic absenteeism rate (Appendix C Table A3). This would suggest that class size and piecemeal policies are insufficient to provide the successful student and ultimately, citizen, standardized education purports. Despite these statistics, three of our schools have an average 90% graduation rate. These statistics warrant deeper scrutiny of the curriculum and metrics for graduation. Although this study combines results from the four schools, focusing on their similarities, notable differences among the schools exist regarding racial demographics and academic achievement. These are most remarkable at schools with the greatest economic disadvantage (Appendix B). This requires discussion of racial and economic inequities beyond the scope of this study; however, it furthers the basis for expanded social capital and mitigating environments for PCEs, provided by the Schools-as-Neighborhoods framework, particularly for vulnerable youth.

The STRYV365 curriculum fosters longitudinal relationships, promotes goal-oriented behaviors, and establishes a structure for self-awareness and positive childhood experiences (PCEs). The *peak team* methodology consisted of trained coach-mentors holding weekly group sessions focused on reframing experiences and interactions, broadening beliefs and dreams, and providing tools for refocusing. Physical activities to foster team building and increase social capital included team sports such as basketball and soccer, multi-player games, reflective writing, and group discussions. The Brain Agents video game similarly fostered resilience in the tasks completed to achieve new game levels and reflections on feelings identified while playing. In Table 2, student participants expressed personal goals and individual characteristics they desired to develop and utilize for social mobility. This additional curriculum offered in schools to students with adverse risk factors supports students not only in their typical education but also in soft skills, which promote the development of the whole individual. Understanding conflict resolution, goal setting, and relationship building are skills that members of a neighborhood use to create safety and growth of the neighborhood and its individuals. Identifying schools as neighborhoods and reframing the current resources and metrics for adolescent success can assist with producing not only informed, but also socially competent and overall healthy graduates [32].

4.2. Schools as Neighborhoods

The impact of the lived environment on adolescents is well documented [9]. Schools, according to the SEM, would be considered one variable in the social context that affects a person. However, since, according to the National Center for Education Statistics, children spend an average of seven hours per day over 180 days in school, these communities can be considered their own neighborhoods [33,34]. Thus, our proposed framework (Figure 1) illustrates that belonging, connection, and supportive relationships function as protective layers within the school environment, reinforcing students' resilience and mental health. Many of the students experienced traumatic life events and prejudices. One student

https://doi.org/10.3390/children13010059

commented: "And I was born here, so I'm like, I know that I'm American, but I'm not white, so I don't feel like I'm validated by white people. It's such a thing with...You have American privilege. I have American privilege for which I'm so grateful, but I don't have white privilege."—FG: *peak team*/8th Grade participant (Quote 15, Table 2). Particularly for students who experience privilege and discrimination outside of school, this framework may help mitigate some of the effects of the lived environment for students, providing an alternative exposure. This furthers the principles outlined in positive childhood experiences (PCEs), explained by Dr. Bethell et. al., which are hypothesized to promote a healthy physical and mental adulthood [35]. Our framework expands the framework for community school transformation (CST). The CST initiative is led by the principal and community school coordinator who develop a vision and goal for the school and student [14]. Our framework also highlights not just family engagement, but student-oriented vision and goals. Additionally, our "integrated systems of support" include school-based health as essential efforts for child physical and mental well-being.

The Schools-as-Neighborhoods framework thrives on the concepts of school-based health and social capital, which would address truancy, safety, wellness, and support scholarly exploration. Improving school climate is associated with academic achievement, especially in middle school-age children [36]. Using the School Climate Measure, Daily et al. determined that feeling more connected to their teachers and schools was important for middle school students [36]. High school students' academic achievement based on these factors was also impacted, although lower than middle school students. Rakesh et al. discuss a restructuring of the child's brain development with stronger relationships improving mental health [35,37]. These areas require more research to address the differences as students develop, and as priorities and interconnectedness change. Neighborhoods grow with the individual; thus, a School-as-Neighborhood model could support the growth of students throughout their education.

4.3. Social Capital Within Schools as Neighborhoods Mitigates Effects of Outside Neighborhood and Promotes Better Learning and Coping Within the School Environment

Social capital is a network of people and resources. An expansive social capital has great impact on an individual's health, wealth accumulation, and social advancement [38]. Education is a way to expand the social network of students and is a major factor in improving public health outcomes and supporting health equity [32,39]. Our students expressed varying visions for their future life. Most students intend to complete high school and pursue higher education, become entrepreneurs, or just get out of their neighborhoods (Table 2). Their current social capital is highlighted by many having had a loved one die or be incarcerated (Table 1). This negatively impacts the students' outcomes through social mechanism of contagion and socialization [12]. Contagion is the influence of one's neighbors on the conduct and beliefs of the individual, while socialization describes the community's response to those who do not ascribe to the norms of the neighborhood. The school as an ideal neighborhood provides a positive outlook, interrupting the previous socialization.

Teachers and school administrators in our study expressed the ways in which social capital, through the trauma-informed care curriculum and sustained coaching, impacted their students. Students appeared more engaged with a substantial difference in emotional regulation and student demeanor after sustained implementation of the trauma-informed curricula. They stated:

"I like those community-building things. I feel like that always just helps the culture... because during the day there's a lot of stressful things going on. Sometimes, things get communicated poorly, and people get frustrated with other people, but then it's at the end of the day, yeah, we're just all human beings. Playing a goofy game, acting out pictures of someone bowling is really funny, and I think has helped me build better relationships with

https://doi.org/10.3390/children13010059

teachers. I think the staff really engaged well with the students. Students were excited to see staff. . .When they saw them even outside of the classroom, they were given high fives and greeting them. They really appreciated the energy that all of the staff from STRYV365 brought into our building."

Teachers noticed differences when the curriculum was paused during summer or winter breaks (Quote 19, 21, Table 3). This suggests that the increase in social capital and a concrete effort to create the culture of the School-as-Neighborhood framework improved behavior and rationale. This may be maintained when students are continuously exposed to a supportive environment. This further shows, as the Robert Wood Johnson Foundation depicts, that a reframing and new environment can have a significant impact on the student. The socialization of the school neighbors can create positive outcomes relationally, but ultimately health-wise, for the student citizens of the school neighborhood [40]. We hypothesize that consistent, relational, trauma-informed interventions help students regulate emotions, feel safer, and engage more deeply in school life. Teachers' testimonies confirm that school climate improved when these supports were active. Further research accounting for confounding variables is warranted to elucidate the direct impact of the curricula.

4.4. School-Based Health as a Form of Connection and Stopgap to Truancy and Low Health Outcomes

Truancy is increased in underserved communities, often due to physical and mental health ailments. It is well documented how the lived environment affects one's health, with those in underserved areas more likely to have diagnoses of asthma, obesity, anxiety, and depression [41,42]. This is further exacerbated by a student's inability to attend scheduled doctor's appointments due to lack of transportation and time constraints [43]. School-based health centers (SBHC) have proven to alleviate these concerns [41]. The Robert Wood Johnson Foundation, a pioneer in public health, first discussed SBH in 1979, piloting nurses in schools to support the success and well-being of children [40]. Lim et al. showed how a visit to a school-based health center increased school attendance, particularly for those who had a mental-health-based visit [2]. Some SBHCs have expanded access to include not only students, but also their families.

SBHCs follow the sentiments of a neighborhood, taking care of the needs of the students and their families, and increasing connectedness [44]. This has proven to increase test scores and graduation rates. However, SBHCs are not present in every state, and in 2023, only 19 states and the District of Columbia had state-allocated funds for SBHCs [44,45]. The ESSA expanded funds to schools based on SBHC as they meet the health and safety goals [3]. Although school-based health is an opportunity to address risk factors for low health outcomes and school performance, Dr. Woolf expresses that healthcare alone does not fully encompass the necessary elements to reduce health inequities [46]. Continuing to identify and create policy impacting the root causes of health inequities ultimately allows for greater success [47]. A reframing of schools as neighborhoods favors a comprehensive view of adolescent education and well-being, building on aspects that have already been proven to support adolescent development, competitiveness, and future goals.

4.5. Policy Implications/Recommendations

Initial federal laws and policies focused on expanded access to quality education [1]. The most recent federal education law, signed in 2015—Every Student Succeeds Act (ESSA)—seeks to empower and give autonomy back to states and local educators on improvement metrics and processes [1,3,5]. Although 20% of the distributed federal funds received by districts are to be used for the safety, health of, and support for versatile and adaptable students [5], the implemented funds should be distributed to flexible, locally tailored approaches such as STRYV365 to promote mental health and equity.

https://doi.org/10.3390/children13010059

State and local policies establish curriculum standards, funding allocation, and daily operations. The addition of social workers and mental health counselors is a state and local practice, which fills support gaps but can sometimes seem disjointed from the school system. There have been various models of schools creating credos and principles that support the values of the whole student. These include charter schools, such as the Knowledge is Power Program (KIPP), and private institutions, Montessori Schools [48,49]. Charter and private schools are given flexibility in classroom methods, which yield positive growth in student reading and math scores, often outperforming traditional public schools. These schools also have on average more days of reading and math learning [31,50]. Although charter schools enroll nearly four million students, this is a fraction of the nearly 55 million students who are registered in K-12 education in the United States [50–52].

In Milwaukee, where our four schools, a mixture of public, charter, and private, are located, a discussion about closing Milwaukee public schools causes contention [53,54]. Due to declining rates of enrollment, many school buildings are unoccupied, with others requiring much renovation and expansion. The approved budget for 2025–2026 has Milwaukee Public Schools receiving $1.5 billion [55]. Per student, MPS spends an average of $23,000 for each student, typically larger than other comparable cities. The return on these funds does not appear to be fully realized. As this is a multifaceted, multisystemic issue, a new approach may provide new results. Local and State governments can prioritize revitalizing schools instead of closure. The Schools-as-Neighborhoods framework can support the endeavor. Funding social–emotional and trauma-informed learning programs, such as STRYV365's curriculum, can create social capital, belonging, and relational safety, making schools a place students want to attend; thus, combating truancy and declining enrollment. Further, school-based health can function as measures of student success and well-being.

4.6. Limitations

This study assessed the implementation of a trauma-informed curriculum model that incorporated coaches, peer support, and gamification. The present manuscript intentionally focused on formative and process-oriented findings rather than on definitive estimates of intervention effectiveness. Accordingly, the quantitative results presented in Table 1 are descriptive and intended to characterize the level of adversity and emotional distress in the student population, rather than to test pre-specified impact outcomes. Thus, the study is limited by less robust quantitative evidence. However, anecdotal evidence from focus groups and interviews showed increased interest in school attendance and activities. Future research is needed to further understand the impact of trauma-informed and comprehensive education on truancy and graduation rates. This study utilizes self-reported survey data, which could be attributed to self-selection bias and social desirability bias. Response rates varied across semesters, and missing data were primarily due to absenteeism and student mobility, which may further affect representativeness. The study can be extrapolated through the principles and concepts of a supportive environment where students spend a significant portion of the day. However, the study has restricted generalizability due to its implementation in a mid-sized Midwestern city with a fixed sample size. Our study focuses on middle and high school education; however, students may require various modalities earlier and throughout their education. Future work should quantify behavioral and academic outcomes, exploring the sustainability of this Schools-as-Neighborhoods framework across diverse educational settings. Despite these limitations, this manuscript contributes to the understanding of how trauma-informed, social–emotional curricula promote well-being, especially in at-risk students.

https://doi.org/10.3390/children13010059

5. Conclusions

Schools can function as micro-neighborhoods that nurture belonging, emotional growth, and resilience—key ingredients for educational and mental health success. By reframing schools as neighborhoods, educators and policymakers can create equitable, holistic environments where children thrive physically, academically, emotionally, and socially. Funding should be reallocated to consider and support trauma-informed and positive experiences curricula.

Author Contributions: Conceptualization, C.R.E. and J.R.M.; methodology, C.R.E., J.R.M. and B.C.; software, T.H.C.; validation, C.R.E., J.R.M. and T.H.C.; formal analysis C.R.E. and T.H.C.; investigation, C.R.E., J.R.M. and B.C.; writing—original draft preparation, C.R.E.; writing—review and editing, C.R.E., C.G., J.R.M., B.C. and T.H.C.; visualization, C.R.E.; supervision, J.R.M.; project administration, C.R.E., J.R.M. and B.C.; funding acquisition, J.R.M. and B.C. All authors have read and agreed to the published version of the manuscript.

Funding: The original study was funded by philanthropist Thomas Hurvis and The Greater Milwaukee Foundation.

Institutional Review Board Statement: The study was conducted in accordance with the Declaration of Helsinki and approved by the Institutional Review Board of the Medical College of Wisconsin (code: PRO00037500, date: 14 April 2020).

Informed Consent Statement: Informed consent was obtained from all subjects involved in the study.

Data Availability Statement: The raw data supporting the conclusions of this article will be made available by the authors on request.

Acknowledgments: We acknowledge the work of the STRYV365 staff who were instrumental in implementing the interventions, conducting the focus groups, and obtaining surveys from all participants.

Conflicts of Interest: Brandon Currie is CEO of the non-profit organization STRYV365, Inc., which developed and delivered the intervention programs. Schools were not charged for the programs.

Abbreviations

The following abbreviations are used in this manuscript:

DoE	Department of Education
SEM	Social Ecological Model
ERIC	Education Resources Information Center
SEL	Social Emotional Learning
EL	Emotional Learning
COPE	Creativity, Optimism, Planning, Expert Information
CRAFFT	Care, Relax, Alone, Forget, Family/Friends, Trouble
NSLP	National School Lunch Program
PCEs	Positive Childhood Experience
SBH	School-based Health
SBHC	School-based health centers
ESSA	Every Student Succeeds Act
KIPP	Knowledge is Power Program

https://doi.org/10.3390/children13010059

Appendix A

Table A1. Literature Review search terms in Pubmed, ERIC, SCOPUS, and Google Scholar for the Schools-as-Neighborhoods conceptual framework.

Pubmed	"School based health centers" "Social capital" AND "adolescent health"; "social capital" AND "school based health" public school education and research"
ERIC	(((DE "Social Capital" OR DE "Social Environment" OR (TI "social environment" OR "social support") OR (AB "social environment" OR "social support")) AND ((TI school*) OR (AB school*) OR DE "Schools" OR DE "Bilingual Schools" OR DE "Boarding Schools" OR DE "Colleges" OR DE "Community Schools" OR DE "Consolidated Schools" OR DE "Correspondence Schools" OR DE "Day Schools" OR DE "Disadvantaged Schools" OR DE "Elementary Schools" OR DE "Experimental Schools" OR DE "Folk Schools" OR DE "Free Schools" OR DE "International Schools" OR DE "Laboratory Schools" OR DE "Magnet Schools" OR DE "Middle Schools" OR DE "Military Schools" OR DE "Montessori Schools" OR DE "Multiunit Schools" OR DE "Neighborhood Schools" OR DE "Open Plan Schools" OR DE "Preschools" OR DE "Private Schools" OR DE "Professional Development Schools" OR DE "Public Schools" OR DE "Racially Balanced Schools" OR DE "Regional Schools" OR DE "Rural Schools" OR DE "Schools of Education" OR DE "Secondary Schools" OR DE "Single Sex Schools" OR DE "Slum Schools" OR DE "Small Schools" OR DE "Special Schools" OR DE "State Schools" OR DE "Suburban Schools" OR DE "Summer Schools" OR DE "Traditional Schools" OR DE "Urban Schools" OR DE "Virtual Schools" OR DE "Vocational Schools" OR DE "Year Round Schools") OR AB (school* n2 neighborhood*) OR TI (school* n2 neighborhood*)) AND(DE "At Risk Students" OR (AB "at risk student*") OR (TI "at risk student*"))) AND (DE "School Policy" OR DE "Policy Analysis" OR DE "Economics" OR (TI policy OR policies OR econ* OR financ* OR cost*) OR (AB policy OR policies OR econ* OR financ* OR cost*))
SCOPUS	"urban schools" AND "truancy"; "urban schools" AND "health outcomes"
Google Scholar	"No Child Left Behind" "History of US Education Reform"

Appendix B

Table A2. Incomplete Block Factorial Design for Academic Years 1 and 2 (Time 1 = early fall, Time 2 = after fall semester; Time 3 = after spring semester; BA = Brain Agents; PT = *peak team;* B = both BA and PT; C = control group; X = no participation.

Academic Year	Grade	Time	School			
			A	B	C	D
2022–2023	5	1	C	C	C	X
		2	BA	C	B	X
		3	C	PT	C	X
	6	1	C	C	C	X
		2	C	BA	PT	X
		3	PT	C	C	X
	7	1	C	C	C	X
		2	B	C	C	X
		3	C	BA	PT	X
	8	1	C	C	C	X
		2	C	PT	C	X
		3	BA	C	B	X
	9	1	C	C	C	C
		2	PT	C	BA	C
		3	C	B	C	BA

https://doi.org/10.3390/children13010059

Table A2. *Cont.*

2023–2024	6	4	C	C	C	X
		5	C	BA	C	X
		6	PT	C	B	X
	7	4	C	C	C	X
		5	BA	C	C	X
		6	C	PT	BA	X
	8	4	C	C	C	X
		5	C	PT	BA	X
		6	B	C	C	X
	9	4	C	C	C	X
		5	PT	C	BA	X
		6	C	BA	PT	X
	10	4	C	C	C	C
		5	C	B	PT	PT
		6	BA	C	BA	C

Appendix C

Table A3. Baseline descriptive statistics of four junior high and high schools.

	School A	School B	School C	School D
Number of students/scholars	616	562	365	83
Race/ethnicity	51% black, 13% Asian, 9% Hispanic, 17% white, 8% mixed	98% black	54% white, 30% Hispanic, 6% black, 3% Asian, 5% mixed	98% black
Economic disadvantage	54%	95%	55%	73%
English/Language Arts	36% below basic, 39% basic, 22% proficient	70% below basic, 26% basic	36% below basic, 38% basic, 22% proficient	94% below basic
Math	50% below basic, 16% proficient	78% below basic, 18% basic	46% below basic, 32% basic, 20% proficient	97% below basic
Chronic absenteeism	21%	42%	20%	17%
Graduation rate	95%	86%	90%	47%

Table A4. Survey Participant Demographics.

RACE/ETHNICITY (Checked all that apply)	$n = 321$
Black or African American	59%
White	35%
Hispanic or Latino	14%
Asian	7%
American Indian or Alaskan Native	5%
Native Hawaiian or Pacific Islander	2%

https://doi.org/10.3390/children13010059

Table A4. *Cont.*

GENDER IDENTITY	n = 321
Boy/man	53%
Girl/woman	41%
Non-binary/gender fluid/gender queer/intersex	3%
Prefer not to answer	2%
Other	1%
CURRENT GRADE LEVEL IN SCHOOL	n = 329
5	14%
6	22%
7	22%
8	16%
9	25%

References

1. United States Department of Education. *Federal Role in Education*; United States Department of Education: Washington, DC, USA, 2025.
2. Lim, C.; Chung, P.J.; Biely, C.; Jackson, N.J.; Puffer, M.; Zepeda, A.; Anton, P.; Leifheit, K.M.; Dudovitz, R. School Attendance Following Receipt of Care From a School-Based Health Center. *J. Adolesc. Health* **2023**, *73*, 1125–1131. [CrossRef]
3. Office of the Press Secretary. *Fact Sheet: Congress Acts to Fix No Child Left Behind*; The White House: Washington, DC, USA, 2015.
4. Klein, A. No Child Left Behind: An Overview. *Education Week*, 10 April 2015.
5. Klein, A. The Every Student Succeeds Act: An ESSA Overview. *Education Week*, 31 March 2016.
6. Ballotpedia. Donald Trump Presidential Campaign 2016/Education. 2016. Available online: https://ballotpedia.org/Donald_Trump_presidential_campaign,_2016/Education (accessed on 27 October 2025).
7. Turner, C.W. *Eric Donald Trump's Plan for America's Schools*; National Public Radio: Washington, DC, USA, 2016.
8. Whitaker, C.; McDaniels, A.; Johnson, S. The Trump Administration's Slow But Steady Undoing of the Department of Education. 2017. Available online: https://www.americanprogress.org/article/trump-administrations-slow-steady-undoing-department-education/ (accessed on 29 October 2025).
9. Healthy People 2030. High School Graduation. 2025. Available online: https://odphp.health.gov/healthypeople/priority-areas/social-determinants-health/literature-summaries/high-school-graduation#cit9 (accessed on 27 October 2025).
10. Swisher, R.R. *Neighbourhood*; Encyclopedia Britannica: Chicago, IL, USA, 2025.
11. Galster, G. Nonlinear and Threshold Aspects of Neighborhood Effects. *KZfSS Kölner Z. Soziologie Sozialpsychol.* **2014**, *66*, 117–133. [CrossRef]
12. Nieuwenhuis, J.; Hooimeijer, P. The association between neighbourhoods and educational achievement, a systematic review and meta-analysis. *J. Hous. Built Environ.* **2016**, *31*, 321–347. [CrossRef]
13. National Center for Chronic Disease Prevention and Health Promotion (U.S.). Division of Nutrition, Physical Activity and Obesity. Health Equity Resource Toolkit for State Practitioners Addressing Obesity Disparities. 2012. Available online: https://stacks.cdc.gov/view/cdc/12033 (accessed on 29 October 2025).
14. Community Schools Forward, Framework: Essentials for Community School Transformation. 2023. Available online: https://learningpolicyinstitute.org/project/community-schools-forward (accessed on 12 December 2025).
15. Dryfoos, J.G. School-based health centers in the context of education reform. *J. Sch. Health* **1998**, *68*, 404–408. [CrossRef]
16. Goldstein, D. Can Trump Really Abolish the Department of Education? *The New York Times*, 20 March 2025.
17. Goldstein, D. Trump Targets K-12. *The New York Times*, 17 April 2025.
18. American Psychological Association. Creativity, Optimism, Planning and Expert Information (COPE). 2011. Available online: https://www.apa.org/pi/about/publications/caregivers/practice-settings/intervention/cope (accessed on 29 October 2025).
19. The Center for Adolescent Substance Use Research. *The CRAFFT 2.1 Manual*; Boston Children's Hospital: Boston, MA, USA, 2018.
20. Stoltenburg, A.; McGuire, M.; Liverman, E.; Lumelsky, P.; Bates, G.; Gundacker, C.; Currie, B.; Meurer, J.R. STRYV365 *peak team* and Brain agents: Teacher perspectives on school impact of a trauma-informed, social-emotional learning approach for students facing adverse childhood experiences. *Front. Psychol.* **2024**, *15*, 1388499. [CrossRef] [PubMed]
21. Liverman, E.; Antognoli, D.; Elaiho, C.; McGuire, M.; Stoltenburg, A.; Navarrete, A.; Bates, G.; Chelius, T.; Gundacker, C.; Lumelsky, P.; et al. Game-Based Social-Emotional Learning for Youth: School-Based Qualitative Analysis of Brain Agents. *JMIR Form. Res.* **2025**, *9*, e67550. [CrossRef] [PubMed]

https://doi.org/10.3390/children13010059

22. Veresov, N.; Veresov, N.; Mok, N. Understanding development through the perezhivanie of learning. In *The Routledge Handbook of Sociocultural Theory and Second Language Development*; Lantolf, J.P., Poehner, M., Eds.; Routledge: New York, NY, USA, 2018; pp. 89–101.
23. Vygotsky, L.S. *The Collected Works of L. S. Vygotsky, Volume 4: The History of the Development of Higher Mental Functions*; Plenum Press: New York, NY, USA, 1997.
24. Harris, P.A.; Taylor, R.; Thielke, R.; Payne, J.; Gonzalez, N.; Jose, G. Conde Research electronic data capture (REDCap)—A metadata-driven methodology and workflow process for providing translational research informatics support. *J. Biomed. Inform.* **2009**, *42*, 377–381. [CrossRef] [PubMed]
25. Collaborative for Academic, Social, and Emotional Learning (CASEL). CASEL Framework. 2023. Available online: https://casel.org/fundamentals-of-sel/what-is-the-casel-framework/ (accessed on 12 December 2025).
26. Hamby, S.; Taylor, E.; Blount, Z. *Resilience Portfolio Questionnaire Manual: Scales for Youth*; Life Paths Research Center: Sewanee, YN, USA, 2018.
27. Richardson, L.P.; Rockhill, C.; Russo, J.E.; Grossman, D.C.; Richards, J.; McCarty, C.; McCauley, E.; Katon, W. Evaluation of the PHQ-2 as a brief screen for detecting major depression among adolescents. *Pediatrics* **2010**, *125*, e1097–e1103. [CrossRef]
28. Mossman, S.A.; Luft, M.J.; Schroeder, H.K.; Varney, S.T.; Fleck, D.E.; Barzman, D.H.; Gilman, R.; DelBello, M.P.; Strawn, J.R. The Generalized Anxiety Disorder 7-item scale in adolescents with generalized anxiety disorder: Signal detection and validation. *Ann. Clin. Psychiatry* **2017**, *29*, 227–234. [CrossRef]
29. United States Department of Agriculture. National School Lunch Program: Feeding the Future with Healthy School Lunches. 2025. Available online: www.fns.usda.gov/nslp (accessed on 29 October 2025).
30. Fischler, J.; Claybourn, C. Understanding Charter Schools vs. Public Schools. *U.S. News & World Report*, 20 August 2025.
31. Stanford, L. Charter Schools Now Outperform Traditional Public Schools, Sweeping Study Finds. *Education Week*, 6 June 2023.
32. Hahn, R.A.; Truman, B.I. Education Improves Public Health and Promotes Health Equity. *Int. J. Health Serv.* **2015**, *45*, 657–678. [CrossRef]
33. National Center for Education Statistics. Table 1.1 Minimum Number of Instructional Days and Hours per Day. 2020. Available online: https://nces.ed.gov/programs/statereform/tab1_1-2020.asp (accessed on 12 December 2025).
34. National Center for Education Statistics. Average Number of Hours in the School Day and Average Number of Days in the School Year for Public Schools, by State: 2007-08. 2025. Available online: https://nces.ed.gov/surveys/sass/tables/sass0708_035_s1s.asp?swcfpc=1 (accessed on 25 May 2025).
35. Bethell, C.; Jones, J.; Gombojav, N.; Linkenbach, J.; Sege, R. Positive Childhood Experiences and Adult Mental and Relational Health in a Statewide Sample: Associations Across Adverse Childhood Experiences Levels. *JAMA Pediatr.* **2019**, *173*, e193007. [CrossRef]
36. Daily, S.M.; Mann, M.J.; Kristjansson, A.L.; Smith, M.L.; Zullig, K.J. School Climate and Academic Achievement in Middle and High School Students. *J. Sch. Health* **2019**, *89*, 173–180. [CrossRef]
37. Rakesh, D.; Zalesky, A.; Whittle, S. The Role of School Environment in Brain Structure, Connectivity, and Mental Health in Children: A Multimodal Investigation. *Biol. Psychiatry: Cogn. Neurosci. Neuroimaging* **2023**, *8*, 32–41. [CrossRef]
38. Putnam, R.D. Who Killed Civic America. 1996. Available online: https://www.prospectmagazine.co.uk/essays/59744/who-killed-civic-america (accessed on 12 December 2025).
39. Liljenquist, K.S.; Coker, T.R. Addressing Risky Health Behaviors Among Vulnerable Youth Through the School Environment: Location, Location, Location. *JAMA Pediatr.* **2018**, *172*, 1119–1120. [CrossRef]
40. Ho, E. The Robert Wood Johnson Foundation School Health Project. *J. Sch. Health* **1979**, *49*, 419. [CrossRef]
41. Love, H.E.; Schlitt, J.; Soleimanpour, S.; Panchal, N.; Behr, C. Twenty Years Of School-Based Health Care Growth and Expansion. *Health Aff.* **2019**, *38*, 755–764. [CrossRef]
42. Atkins, M.S.; Cappella, E.; Shernoff, E.S.; Mehta, T.G.; Gustafson, E.L. Schooling and Children's Mental Health: Realigning Resources to Reduce Disparities and Advance Public Health. *Annu. Rev. Clin. Psychol.* **2017**, *13*, 123–147. [CrossRef] [PubMed]
43. Soleimanpour, S. School-Based Health Centers: At the Intersection of Health and Education. *J. Adolesc. Health* **2020**, *67*, 317–318. [CrossRef] [PubMed]
44. County Health Rankings & Roadmaps. School-Based Health Centers. 2025. Available online: https://www.countyhealthrankings.org/strategies-and-solutions/what-works-for-health/strategies/school-based-health-centers (accessed on 29 October 2025).
45. School-Based Health Alliance. State Relations. 2025. Available online: https://www.sbh4all.org/state-relations/ (accessed on 29 October 2025).
46. Woolf, S.H. Necessary But Not Sufficient: Why Health Care Alone Cannot Improve Population Health and Reduce Health Inequities. *Ann. Fam. Med.* **2019**, *17*, 196–199. [CrossRef] [PubMed]
47. Woolf, S.H. Progress In Achieving Health Equity Requires Attention To Root Causes. *Health Aff.* **2017**, *36*, 984–991. [CrossRef] [PubMed]

https://doi.org/10.3390/children13010059

48. American Montessori Society. History of Montessori. 2025. Available online: https://amshq.org/about-montessori/history-of-montessori/ (accessed on 29 October 2025).
49. KIPP: Public Schools. KIPP Network. 2025. Available online: https://www.kipp.org/about/network/ (accessed on 29 October 2025).
50. Center for Research on Education Outcomes (CREDO). As a Matter of Fact: The National Charter School Study. 2023. Available online: https://ncss3.stanford.edu/wp-content/uploads/2023/06/Credo-NCSS3-Report.pdf (accessed on 29 October 2025).
51. National Alliance for Public Charter Schools. Data. 2025. Available online: https://data.publiccharters.org/ (accessed on 29 October 2025).
52. National Center for Education Statistics. Fast Facts: Back-to-School Statistics (372). 2025. Available online: https://nces.ed.gov/fastfacts/display.asp?id=372 (accessed on 9 September 2025).
53. Hess, C. *Milwaukee Public Schools Considers Closing, Merging Schools*; Wisconsin Public Radio: Madison, WI, USA, 2024.
54. Krejci, C. As anger rises over school closure talks, MPS to consider committees to get more feedback. *Milwaukee Journal Sentinel*, 30 October 2024. Available online: https://www.jsonline.com/story/news/education/2024/10/30/mps-board-to-consider-steering-committees-on-school-closures-upgrades/75907874007/ (accessed on 29 October 2025).
55. City of Milwaukee Department of Administration. Budget Documents Archive. 2025. Available online: https://city.milwaukee.gov/doa/budget/Milwaukee-Budgets (accessed on 29 October 2025).

https://doi.org/10.3390/children13010059

children

MDPI

Article

Laying the Foundation for an Elementary School Sleep Education Program

Alzena Ilie [1,†], Peyton Williams [1,†], Gabrielle Rigney [2], Shelly K. Weiss [3], Sarah Bluden [4] and Penny V. Corkum [1,5,*]

1 Department of Psychology and Neuroscience, Faculty of Science, Dalhousie University, Halifax, NS B3H 4R2, Canada; alzenailie@dal.ca (A.I.)
2 Appleton Institute, School of Health Medical and Applied Sciences, Central Queensland University, Adelaide, SA 5034, Australia
3 Department of Paediatrics, Faculty of Medicine, University of Toronto, Toronto, ON M5S 1A1, Canada
4 School of Education, Monash University, Clayton, VIC 3800, Australia
5 Department of Psychiatry, Faculty of Science, Dalhousie University, Halifax, NS B3H 4R2, Canada
* Correspondence: penny.corkum@dal.ca
† These authors contributed equally to this work.

Abstract

Background/Objectives: Many elementary school-aged children (i.e., 5 to 12 years old) experience sleep difficulties that negatively impact their daytime functioning. Despite this high prevalence, sleep education is rarely included in school curricula and evidence-based interventions are limited. To better understand this gap, a needs assessment was conducted to inform the development of a sleep education program. **Method:** Semi-structured virtual interviews were conducted with 14 elementary school teachers in Nova Scotia, Canada. Participants were asked 20 questions about their students' sleep and its impact, teachers' needs and practices in sleep education, what a sleep education program would look like, and how it could be delivered. During the interview, participants watched the online *ABCs of SLEEPING* storybook as a potential foundation for developing a sleep education program, and interview themes were analyzed using deductive thematic analysis. **Results:** All teachers identified poor sleep as an issue impacting students' behavior and learning, and reported that they had a lack of resources to teach sleep education. Teachers believed the storybook could be used with their students and integrated into the curriculum. Recommended modifications include making the storybook available for families, adding interactive activities and student discussions, providing teacher resources, and tailoring the content to be suitable for both lower and upper elementary school-aged students. Most teachers indicated that the storybook could be adapted for upper elementary students with more age-appropriate vocabulary and visuals. **Conclusions:** The findings from this needs assessment will inform the development of an elementary school sleep education program using the *ABCs of SLEEPING* storybook as the foundation of the program, while noting limitations such as sample diversity.

Keywords: sleep; school-aged children; school-based program; needs assessment; sleep education; elementary school

1. Introduction

Sleep is essential for health and well-being at all ages, especially for elementary school-aged children who are expected to learn, concentrate, and retain new information [1]. Approximately 30% of school-aged Canadian children (i.e., 5 to 12 years old) obtain less than the recommended 10 h of sleep per night, often having difficulties falling or staying asleep, and waking too early in the morning [2–4]. If these sleep difficulties reach clinical levels, they are diagnosed as insomnia, which is defined as frequent (three or more nights per week) and chronic (longer than three months) difficulties with sleep initiation and maintenance despite adequate opportunities [4,5]. Of the 30% of school-aged children with sleep difficulties, 10% have clinically diagnosed insomnia [6]. Both insomnia and insomnia symptoms negatively impact daytime functioning and impair skills needed for school success, including attention, memory, reasoning, and worsening behavioral and emotional problems [1,7]. These sleep problems are often due to poor sleep practices, including night-time screen use, social media, and unhealthy eating, as well as irregular sleep schedules, and poor sleep environments [7–9].

Over the past decade research has focused on developing and evaluating digital parent-implemented sleep interventions for their children [10–12]; however, interventions are often difficult to access, which results in many children not receiving treatment for their sleep problems [13,14]. Given these barriers, alternative strategies should be considered to effectively reach children in need of support. Schools have the ability to reach a large number of children and youth, providing an ideal setting to encourage children to adopt and maintain healthy lifestyles [15]. School programs targeting behavioral health outcomes (e.g., physical activity, dietary habits) have been found to improve both health and overall well-being [16]. Moreover, using the existing system can be an affordable and effective way to deliver health promotion programs [17]. Despite the critical role sleep has on daytime functioning and learning, sleep education is rarely included in school health curricula [18].

To date, research examining school-based sleep education programs has mostly been focused on high school students [18–21]. The *Healthy Sleep for Healthy Schools (HS4HS)* program was developed by Dr. Corkum, Dr. Rigney, and colleagues to be used with junior high and high school students with the goal of providing teachers with the knowledge and resources they require to teach students about healthy sleep. This program includes a teacher professional development component delivered online, in which teachers learn about the importance of sleep and healthy sleep practices. Once the teacher demonstrates mastery of the materials, teaching resources (e.g., PowerPoint slides, lesson plans, parent resources) are unlocked to be disseminated among their students. The program has been found to be useful, comprehensive, and easy to incorporate into school curricula [22,23]. To our knowledge, this is the only sleep education program developed and evaluated in Canada and Australia [22]. Preliminary evidence for effectiveness was demonstrated through positive reviews and improvements in sleep knowledge and practices following participation in the program [22]. During this research, educators indicated a need for a similar program for elementary school-aged students.

Despite the need for sleep education, few school-based sleep education programs for elementary school-aged students exist [18,20]. Evaluation of the six programs reported in the literature [17,24–28] indicated mixed results regarding the effectiveness of these programs. Though these studies show promising results, the findings are mixed regarding the effectiveness of these programs, often due to the lack of evidence-based design and the need for interventions to be developed and tailored for the educational systems they will be used in [24,28,29]. Most of the programs made for elementary schools were not specifically designed for the different grade levels, particularly lower elementary school-aged students (i.e., Grade Primary/Kindergarten to Grade 3) and upper elementary school-aged students (i.e., Grades 4 to 6), despite there being substantial differences in these grades in regard to cognitive functioning, executive functioning, and independence [30,31]. Additionally, educational policies and practices in Canada vary significantly across provinces and dis-

https://doi.org/10.3390/children13010138

tricts [15]. Therefore, the development of sleep education programs should be tailored to the specific characteristics of each education system [15].

Given the feedback from teachers in the Nova Scotia school system who requested an elementary school-based sleep education program, our research team decided to build a program to meet this need. As a first step, a needs assessment was deemed necessary. A needs assessment is critical in program development, as it identifies and prioritizes the needs of key stakeholders [32]. Gathering data from teachers directly ensures that the intervention is relevant and appropriately tailored to the context of the school environment [32]. Without a needs assessment, programs may fail to address the sleep-related needs of students within the school setting, thus leading to ineffective outcomes or irrelevant interventions [33].

The current research aimed to gather foundational information to inform the development of a sleep education program for teachers to deliver to elementary school-aged students. The needs assessment followed Witkin's Three Phases of Needs Assessment, including (1) pre-assessment (exploration), (2) assessment (data gathering), (3) and post-assessment (utilization) [34]. The pre-assessment phase has been completed (e.g., informal discussion with educators in Nova Scotia, comprehensive literature review), while the current study focused on Phases 2 and 3, by conducting in-depth individual qualitative interviews with stakeholders (i.e., elementary school teachers) [33]. As a starting point in the development of an elementary school sleep education program, we explored the use of a children's storybook, the *ABCs of Sleeping* [35], designed to help children learn about the importance of sleep and what healthy sleep practices include. It was originally written as a storybook to be read to children in Grades Primary/Kindergarten to Grade 3, but may be a potential foundation for a sleep education program for elementary school-aged students. The *ABCs of SLEEPING* storybook presents a mnemonic, created by Dr. Corkum and trainees, that encapsulates healthy sleep practices [36]. The mnemonic is: Age-appropriate Bedtimes and wake-times with Consistency, Schedules and routines, Location, Exercise and diet, no Electronics in bedroom or before bed, Positivity, Independence, and Needs met, equal Great sleep.

The research was guided by five key objectives: (1) to gather teachers' perspectives on students' sleep and its impacts on elementary school-aged students in the classroom and at school; (2) to determine the need for sleep education and learn what sleep information teachers are currently delivering in their classroom; (3) to determine if the *ABCs of SLEEPING* storybook can be used as the foundation for a sleep education program for the elementary school context, and if so, what additional supports/resources are needed, (4) to collect elementary school teachers' recommendations for effectively delivering the *ABCs of SLEEPING* storybook in the classroom, and (5) to determine whether the above findings differ for lower elementary school-aged students (i.e., Primary to Grade 3) and upper elementary school-aged students (i.e., Grade 4 to Grade 6).

2. Method

2.1. Participant Selection

Eligibility included that the individual was currently working as an elementary school teacher (Primary to Grade 6) in Nova Scotia, Canada for at least one year and be fluent in English. The sample size was finalized at 14 participants when theme saturation was reached. This smaller sample size was expected as the study population is relatively homogenous, the research objectives narrowly defined, and the sample generated enough diversity of data [37,38].

https://doi.org/10.3390/children13010138

2.2. Measures

Participant enrollment, consent, questionnaires, and interview scheduling were arranged through REDCap [39].

2.2.1. Screening Questionnaire

This is an author-made, 5-item questionnaire that was used to verify that participants are eligible to participate in this study. The questionnaire includes items pertaining to the inclusion criteria of the study. The inclusion criteria are that teachers must teach at the elementary school level (Primary to Grade 6) in Nova Scotia, they must have worked as an elementary school teacher for at least 1 year, and they must be fluent in English. There were no exclusion criteria. The questionnaire took approximately 4 min to complete.

2.2.2. Demographic Questionnaire

This is an author-made, 8-item questionnaire used to collect demographic information about the study sample, including the teachers' age, gender, race/ethnicity, education level, the community where they teach, the grade they are currently teaching, and years of teaching experience. The demographic questionnaire was adapted from a questionnaire used in previous research in Corkum LABS [40]. The questionnaire took approximately eight minutes to complete. The data collected was used to describe the sample and determine the representativeness of the sample.

2.2.3. Sleep Education Experiences (SEE) Questionnaire

This is an author-made, 6-item questionnaire used to collect information about teachers' knowledge about sleep and experience teaching sleep information in the classroom. The questionnaire took approximately three minutes to complete. The data collected was used to describe the sample and their sleep knowledge before completing the interview.

2.2.4. Qualitative Interviews

Virtual semi-structured interviews were held, with video and audio recorded and transcribed using the web-based Microsoft Teams Software (see Supplementary Table S1). The interviews were approximately 30 min long (M = 28.64; SD = 8.55; 18–55 min).

Researchers used a templated summary table, a researcher-created data collection form based on the methods used in previous qualitative studies [41,42]. The templated summary tables assisted in organizing qualitative interview data when note taking, coding, and when extracting themes during data analysis.

The 20 interview questions were divided into five sections. For the first set of questions (n = 3) participants were asked about their students' sleep and the impact of sleep problems. For the second set of questions (n = 4) participants were asked about the need for sleep education and current practices in teaching sleep. Teachers then watched the online *ABCs of SLEEPING* storybook video, which required five minutes. Afterwards, the third set of questions (n = 5) was asked, which focused on how the *ABCs of SLEEPING* storybook could be used as the foundation of a sleep education program. The fourth set of questions (n = 7) focused on how the program could be delivered. Lastly, the fifth section provided participants with the opportunity to share any additional information they thought was important which had not been addressed in the interview.

2.3. Procedure

Recruitment was conducted through the investigators' professional contacts within the education system in Nova Scotia and email invitations to teachers from the Accessible Strategies Supporting Inclusion for Students by Teachers (*ASSIST*) Study (Principal

https://doi.org/10.3390/children13010138

Investigator, P.C.) who had consented to being contacted for future studies coordinated in Corkum LABS.

Potential participants completed an initial screening questionnaire to confirm eligibility. To prevent fraudulent participation the screening questionnaire included a verification item asking what school the participant currently teaches at in Nova Scotia. Participants' responses were cross-referenced with publicly available staff directories from Nova Scotia schools to confirm their names appeared on the listed faculty or staff; additionally, participants were required to provide a school-affiliated email addressed to authenticate participants' status as a current educator within the province. Eligible participants were then automatically directed to an electronic Information and Consent form. Once consent had been provided, participants were automatically directed to complete the demographic questionnaire and questionnaire about their experiences related to teaching sleep. Teachers then provided their availability for the qualitative interview. Participants received reminder emails 24 h and two hours in advance of their interview.

Relevant information from the consent form was summarized during the semi-structured interview. After consent was confirmed, the researchers asked questions based on the interview guide and during the interview participants watched the online video of the *ABCs of SLEEPING* storybook. Throughout all interviews, two researchers were working together (PW, AI). One researcher conducted the interview, while the second researcher wrote summary notes of the participant's answers and provided any support to the first researcher if necessary. To compensate participants for their time, participants who completed all study measures and interview were provided with a $30.00 CAD Amazon.ca online gift card.

2.4. Data Analysis

The demographic and SEE questionnaires were analyzed using SPSS Version 28 (IBM Canada). Descriptive statistics were calculated for the entire sample.

QSR International's NVivo 12 analysis software [43] was used to organize qualitative data from interviews. Deductive Thematic Analysis [44] was applied to identify the key themes and program recommendations identified by participants. The User Experience Honeycomb framework developed by Morville & Sullenger [45] was used to assess seven important domains (see Supplementary Table S2 for a description of these domains) that impact the desire and motivation to use the *ABCs of Sleeping* storybook as the foundation of a sleep education program. Previous studies have shown that the User Experience Honeycomb framework provides a consistent and reliable method for evaluating program usability [40,46]. Once the interviews were completed, each researcher (P.W. and A.I.) independently coded the themes for each interview. The percentage of coding agreement between the coders was 95%. Discrepancies were resolved by discussing them with a senior member of the research team (P.C.).

Ongoing data analysis was conducted simultaneously with the qualitative interviews and data collection ceased upon data saturation of qualitative themes. Thematic saturation in the current study was defined as the point in data collection and analysis when the identification of new themes no longer contributed significant value or resulted in changes to the overall content analysis (i.e., all main themes of the study have already been found) [47]. In the current data analysis procedure, sub-themes had to be identified by three different participants (30%+) to be considered significant to ensure the themes were not isolated opinions but recurring patterns observed in several participants [48]. This approach captures a broader experience and perspective within the study population, enhancing the reliability and validity of the results [48].

https://doi.org/10.3390/children13010138

3. Results

3.1. Sample Characteristics

Out of the 22 participants who consented to participate in the study, 14 completed the study by attending the virtual interview. Of the eight participants who did not participate in the interview, four withdrew due to their limited availability while the remaining four were automatically withdrawn due to a lack of response to follow-up emails.

The majority of participants identified as females (n = 13), while one participant identified as male. All participants identified as White. The majority of the participants (n = 9) resided in towns or rural areas, while the rest (n = 5) lived in a city. Participants had an average age of 40 years old (M = 40.35; SD = 10.94; 26–59 years). Half of the participants (n = 7) taught at the lower elementary level (i.e., Primary to Grade 3), and half (n = 7) taught at the upper elementary level (i.e., Grade 4 to 6). Further demographic information regarding study participants is in Table 1.

Table 1. Teacher Demographic Variables.

Demographic Details	**Total (N = 14; 100%)**
Teacher Gender	
Female	13 (92.9%)
Male	1 (7.1%)
Teacher Ethnicity	
White	14 (100%)
Community	
Rural	5 (35.7%)
Town	4 (28.6%)
City under 500,000 people	4 (28.6%)
City over 500,000 people	1 (7.1%)
Highest Education	
Bachelors/Undergraduate Degree or Teacher's College (e.g., B.A., B.SC., B.Ed.)	7 (50%)
Master's Degree (e.g., M.A., M.Sc., M.Ed.)	7 (50%)
Current Grade Teaching	
Lower Elementary	
Grade 1	1 (7.1%)
Grade 2	1 (7.1%)
Grade 3	3 (21.4%)
Upper Elementary	
Grade 4	0 (0%)
Grade 5	1 (7.1%)
Grade 6	3 (21.4%)
Other (i.e., Split Class)	5 (35.7%) (2 Lower/3 Upper)
What Grade Participant has Taught in Teaching Career	
Elementary (Grades 1–6)	14 (100%)
Junior High School (Grades 7–9)	5 (35.7%)
Senior High School (Grades 10–12)	4 (28.6%)
Demographic Details	**M (*SD*)**
Teacher Age	40.35 (10.94)
Length of Time Teaching	14.64 (9.89)
Number of years Taught in Elementary	13.35 (8.39)

In terms of the teachers' experiences in sleep education, four teachers reported they had 'none' to 'not very much' knowledge regarding the concept of sleep education and its

https://doi.org/10.3390/children13010138

goals, while ten teachers reported they were 'somewhat' to 'very knowledgeable'. Most teachers (n = 9) reported having never taught sleep information in their curriculum, while five teachers reported that they had. All teachers agreed that sleep education is needed. Further information regarding experiences in sleep education is in Table 2.

Table 2. Teacher Experiences in Sleep Education.

Sleep Education Experiences	Total (N = 14; 100%)
Teacher Knowledge Level	
No knowledge of this subject	1 (7.1%)
Not very knowledgeable	3 (21.4%)
Somewhat knowledgeable	8 (57.1%)
Knowledgeable	1 (7.1%)
Very knowledgeable	1 (7.1%)
Experience Teaching Sleep	
Never Taught About Sleep in Curriculum	9 (64.3%)
Taught About Sleep in Curriculum	5 (35.7%)
Sources of Information Accessed on Sleep Education	
No Information Accessed	10 (71.4%)
Accessed Sleep Information	4 (28.6%)
Types of Resources Accessed	
Readings Materials on Sleep Education	4 (28.6%)
Sleep Education Courses	1 (7.1%)
Sleep Education Workshops	1 (7.1%)
Other	1 (7.1%)
Belief in the Need for Sleep Education in Curriculum	
Strongly agree	8 (57.1%)
Agree	6 (49.2%)
Neutral	0 (0%)
Disagree	0 (0%)
Strong Disagree	0 (0%)
Comfort Level with Teaching Sleep Education	
Strongly agree	1 (7.1%)
Agree	6 (42.9%)
Neutral	3 (21.4%)
Disagree	4 (28.6%)
Strongly Disagree	0 (0%)
Teacher Previously Used or Reviewed a Sleep Education Program	
Yes	0 (0%)
No	14 (100%)

3.2. Teachers' Perspectives on Students' Sleep and Its Impacts

At the beginning of the interview, teachers were asked questions about their students' sleep. Responses are presented descriptively rather than thematically. The majority of teachers (n = 12) reported that their students were not aware of the importance of sleep. In terms of sleep problems, teachers reported delayed bedtimes (n = 12), falling asleep in class (n = 7), difficulties falling asleep (n = 5), daytime sleepiness (n = 3), and early morning awakenings (n = 2) in their students. Teachers also reported that, on average, 31% of students do not sleep well.

When asked about the impact of poor sleep, five themes were identified from the data (see Supplementary Table S3 for quotes). The most prevalent theme identified (n = 13) was student tiredness and low energy. Teachers (n = 12) noted negative impacts on their students' mood and behavior (e.g., irritability, emotion regulation, externalizing behaviors), and had difficulties completing schoolwork/tasks when they did not sleep well. Teachers

https://doi.org/10.3390/children13010138

reported reduced focus and attention (n = 8), and learning difficulties among students (n = 7).

3.3. Teachers' Needs and Current Practices in Sleep Education

When asked about their needs and current practices in sleep education, five themes arose from the data (see Supplementary Table S4). The majority of teachers (n = 13) recognized the need for sleep education; however, many teachers (n = 12) identified a lack of accessible evidence-based resources to effectively deliver sleep information. Most teachers (n = 12) reported engaging in informal conversations with students while nine used strategies to help students manage tiredness (e.g., mindfulness, yoga, movement). Of note, many teachers (n = 9) emphasized the need to reinforce sleep education at home.

3.4. Teachers' Thoughts on Program Development

Teachers' feedback on the potential use of the *ABCS of SLEEPING* storybook as a foundation for a sleep education program for elementary school-aged children were organized using the relevant domains of the User Experience Honeycomb framework (Morville & Sullenger, 2010). Their comments were grouped into 16 themes within the five relevant domains: (1) program credibility (one theme), (2) program accessibility (two themes), (3) program desirability (three themes), (4) program valuableness (three themes), and (5) program usefulness (seven themes) (see Supplementary Table S5 for quotes).

All teachers expressed high confidence in the storybook, likely as it is evidence-based and written by clinical sleep researchers. For program accessibility, most teachers (n = 10) emphasized improving accessibility for families (e.g., sending the book home, handouts for parents), and six teachers recommended translating the storybook for non-English-speaking families. All teachers (n = 14) found the storybook to be visually and thematically appealing. Half of the teachers (n = 7) offered suggestions for the illustrations, such as different forms of screen usage and more detailed images. Some teachers (n = 3) also mentioned the need for more diversity in the characters.

When teachers were asked whether the information and content in the storybook would be relevant and helpful for their students, all teachers reported that the impact of electronics on sleep provided valuable information, as most of the teachers (n = 9) identified electronics as the key cause of sleep problems in their students. Half of the teachers (n = 7) reported the content regarding sleeping in the same environment and having a bedtime routine was valuable and relevant, and six teachers appreciated the content on nutrition and exercise. All teachers recommended adding discussion points to facilitate discussions in the classroom about the storybook content. Most teachers (n = 8) recommended incorporating an activity book (i.e., collection of activities including coloring pages, writing activities); some teachers (n = 5) felt activity books may not be helpful, as one may find it overwhelming to have every activity all at once. Furthermore, ten teachers recommended incorporating parent involvement to support and reinforce their child's sleep practices at home.

Teachers provided further suggestions for program usefulness, including adding individual student activities (n = 10), such as goal-setting activities or engaging in an activity for each letter of the *ABCs of Sleeping* mnemonic. Increasing socially sensitive content was emphasized by some teachers (n = 6), pointing out there are some situations that are not addressed, especially for children from lower socioeconomic status (e.g., not having their own bedroom at home, lacking a quiet space to sleep; see Supplementary Table S5).

3.5. Teachers' Recommendations for Program Delivery

When teachers were asked about their thoughts on program delivery, eight themes surfaced and were organized by the remaining two relevant domains of the User Experience

https://doi.org/10.3390/children13010138

Honeycomb framework (Morville & Sullenger, 2010): (1) program findability (two themes) and (2) program usability (six themes) (see Supplementary Table S6 for quotes). In terms of program findability, most teachers (n = 13) reported that a physical copy of the storybook offered advantages (e.g., planning purposes, limiting screen time). Conversely, ten teachers reported the advantages of having a digital version (e.g., accessing through the classroom website, projecting for group viewing). In terms of the program's usability, all teachers believed the program could be effectively integrated and delivered within their current curriculum. When teachers were asked how they would discover a sleep education program, all teachers noted a variety of methods, including through school administration, newsletters, conferences, and colleagues.

The majority of teachers (n = 13) reported needing additional resources and guidance to teach about sleep with the storybook, such as an online learning module, and supplemental teaching resources (e.g., lesson plans, slideshows). A few teachers (n = 5) felt that no additional resources were needed if the program only involved reading the storybook. The majority of teachers (n = 12) suggested varying frequencies for how often they would use the storybook (e.g., twice to three times, every year, daily). Furthermore, some teachers (n = 8) recommended times for incorporating the storybook into the classroom, such as during snack time, integrating it into students' daily schedules, and during silent reading (see Supplementary Table S6).

3.6. Teachers' Needs Based on Lower and Upper Elementary School-Aged Students

When the qualitative data was compared between lower elementary and upper elementary, three themes were identified from the data (See Supplementary Table S7 for quotes). When asked about what grade level for which the storybook would be most appropriate, nine teachers reported it would be most suitable for lower elementary and five teachers reported it would be most suitable for both upper and lower elementary. In terms of the vocabulary level, nine teachers reported the vocabulary is at an appropriate level for their students; two lower elementary teachers reported that it may be too complex and two upper elementary teachers reported it may be too simple. When asked about the age level of the content, six lower elementary teachers and six upper elementary teachers felt it was at an age-appropriate level; however, twelve teachers provided suggestions for presenting the content in a more mature way for upper elementary school-aged students (e.g., illustrations of older students, mature visuals).

4. Discussion

The purpose of the study was to gather foundational insights to guide the development of a sleep education program for elementary school teachers and their students. The researchers collected information through questionnaires and semi-structured interviews to explore teachers' perspectives on their students' sleep, the impact of poor sleep in the classroom/school, current practices in sleep education, what a sleep education program would look like, and how it could be delivered in the classroom. Additionally, teachers reviewed the ABCs of SLEEPING storybook and provided feedback on its potential to be used as the foundation of the sleep education program. The findings showed that all teachers recognized poor sleep as a major factor impacting students' success at school. They all highlighted the need for sleep education but noted a lack of available resources. Teachers found the storybook accessible, credible, desirable, valuable, useful, findable, and usable. Some teachers suggested changes for improvement, including making the storybook accessible to families, adding interactive activities and discussions for students, and providing additional teaching resources for effective delivery.

https://doi.org/10.3390/children13010138

The first research objective aimed to determine teachers' perspectives on students' sleep and its impacts. All teachers identified poor sleep negatively impacting daily functioning at school, including students' energy levels, mood and behavior, learning, schoolwork completion, and focus and attention. Our findings are consistent with previous research, which links sleep problems to greater levels of student conflict, increased inattention, academic difficulties, externalizing symptoms, and more general behavior problems [49,50]. The rates of sleep problems reported by teachers in this study (~31% of students not sleeping well) were representative of the national average of ~30% of Canadian parents reporting sleep problems in their school-aged children [3,4]. Some teachers indicated that as many as 65% of their students do not sleep well. A potential factor to explain this high prevalence of sleep problems could be the increasing use of technology during the evening among children, which is associated with shorter sleep duration and delayed sleep onset [51]. This is consistent with teachers' reports in the current study, which identified the use of electronics as one of the main causes of sleep problems.

The second research objective aimed to determine the need for sleep education, and to learn what teachers are currently doing related to teaching about sleep. All teachers in the current study believed there is a need for sleep education though also noted the challenges in providing such due to the lack of available resources. Gruber and colleagues [15] found that teachers often do not have the opportunity to acquire information on healthy sleep practices or deliver that information to their students due to time constraints. Furthermore, most teachers have not been trained about the importance of sleep or strategies that can help improve sleep [15]. Additionally, the majority of teachers (n=12) reported that informal conversations were their primary method to address sleep issues; informal conversations can build awareness and influence students' perspectives on healthy sleep behaviors though they may not lead to changes in sleep behavior [52]. This contrasts with evidence-based sleep programs, which have been found to change sleep knowledge and behaviors [53,54]. Furthermore, teachers reported the need to reinforce sleep education at home. Research highlights the need for school-based interventions to be supported through a collaborative approach that includes family involvement [21]. Two studies that encouraged parental involvement demonstrated that the effectiveness of sleep interventions increased when parents were involved [17,55]. This supports the notion that incorporating both teacher and parental involvement in sleep education can enhance the effectiveness of such programs.

The third research objective aimed to determine if the *ABCs of SLEEPING* storybook could be used as the foundation for a sleep education program in the elementary school context. All of the teachers found the storybook to be visually appealing and desirable, with the information provided in the storybook presented in a way that contributes positively to the user experience. For example, the teachers interviewed praised the messages in the storybook, as well as the diversity, format, colors, lettering, and illustrations used. Previous research supports the effectiveness of using the *ABCS of SLEEPING* mnemonic with parents to promote healthy sleep practices in their children [10]

Some teachers offered suggestions for improving the *ABCs of SLEEPING* storybook, particularly regarding the illustrations, culturally sensitive information, and diversity of the characters. Teachers noted that they teach a significant number of students from poorer socioeconomic and minority backgrounds and as such programs need to be more culturally sensitive. According to Sosso & Khoury [56], children from lower socioeconomic backgrounds are more likely to experience sleep difficulties than their higher-income peers. These insights suggest that developing educational materials which represent the diverse backgrounds and experiences in a specific regional area may make a sleep education program more applicable and relevant.

https://doi.org/10.3390/children13010138

Furthermore, to support effective implementation of the program, teachers emphasized the need for additional teaching resources and guidance to effectively teach sleep education using the storybook. Findings from the *HS4HS* program designed for junior high/high school showed that incorporating teaching materials and resources made the program more usable and facilitated program implementation [22]. This suggests that similar resources would be valuable and helpful for a sleep education program for elementary school-aged students as well.

The fourth research objective aimed to determine the recommendations elementary school teachers have for delivering the *ABCs of SLEEPING* storybook. Teachers expressed a preference for both physical and digital versions of the storybook, noting different advantages in each format. While there is little evidence suggesting one way of delivery is better than the other in changing sleep behavior, student engagement and improved sleep outcomes likely depend on the teacher's ability to deliver the program effectively [20]. Our study's findings support this, as teachers expressed a preference for a combination of both formats to enhance student engagement and accessibility.

The fifth and final research objective aimed to determine whether the findings from the research differed based on lower elementary versus upper elementary. Most teachers identified that the storybook was most suitable for lower elementary school-aged students and could be adapted for upper elementary school-aged students with adjustments to vocabulary and content. Teachers suggested including illustrations of older students, more mature visuals, and content that resonates with the needs of upper elementary students. As discussed previously, there are significant differences in cognitive and executive functioning between these grades [30,31]. Tailoring a school-based sleep education program to the developmental needs of school-aged children, such as addressing varying levels of autonomy and social stimulation, can increase the effectiveness of the program in promoting changes in sleep behavior [21].

4.1. Strengths

The current study has several strengths, such as its use of theoretical frameworks, which guided and structured the formulation of research questions and the organization of the research data. By adopting a user-centered design approach, following Witkin's Three Phases of Needs Assessment [34], the study ensured that the development of the sleep education program would be effective and useful for teachers. This approach underscores the study's focus on creating an effective intervention that is based on a clear understanding of the specific needs of key stakeholders [34]. Additionally, the use of the User Experience Honeycomb framework [45] is a notable strength, as it assesses seven essential domains of usability. By evaluating these domains, the study ensures that the *ABCs of SLEEPING* storybook meets the needs and preferences of its users, which will enhance the program's potential for successful engagement and retention [45]. By only interviewing lower and upper elementary school teachers, the researchers were able to focus on the needs of the current Nova Scotia elementary school system and gain knowledge to help inform the development of a sleep education program. This distinction is important, as despite being grouped together within elementary education, lower and upper elementary school-aged students exhibit developmental differences, and therefore should be considered separately [30,31]. As such, the findings of this research may have important implications for the adaption or implementation of similar sleep education programs across Canada in other educational systems.

https://doi.org/10.3390/children13010138

4.2. Limitations

This study is not without limitations. First, it is likely that only teachers who believed there was a need for sleep education participated in the study, as reported in the SEE questionnaire. This introduces a potential bias as those who see sleep education as necessary may be more inclined to support the development of a school-based sleep education program. Additionally, as all participants identified as White, and the recruitment of participants was carried out relying on investigators' professional contacts and previous research participants, the current sample may not be representative of a more diverse group of teachers in Nova Scotia. Teachers that are racially diverse may have different perspectives about sleep or sleep education in their students. Lastly, the current study used the approach of requiring themes to be identified by at least three different participants (30%+) to be considered significant. This was done to ensure the identified themes represented recurring patterns observed across multiple participants to capture a broader, shared experience and perspective within the study population [42,48]. However, this approach introduces a potential bias, as it may overlook valuable insights, different perspectives, and experiences that were not shared by a larger portion of the sample [48].

4.3. Implications and Future Research

The first step in advancing this research will be to use the findings from this study, in conjunction with the findings from the Australian study, to develop the *HS4HS Elementary* sleep education program. The Australian study involved focus groups with 15 elementary school teachers who were asked to review and provide feedback on the *HS4HS* for junior high/high school program in order to meet the needs of elementary school teachers. The research will use these findings combined with existing clinical and research knowledge, to develop an elementary school sleep education program. Following this, the program will be tested for its usability and its effectiveness in improving sleep outcomes among elementary school-aged students in Canada and in Australia.

In summary, the findings of this study underscore the critical need for sleep education programs in elementary schools in Canada. Teachers recognize the negative impact of poor sleep on students' academic and behavioral outcomes and expressed the need for evidence-based resources to address this issue. The *ABCs of SLEEPING* storybook, with some modifications, was thought to provide a strong foundation for a sleep education program for elementary school-aged students. It is hoped that this research will help to inform the development of a sleep education program for elementary school teachers in order to improve sleep knowledge, sleep quality, and overall well-being in elementary school-aged students.

Supplementary Materials: The following supporting information can be downloaded at: https://www.mdpi.com/article/10.3390/children13010138/s1, Supplementary Table S1. *HS4HS* Needs Assessment Qualitative Interview Guide; Supplementary Table S2. User Experience Honeycomb Framework Domain Definitions; Supplementary Table S3. Teachers' Perspectives on the Impacts of Poor Sleep on their Students (Themes); Supplementary Table S4. Teachers' Needs and Current Practices in Sleep Education (Themes); Supplementary Table S5. Teachers' Thoughts on Program Development (Themes Organized by User Experience Domains); Supplementary Table S6. Teachers' Thoughts on Program Delivery (Themes organized by User Experience Domains); Supplementary Table S7. Teachers' Needs Based on Lower and Upper Elementary Students Themes.

Author Contributions: Conceptualization, P.W., A.I., G.R., S.K.W., S.B. and P.V.C.; data curation—P.W. and A.I.; formal analysis–P.W. and A.I.; investigation–P.W. and A.I.; methodology, A.I., G.R. and P.V.C.; project administration—P.W. and A.I.; writing—original draft preparation P.W. and A.I.; writing—review and editing, G.R., S.K.W., S.B. and P.V.C.; validation—P.V.C.; resources—P.V.C.;

https://doi.org/10.3390/children13010138

visualization—P.W., A.I. and P.V.C.; supervision–A.I. and P.V.C.; funding acquisition—P.V.C. All authors have read and agreed to the published version of the manuscript.

Funding: The authors acknowledge the funding from CIHR Team Grant: Sleep Research Consortium—Sleep Across the Lifecycle, entitled Better Nights, Better Days for Canadians: An innovative national sustainable strategy to prevent and treat insomnia across the lifespan using digital approaches for sleep promotion, intervention, and provider training (CIHR 472502).

Institutional Review Board Statement: The study was conducted in accordance with the Declaration of Helsinki, and approved by the IWK Research Ethics Board (#1031284, 12 December 2024) for studies involving humans.

Informed Consent Statement: Informed consent was obtained from all subjects involved in the study.

Data Availability Statement: The datasets generated and analyzed during the current study are not publicly available due to keeping participant's identity and information confidential. The researchers do not have ethical approval to share the data.

Acknowledgments: The authors would like to thank the larger Corkum LABS research team with this study and article preparation, and to thank Derek van Voorst for editing the manuscript. We would also like to thank the teachers who took the time to participate in interviews and for sharing their expertise and knowledge with us. Peyton Williams would like to thank Penny Corkum and Alzena Ilie for their supervision.

Conflicts of Interest: The author(s declared no potential conflicts of interest with respect to the research, authorship, and/or publication of this article.

References

1. Liu, J.; Xiaopeng, J.; Pitt, S.; Wang, G.; Rovit, E.; Lipman, T.; Jiang, F. Childhood sleep: Physical, cognitive, and behavioral consequences and implications. *World J. Pediatr.* **2022**, *20*, 122–132. [CrossRef]
2. Chaput, J.; Janssen, I. Sleep Duration Estimates of Canadian Children and Adolescents. *J. Sleep Res.* **2016**, *25*, 541–548. [CrossRef]
3. Michaud, I.; Chaput, J.-P. Are Canadian Children and Adolescents Sleep Deprived? *Public Health* **2016**, *141*, 126–129. [CrossRef]
4. Kahn, M. Insomnia in Infancy, Childhood, and Adolescence. *Sleep Med. Clin.* **2023**, *18*, 135–145. [CrossRef]
5. American Psychiatric Association. *Diagnostic and Statistical Manual of Mental Disorders*; DSM-5-TR; American Psychiatric Association Publishing: Washington, DC, USA, 2022; ISBN 978-0-89042-575-6.
6. Corkum, P.; Weiss, S.; Hall, W.; Brown, C.; Chambers, C.; Constantin, E.; Godbout, R.; Hanlon-Dearman, A.; Ipsiroglu, O.; Reid, G.J.; et al. Assessment and Treatment of Pediatric Behavioral Sleep Disorders in Canada. *Sleep Med.* **2019**, *56*, 29–37. [CrossRef]
7. Buckhalt, J.A. Insufficient Sleep and the Socioeconomic Status Achievement Gap. *Child Dev. Perspect.* **2011**, *5*, 59–65. [CrossRef]
8. Hartley, S.; Royant-Parola, S.; Zayoud, A.; Gremy, I.; Matulonga, B. Do Both Timing and Duration of Screen Use Affect Sleep Patterns in Adolescents? *PLoS ONE* **2022**, *17*, e0276226. [CrossRef]
9. Zhao, Y.; Qu, D.; Liang, K.; Bao, R.; Chen, S. Eating Habits Matter for Sleep Difficulties in Children and Adolescents: A Cross-Sectional Study. *Front. Pediatr.* **2023**, *11*, 1108031. [CrossRef]
10. Allen, S.L.; Howlett, M.D.; Coulombe, J.A.; Corkum, P.V. ABCs of SLEEPING: A Review of the Evidence behind Pediatric Sleep Practice Recommendations. *Sleep Med. Rev.* **2016**, *29*, 1–14. [CrossRef] [PubMed]
11. Johnson, C.R.; Barto, L.; Worley, S.; Rothstein, R.; Alder, M.L. Telehealth Parent Training for Sleep Disturbances in Young Children with Autism Spectrum Disorder: A Randomized Controlled Trial. *Sleep Med.* **2023**, *111*, 208–219. [CrossRef]
12. Schnatschmidt, M.; Lollies, F.; Schlarb, A.A. Can a Parental Sleep Intervention in an Individual Setting Improve the Maternal and Paternal Sense of Competence and Parent–Child Interaction in Parents of Young Sleep-Disturbed Children? Findings from a Single-Arm Pilot Intervention Study. *BMC Psychol.* **2022**, *10*, 243. [CrossRef]
13. Orr, M.; Isaacs, J.; Godbout, R.; Witmans, M.; Corkum, P. A Usability Study of an Internet-Delivered Behavioural Intervention Tailored for Children with Residual Insomnia Symptoms after Obstructive Sleep Apnea Treatment. *Internet Interv.* **2019**, *18*, 100265. [CrossRef] [PubMed]
14. McLay, L.; Sutherland, D.; Machalicek, W.; Sigafoos, J. Systematic Review of Telehealth Interventions for the Treatment of Sleep Problems in Children and Adolescents. *J. Behav. Educ.* **2020**, *29*, 222–245. [CrossRef]
15. Gruber, R.; Somerville, G.; Finn, C. School-Based Sleep Health Education in Canada. *Sleep Med.* **2019**, *56*, 9–15. [CrossRef]
16. Pulimeno, M.; Piscitelli, P.; Colazzo, S.; Colao, A.; Miani, A. School as Ideal Setting to Promote Health and Wellbeing among Young People. *Health Promot. Perspect.* **2020**, *10*, 316–324. [CrossRef]

https://doi.org/10.3390/children13010138

17. Gruber, R.; Somerville, G.; Bergmame, L.; Fontil, L.; Paquin, S. School-Based Sleep Education Program Improves Sleep and Academic Performance of School-Age Children. *Sleep Med.* **2016**, *21*, 93–100. [CrossRef]
18. Rigney, G.; Watson, A.; Gazmararian, J.; Blunden, S. Update on School-Based Sleep Education Programs: How Far Have We Come and What Has Australia Contributed to the Field? *Sleep Med.* **2021**, *80*, 134–157. [CrossRef] [PubMed]
19. Blunden, S.L.; Chapman, J.; Rigney, G.A. Are Sleep Education Programs Successful? The Case for Improved and Consistent Research Efforts. *Sleep Med. Rev.* **2012**, *16*, 355–370. [CrossRef]
20. Blunden, S.; Rigney, G. Lessons Learned from Sleep Education in Schools: A Review of Dos and Don'ts. *J. Clin. Sleep Med.* **2015**, *11*, 671–680. [CrossRef] [PubMed]
21. Gruber, R. School-Based Sleep Education Programs: A Knowledge-to-Action Perspective Regarding Barriers, Proposed Solutions, and Future Directions. *Sleep Med. Rev.* **2017**, *36*, 13–28. [CrossRef]
22. Davis, J., Blunden, S.; BoydPratt, J.; Corkum, P.; Gebert, K.; Trenorden, K.; Rigney, G. Healthy Sleep for Healthy Schools: A Pilot Study of a Sleep Education Resource to Improve Adolescent Sleep. *Health Prom. J. Aust.* **2022**, *33*, 379–389. [CrossRef]
23. Rosenberg, L.E. Healthy Sleep for Healthy Schools: Evaluating the Usability, Effectiveness, and Implementation Potential of a School-Based Sleep Education Program. Ph.D. Thesis, Dalhousie University, Halifax, NS, Canada, 2025.
24. Bavarian, N.; Lewis, K.M.; Acock, A.; DuBois, D.L.; Yan, Z.; Vuchinich, S.; Silverthorn, N.; Day, J.; Flay, B.R. Effects of a School-Based Social–Emotional and Character Development Program on Health Behaviors: A Matched-Pair, Cluster-Randomized Controlled Trial. *J. Prim. Prev.* **2016**, *37*, 87–105. [CrossRef] [PubMed]
25. Blunden, S. The Implementation of a Sleep Education Program in Primary School Children. *Sleep Biol. Rhythms* **2007**, *5*, A31.
26. Chen, S.-J.; Li, S.X.; Zhang, J.-H.; Lam, S.P.; Yu, M.W.M.; Tsang, C.C.; Kong, A.P.S.; Chan, K.C.C.; Li, A.M.; Wing, Y.K.; et al. School-Based Sleep Education Program for Children: A Cluster Randomized Controlled Trial. *Healthcare* **2023**, *11*, 1853. [CrossRef]
27. Rey, A.E.; Guignard-Perret, A.; Imler-Weber, F.; Garcia-Larrea, L.; Mazza, S. Improving Sleep, Cognitive Functioning and Academic Performance with Sleep Education at School in Children. *Learn. Instr.* **2020**, *65*, 101270. [CrossRef]
28. Tamura, N.; Tanaka, H. Effects of Sleep Education with Self-Help Treatment for Elementary Schoolchild with Nocturnal Lifestyle and Irritability: Sleep Education for Children. *Sleep Biol. Rhythms* **2014**, *12*, 169–179. [CrossRef]
29. Uhlig, S.; Jansen, E.; Scherder, E. Study Protocol RapMusicTherapy for Emotion Regulation in a School Setting. *Psychol. Music.* **2016**, *44*, 1068–1081. [CrossRef]
30. Eccles, J.S. The Development of Children Ages 6 to 14. *Future Child.* **1999**, *9*, 30. [CrossRef] [PubMed]
31. Pureza, J.R.; Gonçalves, H.A.; Branco, L.; Grassi-Oliveira, R.; Fonseca, R.P. Executive Functions in Late Childhood: Age Differences among Groups. *Psychol. Neurosci.* **2013**, *6*, 79–88. [CrossRef]
32. Pick de Weiss, S.; Sirkin, J. *Breaking the Poverty Cycle: The Human Basis for Sustainable Development*; Oxford University Press: New York, NY, USA, 2010.
33. Altschuld, J.W.; Watkins, R. A Primer on Needs Assessment: More than 40 Years of Research and Practice. *New Dir. Eval.* **2014**, *144*, 5–18. [CrossRef]
34. Witkin, B.R.; Altschuld, J.W. *Planning and Conducting Needs Assessments: A Practical Guide*; Sage Publications: Thousand Oaks, CA, USA, 1995.
35. Corkum, P.; Weiss, S. *ABCs of Sleeping [Unpublished Storybook]*; to be published; Department of Psychology, Dalhousie University; Department of Paediatrics, University of Toronto: Halifax, NS, Canada, 2026.
36. Bessey, M.; Coulombe, J.A.; Smith, I.M.; Corkum, P. Assessing Parental Sleep Attitudes and Beliefs in Typically Developing Children and Children With ADHD and ASD. *Child. Health Care* **2013**, *42*, 116–133. [CrossRef]
37. Hennink, M.; Kaiser, B.N. Sample Sizes for Saturation in Qualitative Research: A Systematic Review of Empirical Tests. *Soc. Sci. Med.* **2022**, *292*, 114523. [CrossRef]
38. Saunders, B.; Sim, J.; Kingstone, T.; Baker, S.; Waterfield, J.; Bartlam, B.; Burroughs, H.; Jinks, C. Saturation in Qualitative Research: Exploring Its Conceptualization and Operationalization. *Qual. Quant.* **2018**, *52*, 1893–1907. [CrossRef]
39. Harris, P.A.; Taylor, R.; Thielke, R.; Payne, J.; Gonzalez, N.; Conde, J.G. Research Electronic Data Capture (REDCap)—A Metadata-Driven Methodology and Workflow Process for Providing Translational Research Informatics Support. *J. Biomed. Inf.* **2009**, *42*, 377–381. [CrossRef]
40. Rosenberg, L.; Rigney, G.; Jemcov, A.; Van Voorst, D.; Corkum, P. Usability of an eHealth Sleep Education Intervention for University Students. *Digit. Health* **2024**, *10*, 20552076241260480. [CrossRef] [PubMed]
41. Ali, N.; Rigney, G.; Weiss, S.K.; Brown, C.A.; Constantin, E.; Godbout, R.; Hanlon-Dearman, A.; Ipsiroglu, O.; Reid, G.J.; Shea, S.; et al. Optimizing an eHealth Insomnia Intervention for Children with Neurodevelopmental Disorders: A Delphi Study. *Sleep Health* **2018**, *4*, 224–234. [CrossRef]
42. Ilie, A.; Orr, M.; Weiss, S.; Smith, I.M.; Reid, G.J.; Hanlon-Dearman, A.; Brown, C.; Constantin, E.; Godbout, R.; Shea, S.; et al. Optimizing the Better Nights, Better Days for Children with Neurodevelopmental Disorders Program for Large Scale Implementation. *Front. Sleep* **2023**, *2*, 1158983. [CrossRef]
43. *Nvivo: Qualitative Data Analysis Software*, version 12; QSR International: Burlington, MA, USA, 1999.

https://doi.org/10.3390/children13010138

44. Braun, V.; Clarke, V. Using Thematic Analysis in Psychology. *Qual. Res. Psychol.* **2006**, *3*, 77–101. [CrossRef]
45. Morville, P.; Sullenger, P. Ambient Findability: Libraries, Serials, and the Internet of Things. *Ser. Libr.* **2010**, *58*, 33–38. [CrossRef]
46. Ilie, A.; Keys, E.; Weiss, S.; Pencer, A.; Corkum, P. A Mixed-Methods Usability Study of the Promoting Healthy Sleep eLearning Professional Development Program for Healthcare Providers. *JMIR Form. Res.*. Submitted.
47. Glaser, B.; Strauss, A. *The Discovery of Grounded Theory: Strategies for Qualitative Research*; Sociology Press: Mill Valley, CA, USA, 1967.
48. Fugard, A.J.B.; Potts, H.W.W. Supporting Thinking on Sample Sizes for Thematic Analyses: A Quantitative Tool. *Int. J. Soc. Res. Methodol.* **2015**, *18*, 669–684. [CrossRef]
49. Holdaway, A.S.; Becker, S.P. Children's Sleep Problems Are Associated with Poorer Student–Teacher Relationship Quality. *Sleep Med.* **2018**, *47*, 100–105. [CrossRef]
50. Lucas, I.; Mulraney, M.; Sciberras, E. Sleep Problems and Daytime Sleepiness in Children with ADHD: Associations with Social, Emotional, and Behavioral Functioning at School, a Cross-Sectional Study. *Behav. Sleep Med.* **2019**, *17*, 411–422. [CrossRef]
51. Brosnan, B.; Haszard, J.J.; Meredith-Jones, K.A.; Wickham, S.-R.; Galland, B.C.; Taylor, R.W. Screen Use at Bedtime and Sleep Duration and Quality Among Youths. *JAMA Pediatr.* **2024**, *178*, 1147–1154. [CrossRef] [PubMed]
52. Mellon, P.; Montemurro, G.; Yang, S.; Sulz, L.; Torrance, B.; Storey, K. Students', Parents' and Teachers' Perspectives on Comprehensive School-Based Sleep Promotion. *Health Educ. J.* **2024**, *83*, 796–808. [CrossRef]
53. Ashton, R. Does a Universal Sleep Education Programme Improve the Sleep Habits of Primary School Children? *Sleep Biol. Rhythms* **2017**, *15*, 143–151. [CrossRef]
54. Gaskin, C.J.; Venegas Hargous, C.; Stephens, L.D.; Nyam, G.; Brown, V.; Lander, N.; Yoong, S.; Morrissey, B.; Allender, S.; Strugnell, C. Sleep Behavioral Outcomes of School-Based Interventions for Promoting Sleep Health in Children and Adolescents Aged 5 to 18 Years: A Systematic Review. *Sleep Adv.* **2024**, *5*, zpae019. [CrossRef] [PubMed]
55. Flint Bretler, O.; Tzischinsky, O.; Asraf, K.; Shochat, T. The Effects of Parental Intervention on Sleep Patterns and Electronic Media Exposure in Young Adolescents. *Clocks Sleep* **2022**, *4*, 129–144. [CrossRef] [PubMed]
56. Sosso, F.E.; Khoury, T. Socioeconomic Status and Sleep Disturbances among Pediatric Population: A Continental Systematic Review of Empirical Research. *Sleep Sci.* **2021**, *14*, 245–256.

https://doi.org/10.3390/children13010138

MDPI AG
Grosspeteranlage 5
4052 Basel
Switzerland
Tel.: +41 61 683 77 34

Children Editorial Office
E-mail: children@mdpi.com
www.mdpi.com/journal/children

www.ingramcontent.com/pod-product-compliance
Lightning Source LLC
Chambersburg PA
CBHW061618210926
51850CB00009B/2360
* 9 7 8 3 7 2 5 8 7 8 3 7 6 *